ALZHEIMER'S DISEASE

Cause(s), Diagnosis, Treatment, and Care

ALZHEIMER'S DISEASE

Cause(s), Diagnosis, Treatment, and Care

Edited by

Zaven S. Khachaturian
Teresa S. Radebaugh

CRC Press

Boca Raton   New York   London   Tokyo

Senior Acquisitions Editor: Paul Petralia
Editorial Assistant: Cindy Carelli
Project Editor: Carrie L. Unger
Marketing Manager: Susie Carlisle
Direct Marketing Manager: Becky McEldowney
Cover design: Denise Craig
PrePress: Carlos Esser
Manufacturing: Sheri Schwartz

Library of Congress Cataloging-in-Publication Data

Alzheimer's disease: cause(s), diagnosis, treatment, and care / edited by Zaven S. Khachaturian, Teresa S. Radebaugh
     p. cm.
    Includes bibliographical references and index.
    ISBN 0-8493-8997-6
    1. Alzheimer's disease.   I. Khachaturian, Zavin S. II.Radebaugh, Teresa S.
    [DNLM: 1. Alzheimer's Disease. WT 155 A4785 1996]
  RC523.A3792 1996
  616.8′31—dc20
  DNLM/DLC
  for Library of Congress   96-16043
                                        CIP

Zaven Khachaturian, Ph.D., is widely regarded as the architect of the many successful and international scientific programs in neurobiology and Alzheimer's disease which were launched from the National Institute on Aging, National Institutes on Health, where he served as the Associate Director, Neuroscience and Neuropsychology of Aging Program. Dr. Khachaturian is a cofounder of Khachaturian, Radebaugh & Associates, Inc., an international consulting group focused on the conceptualization, development, and management of large scale research programs in Alzheimer's disease. He is also the Director, The Ronald and Nancy Reagan Institute, of the Alzheimer's Association.

In 1984, Dr. Khachaturian formulated a unifying theory of brain aging which is now referred to as the "Calcium Hypothesis of Brain Aging." Since its initial formulation, this hypothesis has received substantial scientific support and has been important in stimulating the field of aging research to shift from descriptive studies to those exploring biological mechanisms of brain aging. His research interests have focused on the neurophysiology and neuropharmacology of learning and memory.

Teresa Sluss Radebaugh, Sc.D., is a psychiatric epidemiologist with a long history of research and research support work in the dementias, Alzheimer's disease, and gerontology. Her particular research interests include epidemiological methods, cross-cultural epidemiological research, and the social and behavioral issues in Alzheimer's disease. Dr. Radebaugh, formerly the Director of Extramural Programs, National Institute of Nursing Research, National Institutes of Health, also served as the Chief, Dementias of Aging Branch, National Institute on Aging. Dr. Radebaugh is also a cofounder of Khachaturian, Radebaugh & Associates, Inc.

John P. Blass, M.D., Ph.D.
Cornell University Medical College
White Plains, New York

Kathleen C. Buckwalter, Ph.D., R.N.
University of Iowa
College of Nursing
Iowa City, Iowa

Thomas F. Budinger, M.D., Ph.D.
Lawrence Berkeley Laboratory
University of California
Berkeley, California

Jiska Cohen-Mansfield, Ph.D.
Department of Psychiatry
Georgetown University Medical Center
Washington, D.C. and
Research Institute
Hebrew Home of Greater Washington
Rockville, Maryland

Barbara J. Crain, M.D., Ph.D.
The Johns Hopkins University
Baltimore, Maryland

Kenneth L. Davis, M.D.
Department of Psychiatry
Mount Sinai School of Medicine
New York, New York

Denis A. Evans, M.D.
Rush Alzheimer's Disease Center
Rush University
Rush-Presbyterian-St. Luke's Medical Center
Chicago, Illinois

Steven H. Ferris, Ph.D.
Aging and Dementia Research Center
New York University Medical Center
New York, New York

Douglas Galasko, M.D.
Department of Neurology
Veterans Affairs Medical Center
San Diego, California

Sid Gilman, M.D.
Department of Neurology
University of Michigan
Ann Arbor, Michigan

Barry J. Gurland, M.D., F.R.C. Physicians, F.R.C. Psychiatry (London)
Straud Center
Columbia University
New York State Psychiatric Institute
New York, New York

Lisa P. Gwyther, M.S.W.
Bryan Alzheimer's Disease Research Center
Duke University Medical Center
Durham, North Carolina

Albert Heyman, M.D.
Duke University Medical Center
Durham, North Carolina

Robert Katzman, M.D.
Department of Neurosciences
University of California
La Jolla, California

Zaven S. Khachaturian, Ph.D.
Khachaturian, Radebaugh & Associates, Inc.
Potomac, Maryland

William R. Markesbery, M.D.
Departments of Pathology and Neurology
Sanders Brown Center on Aging
University of Kentucky
Lexington, Kentucky

George M. Martin, M.D.
Departments of Pathology and Genetics
University of Washington
Seattle, Washington

Richard Mayeux, M.D., M.S.E.
Gertrude H. Sergievsky Center
Columbia University
College of Physicians and Surgeons
New York, New York

Suzanne Mirra, M.D.
Department of Pathology and Laboratory
  Medicine
Veterans Affairs Medical Center
Emory University
Atlanta, Georgia

Edith G. McGeer, Ph.D.
Kinsmen Laboratory of Neurological Research
University of British Columbia
Vancouver, British Columbia, Canada

Patrick L. McGeer, M.D.
Kinsmen Laboratory of Neurological Research
University of British Columbia
Vancouver, British Columbia, Canada

Mary S. Mittelman, Dr. P.H.
Aging and Dementia Research Center
New York University Medical Center
New York, New York

Richard C. Mohs, Ph.D.
Psychiatry Service
Veterans Affairs Medical Center
Bronx, New York

Rhonda J. V. Montegomery, Ph.D.
Department of Sociology
University of Kansas
Kansas City, Kansas

John C. Morris, M.D.
Department of Neurology
Washington University School of Medicine
St. Louis, Missouri

Donald L. Price, M.D.
The Johns Hopkins University
Baltimore, Maryland

Teresa S. Radebaugh, Sc.D.
Khachaturian, Radebaugh & Associates, Inc.
Potomac, Maryland

Allen D. Roses, M.D.
Departments of Medicine (Neurology)
  and Neurobiology
Duke University School of Medicine
Durham, North Carolina

Lina Shihabuddin, M.D.
Department of Psychiatry
Mount Sinai School of Medicine
New York, New York

Sangram S. Sisodia, Ph.D.
The Johns Hopkins University
Baltimore, Maryland

Linda Teri, Ph.D.
Department of Psychiatry and Behavioral
  Sciences
University of Washington Medical School
Seattle, Washington

Robert D. Terry, M.D.
Department of Neurosciences
University of California
La Jolla, California

Leon J. Thal, M.D.
Department of Neurosciences at the
  University of California/San Diego and
Neurology Service
Veterans Affairs Medical Center
San Diego, California

Juan C. Troncoso, M.D.
The Johns Hopkins University
Baltimore, Maryland

Anne B. Young, M.D., Ph.D.
Neurology Service
Massachusetts General Hospital
Boston, Massachusetts

TABLE OF CONTENTS

To President and Mrs. Ronald Reagan
For their efforts on behalf of Alzheimer's
disease patients and families

INTRODUCTION

Chapter **1**

SYNTHESIS OF CRITICAL TOPICS IN ALZHEIMER'S DISEASE*

Zaven S. Khachaturian
Teresa S. Radebaugh

CONTENTS

---

* Reprinted with permission from the 1995 *Medical and Health Annual*, ©1994 by Encyclopaedia Britannica, Inc.

I. INTRODUCTION

Alzheimer's disease (AD), a degenerative disorder that attacks the brain and leads to dementia, is one of the most common dementing disorders of old age, affecting nearly 4 million individuals in the U.S. alone. If a cure is not found and current demographic trends continue, it is estimated that the number of persons affected by AD will double every 20 years.

Dementia is a group of symptoms characterized by an insidious decline in intellectual functioning of sufficient severity to interfere with normal daily activities and social relationships. The most serious aspect of the loss in intellectual functioning is in the domain of cognitive ability. The dementia of AD is distinguished from that seen in such conditions as age-associated memory impairment and benign senescent forgetfulness in that it is inevitably marked by progressive, irreversible declines in memory, performance of routine tasks, time and space orientation, language and communication skills, abstract thinking, and the abilities to learn, carry out mathematical calculations, and construct an object with blocks. In addition, AD is distinguished by personality changes and impairment of judgment. The rate of deterioration varies, but invariably the disease eventually renders patients unable to care for themselves. The time from the onset of symptoms to the end of the life can vary from 2 to 20 years. The chapters in the section on diagnosis by Drs. John C. Morris, Sid Gilman, Richard Mohs, and Albert Heyman provide a comprehensive definition and characterization of the concept of dementia and in particular AD.

The increasing visibility of AD, evidenced by the amount of attention it receives in both the scientific community and the lay community, may create the impression that it is now being more widely or perhaps inappropriately diagnosed. There is, however, no evidence to indicate that the incidence of the disease — that is, the rate of occurrence of new cases — has increased over the years. (Incidence is distinguished from prevalence — the percentage of a population that is affected with a particular disease at a given time.) In fact, ancient Greek and Roman writers as well as Elizabethan chroniclers accurately described the symptoms of AD, thus suggesting that it or very similar dementing disorders have long been part of the human condition.

Because dementia typically makes its appearance in the later years of life, its signs and symptoms have been mistakenly assumed to be indicators of old age. In fact, the term senile was once used almost interchangeably to describe the condition of being demented or being aged. In recent years, however, as scientists have learned more about the processes of the aging brain, it has become apparent that the aging process does not, by itself, lead to dementia or neurodegenerative disease. AD and other dementing disorders of old age are caused by specific pathological conditions. In the absence of disease, the human brain can and does continue to function unimpaired — often well into the 10th decade of life. The chapters in the section on Overview and Historic Perspectives by Drs. Robert Katzman and Robert D. Terry, written by two of the pioneers of AD research in the U.S., provide an excellent review of the recent history and the evolution of current knowledge on this disease. Chapter 14 by Dr. George M. Martin gives the reader a clearer picture of the relationship between the biology of aging and pathological processes associated with diseases such as AD.

II. WHO IS AT RISK?

Although aging per se causes neither dementia nor Alzheimer's disease, it is the most strongly associated risk factor for AD. Family history, or genetic predisposition, is another important risk factor; a history of AD in a first-degree relative (parent or sibling) increases the odds of developing AD three- to fourfold. A history of severe head injury that leads to brief loss of consciousness doubles the risk of developing AD. These three risk factors — age, genetic predisposition, and head trauma — meet the accepted epidemiological criteria for causal factors: (1) they provide a plausible biological explanation and (2) their effects are strong and consistent. Other risk factors that have been investigated — such as maternal age, hypothyroidism, and exposure to environmental toxins such as aluminum or to chemicals such as benzene and toluene — have not been shown to meet the above criteria.

Factors that apparently decrease a person's risk for AD have also been identified. Among these, the most important appears to be educational and occupational attainment. People who achieve only a low level of education have double the risk of developing AD compared with those who have had 6 to 8 or more years of schooling. Education presumably increases the brain's reserve capacity such that the clinical manifestations of AD are delayed or become more difficult to detect. Other factors that have been implicated as having a protective effect — but need to be confirmed by further and more careful studies — include postmenopausal estrogen replacement therapy, long-term use of antiinflammatory drugs, and cigarette smoking.

As an increasing proportion of the population survives beyond the age of 85 years, more people will be at risk for developing a dementing disorder. Recent well-designed epidemiological studies have assessed the prevalence of all dementias (including Alzheimer's disease) in diverse communities around the world. These surveys indicate that 25 to 35% of those 85 and over are affected by some form of dementia. In one such study conducted in East Boston the prevalence of AD alone in the 85-and-over age group was found to be 47%. The variations in prevalence rates are due primarily to differences in the criteria used by investigators to identify individuals with dementia and, more specifically, with AD. One of the major problems in all such community surveys of dementia is that 15 to 30% of the sample population may be unwilling, unable, or unavailable to participate. Because it is possible that dementia might be more frequent among those who do not participate, the reported prevalence rates may actually underestimate the true prevalence.

Regardless of these problems in methodology and the differences in the estimates, two important facts have emerged from the epidemiological studies conducted during the past several decades:

- The prevalence of dementia increases in an exponential fashion with increasing age; that is, the percentage of the population affected doubles for every decade people live beyond the age of 65. Thus, if 10% of all people 65 and older have AD, 20% of the over-75 population will be affected and 40% of all those over age 85.
- Since the Industrial Revolution, but particularly starting at the turn of the last century, life expectancy has been increasing. During the past 3 decades, improvements in public health measures, diet, and health behavior have brought about dramatic demographic changes, including a lower birthrate. Thus, today in most industrialized countries, the 85-and-older age group is the fastest-growing segment of population.

These two facts, the growing number of older people and the increasing incidence of dementia with age, point to an ever larger group of those at risk for Alzheimer's disease.

The chapters in the section on Epidemiology by Drs. Richard Mayeux, Dennis A. Evans, and Barry J. Gurland discuss in greater detail risk factors, prevalence, incidence and the methodological problems in conducting survey studies on dementia.

III. NEUROBIOLOGICAL BASIS OF ALZHEIMER'S DISEASE

Although AD is a distinct disease defined by its characteristic clinical course and pathology, it is a heterogeneous condition with varied manifestations. The rate of cognitive impairment, for example, differs markedly among individuals. The characteristic features of AD brain pathology also differ sharply among people. Though the onset, course, and sequence of events may vary widely, it seems likely nonetheless that the destructive forces involved ultimately converge to cause nerve cell (neuron) dysfunction, loss of connections between nerve cells, and death of some nerve cells. The quest for mechanisms by which neurons lose their ability to communicate with each other and the reasons for selective neuronal death are at the heart of the worldwide scientific effort to discover the cause — or causes — of AD.

It has been known for some time that the survival of nerve cells in the brain depends on the proper functioning of many interrelated systems. These systems can be characterized by the three aspects of neuronal activity they modulate: *communication, metabolism,* and *repair.*

The communication system used by most neurons relies on a vast array of chemicals to carry information between and within nerve cells as well as to cells outside the nervous system. Through this complex chemical signal transduction system, the brain functions as a master control center for the whole body. Depletion or absence of any of these chemicals disrupts cell-to-cell communication and interferes with normal brain function.

The metabolic activity of neurons depends on the blood circulation provided by a complex system of both large and extremely small blood vessels in the brain. The supply of oxygen, glucose, and other nutrients to nerve cells is critical to the health, survival, and normal functioning of the brain. A sustained reduction in the supply of oxygen can lead to cell death.

The third system involves the repair and cleanup functions of the neuron. Unlike other types of cells in the body, nerve cells do not replicate after birth. Instead, they constantly degrade or digest old, worn-out parts of themselves and synthesize new proteins for replacement parts. This system of continuous protein synthesis and degradation is finely regulated, and any disruption can have disastrous consequences for nerve cell function.

These three interrelated systems normally work in synchrony. Sometimes, however, internal (endogenous) factors, such as changes in an individual's nutritional, immune, or neuroendocrine status, interfere with the normal functioning of one of these systems, thus disrupting the delicate balance. Alternatively, external (exogenous) factors such as toxins, trauma, or infectious agents might disrupt the equilibrium. There is evidence that the pathology seen in AD is associated with changes in all three systems. The chapters by Drs. George M. Martin, John P. Blass, Allen D. Roses, Patrick L. McGeer, Edith G. McGeer, Anne B. Young, and William R. Markesbery in the section on Cause(s) provide more accurate and detailed accounting of our knowledge on the biology of this disease. The following is a general sketch and a simplified overview of what is known with respect to each of these systems in AD.

A. CELL-TO-CELL COMMUNICATION

Changes in the brain's communication systems ultimately affect the individual's behavior. The behavioral effects of alcohol consumption, for example, are mediated through changes in the signal transduction pathways of large numbers of nerve cells. In the case of specific behaviors seen in AD patients — namely, cognitive impairment and performance decline — the most immediate precipitating events in the brain are alterations in the chemical communication pathways within and among neurons.

A vast repertoire of chemicals — including neurotransmitters, neuroendocrine peptides, growth-promoting factors, metal ions, and many others — is used by each neuron for different kinds of communication, much as multilingual individuals in a cosmopolitan community may use different languages for different conversations. In the mid-1970s, AD researchers found that an enzyme necessary for the synthesis of one such chemical, the neurotransmitter acetylcholine, was deficient in the brains of AD patients. This was an important discovery in that it provided the first link between AD and specific biochemical defect in the brain.

The scientific community was particularly ready to accept the challenge of AD at this time because, in the preceding few years, research in neurotransmitter chemistry had revealed that acetylcholine-containing neurons (i.e., cholinergic neurons) play an important role in memory. Since the initial discovery of a cholinergic deficit in AD, it has been shown that the disease also involves abnormalities in other neurotransmitters as well as in other chemical signals that modulate neuronal activity. However, over the years, animal studies and analysis of human brain tissue obtained at autopsy have consistently confirmed the relationship between cholinergic deficits and memory impairments.

In the early 1980s, the "cholinergic hypothesis" of AD engendered great optimism that the cholinergic deficits could be corrected — and the disease cured — through pharmacological manipulations. The confidence that many scientists placed in this approach was based on the apparent similarity between AD and another neurodengerative disorder, Parkinson's disease, in which neurotransmitter deficits can be ameliorated by an increase in the supply of the deficient chemical. In subsequent years a number of strategies were tried for correcting the cholinergic deficits in AD, all designed to maintain or improve the availability of acetylcholine by increasing its synthesis, facilitating its release at the synapse (the contact point between nerve cells), or slowing the rate of its breakdown. Generally, these approaches have not fulfilled their initial promise, in spite of modest successes in some patients for short periods.

1. Promise and Problems of Tacrine

One of these experimental efforts involved a multicenter clinical trial of tetrahydroaminoacridine (THA). This substance was approved as a treatment for AD by the U.S. Food and Drug Administration in September 1993 under the name of tacrine (Cognex), despite controversy about its effectiveness. Tacrine is a cholinesterase inhibitor, one of a class of compounds that slow the degradation, or breakdown of acetylcholine, thus allowing the small amounts of neurotransmitter that are released to remain at the synapse a bit longer than usual. The rationale was that prolonging acetylcholine availability at the synapse would effectively facilitate the transmission of information from one cell to the other. A number of studies with various cholinesterase inhibitors have shown that in some AD patients these compounds do slightly slow the rate of decline in performance on some neuropsychological tests. Tacrine is not without drawbacks, however. It does not appear to help all patients, and it can cause liver toxicity, although this can be controlled. Studies are being conducted continually to improve the optimal dosage of tacrine and to identify subgroups of patients who stand to benefit most from the drug. More important, however, the search continues for more effective treatments with fewer side effects that would help more AD patients for longer periods. At present many laboratories at university medical centers as well as pharmaceutical companies are searching for a more effective and longer lasting agent that would correct this neurotransmitter defect. Some of these compounds are at various stages of testing for approval by the FDA.

There are several possible reasons why treatment strategies directed at correcting cholinergic deficits have not been as successful as expected. One is that the most effective compound for correcting the chemical deficiency or the appropriate molecular target has not yet been found. Another potential reason is that the cholinergic neurons are selectively vulnerable in AD and are dying; therefore, therapy to increase available acetylcholine is too little too late. Still another distinct possibility is that some other biochemical abnormalities may occur first, placing the cholingergic system at risk; this antecedent event, therefore, should be the target of treatment. Finally, it is highly likely that an effective treatment for AD would need to select multiple targets since it is known that the disease affects many biochemical systems, all of which influence the neuronal signal transduction pathway.

2. Multiple Therapeutic Targets

Many groups of researchers at major universities and at biotechnology and pharmaceutical companies around the world have become interested in the problems of AD and committed to developing active agents to intervene at various stages of the signal transduction process. Neuroscientists have made significant advances in discovering the details of molecular mechanisms in cell-to-cell communication and the intricate signal transduction pathways within a neuron. This knowledge now provides a vast array of molecular targets for intervention. To promote and facilitate drug-discovery efforts at academic institutions and to accelerate the testing of promising compounds, the Alzheimer's Disease Cooperative Study Unit (ADCSU), a 33-site U.S. consortium, was established. It represents a major national resource for developing improved technologies for clinical trials, for conducting clinical trials, and for testing new diagnostic procedures. At present, many potential treatments aimed at enhancing neuronal communications are in various stages of planning for testing. The chapters by Drs. Leon J. Thal, Douglas Galasko, Linda Shihabuddin, Kenneth L. Davis, Marry S. Mittelman, and Steven H. Ferris in the section on Treatment provide more thorough descriptions of the issues concerning cell-to-cell communication, clinical trials, and the various strategies and targets for treatments that are being developed. These authors are some of the pioneers in the development and testing of treatments for Alzheimer's disease in the U.S.

B. METABOLIC STRESS: CAUSES AND EFFECTS

The second system that is important for neuronal survival consists of the structural and functional elements that regulate nerve cell metabolism. Scientists have known for some time that, without an adequate supply of oxygen and glucose, neurons will die. Moreover, these cells are extremely demanding and fussy about the metabolic fuel they consume; they need an abundant supply of pure glucose, and any sustained depravation, as occurs in asphyxiation or stroke, has disastrous consequences. The chapter by Dr. John B. Blass in the section on Cause(s) is an exceptionally good review of the problems associated with brain metabolic deficits. A number of studies have demonstrated that vascular changes in the brain are intrinsic to the pathology of AD. Profound structural and biochemical alterations in tiny blood vessels in the brain can lead to chronic deprivation of blood flow, resulting in a progressive decline in neuronal function in selected brain areas. Pathological changes in the capillaries of the brain imply that the function of the blood-brain barrier (BBB) is altered in AD. The BBB allows oxygen, glucose, and other essential nutrients and chemicals to pass from the capillary circulation into brain tissue while at the same time preventing the passage of undesirable compounds such as environmental toxins, pathogens, and drugs. The association of severe head trauma with an increased risk for AD is probably related to damage to the brain microvessel system and possible failure of the BBB.

In recent years the application of sophisticated imaging techniques to the study of the brains of AD patients has yielded insight into metabolic abnormalities. The chapter by Dr. Thomas F. Budinger in the section on Biological Markers provides an excellent comprehensive overview of the potentials and limitations of different imaging approaches. One such technique, positron emission tomography (PET), has shown that in AD patients certain parts of the brain involved in cognitive functioning are unable to utilize glucose properly. Scientists are not certain whether these deficits are due to microvessel pathology or dysfunction in other parts of the metabolic cascade, such as a defect in the protein that transports glucose. The end result, however, is that in AD certain parts of the brain are under a condition of chronic metabolic stress. Continuous malnutrition of neurons, for whatever reason, could have several important implications for understanding of the pathologies associated with AD. The synthesis of acetylcholine, the key neurotransmitter for memory, is highly dependent on glucose metabolism in the brain. Thus, selective vulnerability of cholinergic neurons might actually be a consequence of inadequate blood circulation to those parts of the brain, resulting in a gradual starvation of these cells. The cholinergic deficits and associated cognitive decline could be the result of metabolic abnormalities that may have proceeded unnoticed for a long period before the onset of obvious, disabling cognitive changes.

Another consequence of chronic glucose insufficiency in the brain is the conversion of a harmless and essential neurotransmitter, glutamate, into a potent killer of neurons. Glutamate is an excitatory amino acid; in appropriate amounts it is essential for development and normal functioning of neurons but, as with other excitatory amino acids, in excessive amounts it can become toxic to the very neurons it normally stimulates. Glutamate becomes neurotoxic when too much of it is present at a synapse or when, in normal amounts, it stimulates a glucose-deprived neuron. Glutamate toxicity is mediated by the influx of calcium into the cell, and it is the excessive internal concentration of calcium that eventually kills the cell.

In recent years scientists have become especially interested in the biochemical mechanisms of neurotoxicity for two reasons. First, it has been shown that a wide variety of toxic compounds, some present in the environment (exogenous toxins), such as aluminum, and others naturally present in the body (endogenous toxins), such as glutamate, can lead to selective neuronal dysfunction and death. Second, neurotoxins have become an important analytical tool, allowing neuroscientists to study different characteristics of nerve cells as reflected by their selective vulnerability.

Among the many potentially neurotoxic compounds in the environment, aluminum has captured the most attention. Aluminum is a ubiquitous element. While autopsy analyses of the brains of AD patients have produced conflicting results depending on methods used, there appears to be a modest accumulation of aluminum in the brain lesions — the neuritic plaques and neurofibrillary tangles — that are characteristic of the disease. The chapters by Drs. Anne B. Young and William R. Markesbery in the section on Cause(s) cover the general topic of neurotoxicity and the specific subject of the role of aluminum in the etiology of A.D.

C. SYNTHESIS AND DEGRADATION: A DELICATE BALANCE

The third essential system for maintaining the health of a neuron is its ability to control and balance two opposing biochemical events, one involving the mechanisms of protein and membrane synthesis, the other involving the processes that degrade or digest proteins. It is through this complex balancing act that neurons repair and renew themselves and drive their unique ability for self-modification in response to stimuli, experiences, or injuries.

Most nerve cells, once fully developed, are designed to provide a lifetime of service. A neuron, to function properly, must renew between 50,000 and 100,000 different types of proteins. A mistake in the synthesis of any one of these proteins could interfere with an essential cellular function and lead to a failure in a neuron's ability to communicate vital information. Such errors could result in too much or too little of a protein or one with the wrong sequence of amino acids (the building blocks of protein), something like a string of words with spelling and grammatical errors. Errors in amino acid sequence, in turn, could influence the three-dimensional structure of the protein, thus affecting how well it does the job. What might appear to be a minor change in the position of one or two amino acids could become the cause of a disease such as AD. Errors in protein degradation can have equally disastrous consequences. Proteins that are not properly digested or broken down could accumulate, forming new, harmful aggregates.

As mentioned above, the neuropathological hallmarks of AD are two kinds of microscopic lesions, called neuritic (or senile) plaques and neurofibrillary tangles, which are found in the brains of AD patients at autopsy. Both are consequences of abnormalities in the processing of different types of proteins. The major constituent of the tangles is a protein called tau, which is present in normal brain tissue. Tangles apparently form as a result of abnormal phosphorylation (the addition of phosphate molecules) of tau, a process that interferes with the protein's role in the construction of vital intracellular transport structures known as microtubules.

The other major lesion associated with AD, the neuritic plaque, has as its principal constituent beta-amyloid protein. Amyloid is derived from a larger protein, called the amyloid precursor protein (APP), which is normally found partially embedded in the membrane of the neuron. The exact function of APP and how it is related to the clinical signs of dementia is not known. It is believed that it may play an important role in stabilizing synaptic contact points. It is very likely that APP is critical to the plasticity of the nervous system, thus being of great importance for understanding the neurobiology of cognitive functioning. It must also play other, undiscovered roles in the normal functioning of neurons because there are many different forms of APP, each with a slightly different amino acid sequence; they have been found in all kinds of animals, from fruit flies to humans.

Amyloid protein has the unusual characteristics of being highly insoluble and resistant to degradation, thus readily accumulating within the nervous system. How it interferes with cell functioning is not totally clear, but there are some suggestions that aggregations of beta-amyloid become highly toxic in neurons in a way similar to glutamate. In fact, both of these substances may inflict their damage by disrupting the internal homeostasis of calcium ions. Recent discoveries concerning the nature of amyloid protein, how it is formed and processed, what it does to a cell, and the genes that determine its structure have created tremendous excitement among neuroscientists. Many believe that pursuit of this clue will lead to discovery of the specific causes of AD. The chapter by Drs. Suzanne S. Mirra, William R. Markesbery, Juan C. Troncoso, Barbara J. Crain, Sangram S. Sisodia, and Donald L. Price in the section on Biological Markers provides a more detailed overview of the neuropathological lesions and other abnormalities associated with AD.

D. GENETIC KEYS?

The scientific enthusiasm about the possible role of amyloid protein in the pathology of AD has been further fueled by the results of molecular genetics studies that have identified genes associated with familial (inherited) AD on chromosomes 21, 14, 1, and 19. The first specific gene linked with familial AD was the APP gene on chromosome 21, which is responsible for producing amyloid protein. After the initial report, several other mutations were found in the region of the APP gene in members of families that had a history of AD onset at a relatively young age. How these mutations alter the behavior of APP and their significance to normal cell functioning are not known, but are being actively studied. Subsequently, a region on chromosome 14 was also linked to an early-onset form of the disease. Recently the exact locus of this gene was pinpointed. The exact function of this gene is still unknown, but it is only a matter of time when this will be no longer be a mystery. Within a short period following the discovery of the of the locus of chromosome 14, a locus on chromosome 1 was linked to a family with an unusually high incidence of AD, known as the Volga-German families.

The fourth and perhaps the most important recently discovered gene linked to AD is the Apolipoprotein E (ApoE) gene on chromosome 19, which has been associated with many late-onset familial cases of AD as well as sporadic cases in the over-60 age group. (Sporadic cases are those occurring in individuals who have no strong family history of the disease.) The ApoE gene directs the synthesis of a cholesterol-transporting blood protein. The gene occurs in three different forms: apoE2, apoE3, and apoE4. One of these, apoE4, is found in 14% of control populations but is present in 30 to 40% of the late-onset sporadic cases of AD before age 85 and rises to 90% for individuals who are homozygous for apoE4, which means they have inherited this form of the gene from both parents. These people have a 5:1 odds of developing AD, compared with the 15:1 odds in individuals who have a single ApoE4 gene. It has been estimated that between 25 and 40% of AD cases can be attributed to the presence of this form of the gene.

Not only does the ApoE gene have a strong and consistent relationship with the disease, but, within a few months after it was identified, researchers postulated a plausible biological explanation for its role in the pathological processes of AD. It has been shown that the protein encoded by the ApoE gene has a high affinity for and binds with beta-amyloid in the plaques. Among Alzheimer's patients, those who have the gene for apoE4 have larger plaques than those who lack the gene. It appears that ApoE4 acts as a chaperone to APP and, in some unknown way, promotes the formation of neuritic plaques. It has also been postulated that it plays an important role in the formation of neurofibrillary tangles. In the brain ApoE proteins are taken up by neurons in large quantities after neuronal injury and appear to play an important role in various recuperative processes and in neuronal plasticity. The chapter by Dr. Allen D. Roses in the section on Cause(s) provides a more detailed description of the possible roles of ApoE in AD.

The excitement and optimism generated by the discovery of a relationship between AD and ApoE is well warranted; epidemiological studies of AD will now have a biological marker for sorting patients into homogenous groups and studying them with the hope of finding other contributing factors. At the same time, this research has begun to provide new opportunities for developing alternative treatment strategies.

IV. CARE AND MANAGEMENT

One of the most critical dilemmas of the recent history of AD is the search for a balance between the excitement generated by the advances in understanding the biological underpinnings of the disease and the frustration of families created by the slow pace of progress in developing the practical knowledge to reduce the burdens of care. On one side of the balance, a growing number of scientists have the firm conviction that the present investment in research on the etiology and pathogenesis will lead to the development of safer and more-effective treatments. Many family members, policy formulators, and the general public share with the scientist a strong belief and hope that the current research efforts will lead to development of treatments to delay the onset of disabling symptoms, restore function for ill people, and prevent the loss of function for those not yet impaired. There is no doubt that during the last 15 to 20 years we have made impressive strides in understanding the neurobiology of AD, and excitement about these accomplishments is well warranted, while work continues on the neurobiological basis of AD. However, for many who have to take care of a family member, this work remains a promissory note. While they share the excitement of progress, they experience the pain and frustration of the reality they face every day in their home. At present, 4 million people and their families and care providers are currently in the grips of the illness and want help in managing their day-to-day difficulties.

Although research on the behavioral, social, and environmental aspects of AD may not be as glamorous or as well publicized as some of the biomedical studies, during the last few years this area of investigation has been making impressive progress steadily. It is very likely that the advances being made in this arena will find immediate practical applications and thus provide families with the help they need so desperately.

The early research on the social and behavioral aspects of AD focused on such broad questions as: what happened to patients and to families? what were the stresses? what were the burdens? who were the caregivers and what happened to them? Some of these early works have demonstrated that AD is a heterogeneous disease. It is now well accepted that this heterogeneity is present not only among the people who suffer from the disease but their families as well. Research to understand the diversity, complexity, and consequences of caregiving, the precise nature of the problems confronting caregiving through the course of the disease, and the types and nature of effective interventions are of great importance. It has been clearly established and widely accepted that the consequences of the disease are very difficult but vary by social structural and environmental characteristics. The stresses have been demonstrated to be enormous with implications for the health of primary caregivers. The families of patients suffer substantial and varied, but negative, consequences from the disease including financial burdens.

Investigators have moved beyond the establishment of and general characterization of care and management issues to a more refined dissection of the circumstances and reverberations leading to requirements for care and management. The goal is to provide carefully delineated targets and timetables for interventions and for the development of interventions and supportive services which will maintain patients and their families in dignity and independence for as long as possible. An understanding of some of the behavioral disturbances, the changes occurring across the course of disease, and the experiences of families have provided us with guidelines for navigating patients and families through the course of illness. The chapters in the section on Care and Management by Drs. Kathleen C. Buckwalter, Rhonda J.V. Montgomery, Linda Teri, Jiska Cohen-Mansfield, and Ms. Lisa P. Gwyther address the psychosocial factors contributing to the stress of families, the environmental and social factors influencing requirements for care, and behavioral management problems in home and institutional settings. The authors are eminent leaders in this area of research. Their research and clinical efforts have made very important differences in how patients and families are cared for in this country.

A. THE CAMPAIGN AGAINST ALZHEIMER'S DISEASE

The crisis in U.S. health care system stemming from the rising cost of care, the rapidly growing number of older people in the population, and the devastating toll of AD has led to the formulation of a public-private working proposal for a major campaign against the disease. The goal is to slow the rate of deterioration in AD patients by 5 years during the next 5 years and by 10 years within 10 years. The overriding aim of this initiative is to discover treatments that will allow patients to continue to function independently. Importantly, this approach will target not only the cognitive dysfunction associated with AD but also the behavioral disturbances that often leave some families with no choice but to institutionalize their loved ones.

The progress made to date is, in large measure, due to the successful partnership between family-support groups such as the Alzheimer's Association and government-sponsored researchers. Now such partnerships are being expanded under the umbrella of The Ronald and Nancy Reagan Research Institute of the Alzheimer's Association to include academia, industry, private foundations, and individual philanthropists. This collective effort is certain to yield results.

OVERVIEW AND
HISTORICAL PERSPECTIVES

Chapter 2

CURRENT RESEARCH ON ALZHEIMER'S DISEASE IN A HISTORICAL PERSPECTIVE

_____ Robert Katzman

CONTENTS

0-8493-8997-6/97/$0.00+$.50
© 1996 by CRC Press, Inc.

I. INTRODUCTION

"Alzheimer's disease" is now so universally recognized as the major dementing disorder of aging that the term has become part of everyday speech. This recognition reflects the reality of late 20th century demography: Alzheimer's disease epitomizes the age-dependent disorders of late life with the prevalence doubling every 5 years of age, at least between ages 65 and 85.

Yet one is faced with the historical anomaly that the eponymic case, described in 1907, was in her fifties, and that for decades Alzheimer's disease was considered to be a "presenile" dementia. In part this might be attributed to the fact that life expectancy at the turn of the century was under 50 years and there were relatively fewer elderly. However, the story is more complicated than this.

II. ALOIS ALZHEIMER 1907 REPORT OF THE CLINICAL AND NEUROPATHOLOGICAL FEATURES OF HIS EPONYMIC CASE; UNIVERSALLY ACCEPTED AS A SPECIFIC FORM OF PRESENILE DEMENTIA

At the turn of the century, psychiatrists were engaged in subclassifying the "insane". Alois Alzheimer worked in a laboratory dedicated to identifying changes in brain tissue that might accompany these newly described mental disorders. (An excellent description of the circumstances under which Alois Alzheimer described his original case is given by Bick.[1]) At this time, the dominant "organic" mental disorder was the "dementia paralytica" (general paresis), a form of neurosyphilis that develops decades after the initial infection. The overriding importance of neurosyphilis at the turn of the century is evident in contemporaneous neurological and psychiatric texts. It had thus become important for these pioneering psychiatrists to differentiate cases of neurosyphilis from other conditions that produce dementia in middle-aged individuals. Alzheimer, in his role as physician and psychiatrist, reported in 1907 the case of a patient in her fifties with an aggressive dementia including memory, language, and behavioral deficits; Alzheimer, in his role as a neuroanatomist, described the atrophy of the brain and loss of nerve cells observed at the autopsy of his patient. New silver stains developed by the German photographic industry at the turn of the century had just become available, and Alzheimer was able to visualize the pathological changes that characterize this disease. His vivid line drawings of these neuritic plaques and neurofibrillary tangles were especially compelling. The existence of this new entity was quickly confirmed by other investigators and by 1910 there was a consensus to name this "novel" form of presenile dementia "Alzheimer's disease", the "senium" then considered to begin at age 60!

A. ULTRASTRUCTURAL STUDIES RESOLVE THE HALF-CENTURY DEBATE AS TO WHETHER "SENILE DEMENTIA" IS THE SAME ENTITY AS ALZHEIMER'S PRESENILE DEMENTIA AND PROVIDE THE BASIS OF SUBSEQUENT MOLECULAR CHARACTERIZATION OF THE ABNORMAL FIBROUS PROTEINS CHARACTERISTIC OF ALZHEIMER'S DISEASE

According to Bick[1] the question of whether this newly discovered disorder was also responsible for so-called "senile dementia" was argued within Alzheimer's laboratory. His colleague, Simchow-isz, said yes. Alzheimer was unsure in part because Alzheimer's laboratory actually had few cases of senile dementia to study; in part because demented elderly were confined to "asylums" to which Alzheimer did not have direct access, in part due to the paucity of the very elderly. In the U.S., for example, the percentage of the population over age 65 at the turn of the century (4.1%) was one third that of 1990 (12%). Thus, the lack of a consensus in regard to the role of Alzheimer's disease in the dementias of the elderly continued as a muted debate over the first half of the 20th century, but did not rouse much passion. By 1960 the number of those over age 65 had increased to 16.6 million (9.2% of the population) with 2.5 million over the age of 80, and the reality of a growing elderly population began to draw the attention of the medical profession to senile dementia.

For research to progress, the question of the identity of Alzheimer's disease as a presenile disorder and senile dementia had to be established. In 1948, Newton[2] argued that one could not distinguish clinically cases of Alzheimer's disease with a presenile onset from senile dementia and thus that the two should be considered to be identical. Similar data were presented by Neuman and Cohn in 1953.[3] For this argument to be accepted, however, biologically based data needed to be obtained. Although it was recognized that the pathology in most cases of senile dementia was the same as in the presenile form of Alzheimer's disease, the situation was confused by evidence of some plaques and tangles in the brains of apparently nondemented elderly and by the coexistence of Alzheimer and vascular changes in brains of a significant number of elderly demented patients. In the late 1950s and early 1960s, Terry began to apply the newly developed electron microscope to investigation of degenerative diseases of the brain. In 1963, Terry,[4] located in New York, and Kidd,[5] working independently in Great Britain, reported that on the ultrastructural level a single neurofibrillary tangle contained masses of submicroscopic fibers with a periodic structure, the paired helical filaments.

In 1947 Divry[6] had obtained histochemical evidence that the core of the Alzheimer plaque contained a substance then considered to be starch-like or "amyloid" on the basis of its staining properties. "Amyloid" deposits in biological tissues are now known to consist of collections of protein fibrils rather than a starch-like material, with staining properties resulting from the β-pleated structure of the specific proteins that can form amyloid. Terry and colleagues[7] identified the ultrastructure of the amyloid core of the Alzheimer plaque and showed that it had the typical structure of extracellular amyloid fibrils. Moreover, they demonstrated that surrounding this amyloid core were swollen degenerating neurites, some dendritic, some axonal with synaptic thickenings and synaptic vesicles still discernible, containing abnormal elements such as mitochondria, lyso-somes, and other densely staining bodies. Hence, this plaque was renamed the "neuritic" plaque.

These dramatic ultrastructural changes were identical in subjects whose onset of their dementia was in the presenium and in subjects whose onset of dementia occurred in the senium. Molecular chemistry has since confirmed that the chemical constitution of the amyloid fibril and the paired helical filament is identical in brains of Alzheimer patients with onset in the presenium and in the senium. Thus, the identity of Alzheimer's disease in "presenile" and "senile" patients became established. (These findings are discussed in greater detail in Chapter 3.)

III. THE ULTRASTRUCTURAL IDENTIFICATION OF THE AMYLOID CORE OF THE PLAQUE AND THE PAIRED HELICAL FILAMENTS IN THE TANGLES HAS LED TO THE MOLECULAR CHARACTERIZATION OF THESE ABNORMAL FIBROUS PROTEINS DURING THE PAST DECADE

The identification of two fibrous proteins that appear to be central to the pathogenesis of Alzheimer's disease was a direct result of these initial ultrastructural studies. Methods of isolating plaques, neurofibrillary tangles, and preparations enriched in paired helical filaments, which were developed during the next 2 decades, depended upon ultrastructural identification of the purity of enriched fractions. However, more sophisticated immunological and molecular tools had to be created before these proteins could be chemically characterized.

A. THE β-AMYLOID PEPTIDE AND THE AMYLOID PRECURSOR PROTEIN GENE

The unique molecule at the core of the neuritic plaque in Alzheimer's disease has been shown to be a small protein or peptide, 38 to 42 amino acids long, which has been termed A/β-amyloid. The A/β-peptide is produced by neurons as a soluble breakdown product of a much larger and complex protein, the amyloid precursor protein (APP). The A/β-peptide secreted into the extracellular space interacts with proteins such as α_1-antichymotrypsin, apolipoprotein E, and complement, among others, and assumes the insoluble β-pleated amyloid configuration, thus serving as the nidus for the neuritic plaque. These associated proteins that may accelerate the precipitation of the A/β-peptide are sometimes considered to be "acute phase reactant" proteins because they are released by supporting cells or astrocytes in response to injury.

The first successful isolation of β-amyloid was reported in 1984 by Glenner and Wong.[8] George Glenner, both a protein chemist and a pathologist, recognized that in Alzheimer's disease amyloid was found not only in the core of the neuritic plaque but was often present in cerebral blood vessels, including the blood vessels in the tissue surrounding the brain (the meninges). Glenner and Wong[8] were able to isolate and purify this peptide and obtain a partial amino acid sequence, using as starting material the meninges from cases with extensive vascular amyloid. In 1984 Glenner and colleagues[9] reported the isolation of an almost identical peptide from brains of individuals who had Down's syndrome. Down's syndrome was of particular interest because it was known that individuals with this syndrome (which is due to a triplication of chromosome 21) develop Alzheimer-like plaques in their brains by age 30 and neurofibrillary tangles by age 40. By 1987 three laboratories[10-12] independently reported the chromosomal localization of the gene coding for the precursor protein of A/β-amyloid on chromosome 21, and in the same year the complete sequence of the APP and the structure of its gene was announced.[13] Since 1987 our knowledge about the processing, secretion, metabolism, and putative toxicity of A/β-amyloid has exploded as many scientists believe that the accumulation of this peptide in brain tissue represents one of the first steps in the pathogenesis of Alzheimer's disease.

B. PAIRED HELICAL FILAMENTS AND TAU

The second fibrous protein characteristic of Alzheimer's disease is tau, the protein that constitutes the paired helical filament. Iqbal and colleagues[14] had obtained small amounts of a soluble protein with a molecular weight near 50 kilodaltons from purified preparations of paired helical filaments in the early 1970s, but did not yet have the tools to characterize this molecule. As was determined later, most of the paired helical filament protein was relatively insoluble and did not migrate on the gels used.[15] The chemical identification of the protein, however, occurred after it was shown by Brion in 1985 that antibodies to a newly characterized protein, tau, stained neurofibrillary tangles.[16] It was quickly confirmed that paired helical filaments are composed largely of hyperphosphorylated tau. Tau is a group of closely related proteins normally associated in adult brain with axonal microtubules, structures which it helps stabilize. When tau becomes phosphory-lated at specific sites, it breaks off of the microtubule; the microtubules, essential in the transport of proteins along the axon to the nerve terminal, are then destabilized, and the axonal transport process is impaired as had been predicted decades earlier on the basis of the morphological changes in the neuritic terminals seen in Alzheimer's disease.[17]

IV. A PROSPECTIVE CLINICAL–PATHOLOGICAL STUDY CLARIFIES THAT ALZHEIMER'S DISEASE, AS MEASURED BY THE NUMBER OF NEURITIC PLAQUES PRESENT, CAUSES DEMENTIA IN THE VERY ELDERLY

Among the neurodegenerative diseases, β-amyloid plaques only occur in Alzheimer's disease and Down's syndrome. Neurofibrillary tangles with paired helical filaments occur primarily in Alzheimer's disease and Down's syndrome, but also in several rather uncommon neurodegenerative disorders.[18] Both, however, are found in the brains of some nondemented elderly individuals. While these are now thought to represent preclinical stages of Alzheimer's disease, the presence of such findings led some investigators during the first half of this century to cast doubt on the importance of Alzheimer changes in the elderly. The question was raised as to whether Alzheimer changes were simply those of normal aging: put another way, was "senile dementia … an accentuation … of normal senescence" (Blessed and colleagues,[19] p. 798).

This issue was addressed directly by Blessed, Tomlinson, and Roth in their prospective study of a group of 60 demented and nondemented elderly (mean age 76.6 years) in a geriatric hospital, selected only to be free of significant cerebrovascular disease. These investigators obtained quan-titative measures of cognitive and functional impairment in these subjects during life and correlated these scores with quantitative estimates of the number of plaques in the brain at autopsy. The nondemented elderly included subjects with physical illness, depression, and paraphrenia. In each case, the plaque number was based on the average of counts obtained from five fields in each of 12 cerebral cortex sections. In these subjects the correlation of plaques with a dementia score based on ability to perform everyday tasks was 0.77 ($p<0.001$) and the correlation of plaques with a measure of memory and cognition (the information–memory–concentration test was 0.59, also with a $p<0.001$). Thus, dementia in the elderly, whether measured functionally or cognitively, was unequivocally related to the number of plaques in cerebral cortex.

A. SYNAPSE LOSS IS A BETTER CORRELATE OF COGNITIVE LOSS IN ALZHEIMER'S DISEASE THAN PLAQUE COUNT

The study of Blessed et al. described above unequivocally showed that a major marker of Alzheimer's disease, the neuritic plaque, differentiated *demented from nondemented* elderly. Among the demented subjects, however, the correlation of plaque count and the measures of dementia severity used was much reduced.

It is now apparent that the major determinant of cognitive loss is the loss of synaptic connec-tions. An ultrastructural study carried out by Hamos and co-workers[20] showed a marked loss of synapses in the hippocampus of Alzheimer brains. Masliah and co-workers,[21] using an antibody to the synaptic vesicle component called synaptophysin, showed that the loss of synapses is present in all layers of the neocortex (see also Terry and Katzman[22]). Other studies have confirmed the marked reduction in neocortical synapses in Alzheimer's disease. In a series of cases of "pure" Alzheimer's disease in the elderly, Terry and associates[23] showed that the loss of synapses was about 50% below normal in each layer of the cortex, indicating that presynaptic terminals are markedly diminished in Alzheimer neocortex. Terry notes that "the decrease is even greater than that of the pyramidal neurons within the same cortical areas." The correlations of synaptic density with cognitive measures obtained during the last 18 months of life "were higher here than with any other morphologic assay such as plaque or tangle density, brain weight, and the like."[22] There is now widespread agreement that the loss of synapses is the major correlate of cognitive loss in Alzheimer's disease, although there have not been studies to show the relative importance of neocortical and hippocampal synaptic loss at various stages of the disease.

V. THE SPECIFIC VULNERABILITY OF THE NEURONAL SYSTEMS IN ALZHEIMER'S DISEASE: THE MAJOR LOSS OF CHOLINE ACETYLTRANSFERASE (ChAT) IN ALZHEIMER CEREBRAL CORTEX IS REPORTED INDEPENDENTLY BY THREE BRITISH RESEARCH GROUPS IN 1976

This awakening interest in Alzheimer's disease in 1976 was further fueled by reports of the selective vulnerability of cholinergic neurons in the brain of Alzheimer's disease patients independently emanating from three different laboratories in Great Britain.[24,25] A putative role of acetylcholine in memory was provided by the knowledge that a cholinergic antagonist, scopolamine, had been used for decades as an amnesic drug by anesthesiologists, particularly in producing "twilight sleep" during childbirth so that the pain of childbirth would be forgotten. In 1974 Drachman and Leavitt[26] had shown that scopolamine produced memory deficits in young volunteers not dissimilar from that observed in Alzheimer's disease. Thus, measurement of the level of the acetylcholine biosynthetic enzyme choline acetyltransferase in Alzheimer's disease brain became of interest. The marked reduction of choline acetyltransferase in cerebral cortex of Alzheimer patients reported by these groups was the first specific biochemical change reported for this disease. The reduction of choline acetyltransferase contrasted with the rather stable level of cholinergic receptors in the cerebral cortex of these same brains.

At the time of these discoveries, the site of origin of the cells that contained choline acetyltransferase was not known. Within a few years Coyle and colleagues[27] showed in the rat that most of the cerebral cortical cholinergic terminals originated from neurons in the basal forebrain, and shortly thereafter Whitehouse and colleagues[28] demonstrated the marked loss of basal forebrain cholinergic neurons in Alzheimer's disease. Subsequently, it was shown that there was also extensive involvement of the noradrenergic and serotonergic systems in Alzheimer's disease.[29] This led Rossor to postulate that a major feature of Alzheimer's disease was the involvement of the ascending cortical projection system — subcortical neuronal systems whose axons projected to the cerebral cortex and hippocampus. Indeed if one adds the glutaminergic projection systems (cortical–cortical or hippocampal–cortical–hippocampal) that use glutamate as a neurotransmitter, this is still a reasonable generalized description of Alzheimer's disease.

VI. ALZHEIMER'S DISEASE BECOMES A PUBLIC HEALTH ISSUE

A. THE 1976 KATZMAN EDITORIAL[30]

Early epidemiological studies such as that by Gruenberg[31] indicated that senile dementia increased exponentially with age, afflicting perhaps 4 to 5% of those over the age of 65, if one defined dementia in terms of impairment so severe that the individual can no longer live independently, and perhaps another 5 to 10% with very mild impairment. Once the identity of the senile and presenile forms of Alzheimer's disease were recognized, and autopsy series showed that at least the majority of cases of dementia were due to Alzheimer's disease — even in the series of over 1000 autopsies reported by Jellinger[32] in 1976 — it became evident that Alzheimer's disease was a major public health problem. I had the opportunity of arguing for the importance of the prevalence and malignancy of Alzheimer's disease in a 1976 editorial in the *Archives of Neurology*[30] This editorial struck an immediate response, and widespread interest began to develop in the disorder. This interest was further fueled by the 1976 reports of the selective vulnerability of cholinergic neurons in the brain of Alzheimer's disease patients as described above, the first specific neurochemical change reported in this disorder.

B. THE 1977 NIH WORKSHOP–CONFERENCE

In 1977 in response to a formal suggestion by Dr. Robert Terry and Dr. Robert Katzman, three of the National Institutes of Health — that is, the National Institute of Neurological and Communicative Disorders and Strokes, the National Institute of Mental Health, and the then newly formed National Institute of Aging — jointly sponsored a "Workshop Conference on Alzheimer's Disease–Senile Dementia and Related Disorders" designed to interest scientists in investigating Alzheimer's disease. Although the Workshop–Conference had the unique advantage of being the first conference sponsored by three of the National Institutes, the newly formed National Institute on Aging, under the direction of Dr. Robert Butler, a Washington D.C. psychiatrist and gerontologist, whose book, *Why Grow Old?* had won a Pulitzer Prize, was the institute that subsequently focused on Alzheimer's disease. Over the course of the next 16 years, the total federal support for extramural research in Alzheimer's disease grew from under 5 million dollars per year to over 300 million dollars with the major portion of this growth represented by appropriations for the Alzheimer research program of the National Institute on Aging. The skilled direction of this research support by Dr. Zaven Khachaturian at the National Institute on Aging played an important role in converting these moneys into dramatic research results.

C. THE RISE OF THE ALZHEIMER'S ASSOCIATION IN THE UNITED STATES

Simultaneously with these events in Washington there developed spontaneously intense interest in Alzheimer's disease by family members in several different parts of the U.S. Seven organizations with a primary focus on Alzheimer's disease, or dementing disorders more broadly defined, developed quite independently in the late 1970s. All of these organizations were driven by the anguish or concerns of family members. In particular, Bobbie Glaze, a founder of the Minneapolis-based Alzheimer Association, recounted to groups throughout the country the story of her husband's disease, the difficulty in getting a proper diagnosis, and the obstacles in obtaining help for him from the Veterans Administration. During the prior decade state governments had begun closing state mental hospitals which had traditionally cared for persons with severe dementia, and the Veterans Administration and voluntary chronic disease hospitals were being reformatted as acute-care hospitals, making it increasingly difficult for families to obtain assistance in the care of Alzheimer's disease victims.

In late 1979, Dr. Butler brought the officers of these seven organizations together at the National Institutes of Health and persuaded them to unite into a single organization (see excellent descriptions by P. Fox[33] and N. Lombardo[34]). The Alzheimer's Disease and Related Disorders Association (ADRDA), later to become the Alzheimer Association, was formed in 1980. Today there are chapters throughout the U.S.; the national organization has played a major role in education and public awareness of the disorder, to the point that what had been a technical term is now part of the ordinary vocabulary; local chapters maintain hundreds of support groups and dozens of day care centers, with emphasis on helping the caregiver as well as the patient. However, the national organization has also played two major roles in regard to Alzheimer's disease research: first, by successfully lobbying for increased dollars for Alzheimer research and, second, by emphasizing to its members the importance of autopsy for definitive diagnosis.

VII. THE CLINICAL DIAGNOSIS OF ALZHEIMER'S DISEASE

During this same period, a major advance occurred in the ability of clinicians to diagnose Alzheimer's disease. Retrospective studies in the 1970s showed that there was often a 30 to 50% error rate simply in deciding whether a patient did or did not have dementia, let alone what kind of dementia the patient might have. For example, in an institution as sophisticated as the Maudsley Hospital, the major psychiatric hospital in Great Britain, it had been found that the diagnosis of the presenile form of Alzheimer's disease was in error by 30%, most of the patients misdiagnosed as having been depressed.[35]

A. LEARNING TO DIFFERENTIATE DEMENTIA FROM DEPRESSION

The misdiagnosis of depression as dementia was first described by Kiloh[36] in 1961 as "pseudodementia". During the 1970s differentiation of the dementia syndrome based on studies from major depression were undertaken by a number of psychiatrists,[37,38] and, in 1980, the American Psychiatric Association, in the third edition of its *Diagnostic and Statistical Manual* (DSM-III),[39] set forth clear-cut operational criteria for the two disorders. These criteria limited the diagnosis of dementia to individuals who were alert and awake and who had experienced a decline in functional abilities secondary to cognitive impairment, with evidence of such cognitive impairment in at least two areas of cognition. This powerful definition separated not only dementia from depression but also dementia from amnestic syndromes (in which only memory is involved) and delirium (which occurs with acute medical conditions and in which there is a fluctuating state of awareness). In contrast to the very low accuracy rate of diagnosis of dementia syndrome in the 1970s, by the mid-1980s, clinicians using DSM-III criteria were able to diagnose the dementia syndrome with greater than 95% accuracy.[40]

B. THE DEVELOPMENT OF MENTAL STATUS AND FUNCTIONAL MEASURES OF DEMENTIA SEVERITY

The decline in cognitive and functional abilities in dementia can be usefully measured as a first approximation by use of mental status and functional instruments. An additional major contribution of the 1968 Blessed, Tomlinson, Roth study[19] described above was their validation of formal scales for testing cognitive status and function against autopsy diagnosis. Their initial information–memory–concentration (IMC) test is still a widely used mental status test, and a brief version[41] is now widely used in nursing homes and as part of the test battery used by the multicenter group the Consortium to Establish a Registry for Alzheimer's Disease (CERAD). This test was developed after decades of investigation by psychiatrists interested in identifying test items that differentiated functional from "organic" mental syndromes; the final version was dependent on work by Roth[42] and associates and Shapiro and associates.[43] Subsequently, the Mini-Mental State Examination (MMSE) was described by Folstein et al.[44] and the MMSE has enjoyed wider usage than the IMC test. The two tests have many items in common; they differ in that the MMSE tests a broader range of function with items that test reading, writing, and manipulation of objects, whereas the IMC is entirely verbal but includes items of greater difficulty than those in the MMSE, items that are useful in testing subjects in the earliest stages of Alzheimer's disease. The items include the recall of a five-part name and address and recitation of the months of the year backward.

Mental status tests — and many variations of the above tests have been proposed and field tested — are relatively easy to administer and dominate both clinical and epidemiological studies. Such tests, however, are subject to a variety of problems including the effect of education and culture on the response.

Perhaps a more universal measure of the presence of dementia and dementia severity are questionnaires that quantitate impairment of so-called instrumental activities of daily living, such as the ability to handle money or shop independently, and, in late stages of dementia, instruments that estimate impairment of activities of daily living, such as dressing, eating, or toileting. Both types of activities of daily living were included in the dementia score that had been validated by the Blessed, Tomlinson, and Roth study.[19] Alternate forms of these tests, particularly the scales of Lawton and Brody,[45] Katz,[46] and Pfeffer[47] are more often used today. All of these functional questionnaires depend on the availability of a reliable informant, but when used together with a mental status test are excellent indicators of the presence of a dementing illness and hence are especially useful in epidemiological studies.

C. DIAGNOSTIC CRITERIA FOR ALZHEIMER'S DISEASE

The success of the DSM-III criteria for the diagnosis of dementia led to the formation of a task force by the National Institute of Neurological and Communicative Disorders and Strokes (NINCDS) and the ADRDA to establish criteria for the diagnosis of Alzheimer's disease.[48] The task force agreed that the definitive diagnosis of Alzheimer's disease depends on neuropathological confirmation. However, their criteria for "probable" Alzheimer's disease has turned out to have an accuracy of 85 to 95% based on subsequent clinical–pathological analyses.

This high degree of accuracy was attained by the widespread adoption of an intensive clinical evaluation that required a careful clinical history, mental status testing, and neuropsychological and neuropsychiatric examination, all office procedures. In addition, this evaluation required blood tests to rule out various unusual but important metabolic disorders that might produce cognitive impairment, and an imaging procedure (such as a CT scan) to rule out the rare dementias secondary to hydrocephalus or midline tumors that do not present with focal signs. In addition, the imaging procedure assists in the diagnosis of vascular dementia by confirming the presence of cerebral infarcts. However, neither biopsies nor more complicated procedures such as positron emission tomography (PET) were needed to achieve these accuracy rates. This is perhaps remarkable among the major diseases of our time. Definitive diagnosis was recognized to require autopsy confirmation. The many families who actively participated in giving autopsy permission for their loved ones with presumed Alzheimer's disease were rewarded in most cases with a definitive diagnosis and, in some cases, a diagnosis of important but less common neurodegenerative diseases such as Pick's disease.

D. A REMAINING PROBLEM: DIFFERENTIATING ALZHEIMER'S DISEASE AND CEREBROVASCULAR DEMENTIA IN SUBJECTS WHO HAVE HAD A STROKE OR OTHER EVIDENCE OF SEVERE CEREBROVASCULAR DISEASE

The nosology of dementia is complicated by the existence of a progressive dementia in some individuals with strokes, a relationship that was recognized during the 19th century [Alzheimer published a paper on atheroma and dementia in 1898 (described by Bick[1])]. Strokes, like Alzheimer's disease, are age-dependent disorders which increase exponentially during the same period of life. Hence, there is a significant number of brains in the very elderly that contain evidence both of Alzheimer changes and of cerebrovascular disease. How can the clinician dissociate what role, if any, vascular or Alzheimer changes play in the development of dementia in an elderly patient?

Historically, great confusion was caused by the assumption of some earlier investigators that progressive dementia in the elderly had a single cause, and they could not decide between these two pathologies. The diagnosis of vascular dementia achieved a vogue in the 1940s and 1950s when Dr. Walter Alvarez, a highly respected physician from the Mayo Clinic, ignoring the extant neuropathological literature, speculated that most cases of progressive cognitive symptoms in the elderly were due to multiple small strokes. He was a persuasive writer, and families of elderly dements were told that the condition was due to rigid arteries. It should be noted that, at the middle of the 20th century, there was still not adequate treatment for hypertension, and major stroke was four times more common than today. One can therefore assume that vascular dementia was undoubtedly more common than today, but in our own opinion most of the cases of progressive dementia even in the 1960s were likely due to Alzheimer's disease.

It was the prospective clinical–pathological study of Blessed and colleagues[19] described above that led to an initial, but not fully satisfying, resolution of this problem. Tomlinson and colleagues[49] described in detail the neuropathological changes in the brains of the 17 patients in this study who were thought to have vascular dementia. All had multiple cerebral infarcts — areas of dead brain tissue secondary to strokes — with a total volume greater than 50 ml and in most cases with a volume in excess of 100 ml of infarcted brain. It was the infarcted brain tissue, not the presence of atheromatous plaques in blood vessels, that caused the dementia in these cases.

The concept that most cases of cerebrovascular dementia are due to multiple large infarcts became widely accepted. However, with the successful prevention of stroke by control of hypertension, the type of patient with large multiple infarcts described by Tomlinson et al.[49] in their original clinical pathological description is seldom seen today. Indeed, large cerebral infarcts occur with only one fourth the number that occurred in the 1960s. Nevertheless, as Tatemichi[50] has recently shown, there are patients who have a single major infarct who develop progressive dementia without additional infarcts and others with multiple small infarcts or lacunes who develop dementia secondary to these vascular events. The problem has been further complicated by the overreading of hyperintense spots on the T_2 image of the MRI which have been interpreted by some radiologists as indicative of ischemic disease but which are also seen in normal elderly and in Alzheimer's disease.

A further diagnostic complication is that the amyloid angiopathy of Alzheimer's disease can, if severe, lead to cerebral infarcts, particularly in patients who also are hypertensive.[51] Thus, we are at an impasse today. We do not understand the pathogenesis of vascular dementia. As a consequence we continue to make diagnostic errors. It is now evident that scoring systems based on the original concept of a true multi-infarct dementia — the Hachinski ischemic score[52] or the Rosen modification[53] thereof — lead to only about a 50% accuracy of diagnosis of vascular dementia based on post-mortem findings. Recent attempts[54-56] to develop better criteria for the diagnosis of vascular dementia are now being evaluated. The question of whether diagnosis can improve prior to an improvement in our basic understanding of this type of dementia is yet to be determined.

VIII. EPIDEMIOLOGY AND RISK FACTORS
FOR ALZHEIMER'S DISEASE

A. HOW MANY PERSONS HAVE ALZHEIMER'S DISEASE?
AGE AS A MAJOR DETERMINANT

Can the prevalence of Alzheimer's disease be measured? The diagnostic criteria for dementia that were introduced by the American Psychiatric Association in 1980 as the DSM-III criteria[39] required that there be loss of intellectual abilities of sufficient severity to interfere with social or occupational functioning as well as impairment of memory and at least one other area of cognition in an individual who is alert and awake. In clinical experience, many individuals begin symptomotology with cognitive deficit in just one area, often but not always memory, and do not reach the point at which this deficit interferes with life activities for some period of time, thus making the diagnosis quite conservative. The impact of these conservative diagnostic criteria on community studies may be considerable since elderly persons with impairment of only memory or who are still functioning well despite mild cognitive changes in two areas of cognition would not be counted as demented even if in the early stage of Alzheimer's disease. Thus, the figures for Evans and associates[57] for the prevalence of dementia in East Boston were almost double those obtained in the Shanghai study of dementia described below. These differences may be real differences between communities, but may also reflect of the impact of DSM-III criteria which were used in the Shanghai study whereas, in the East Boston study, the requirement for demonstration of functional impairment was not used.

Despite these problems there is universal agreement between studies that when one plots the log of age-specific prevalence of dementia against a linear plot of age in years a straight line can be obtained over the range of ages between 65 and 85 years, indicating that dementia doubles every 4.9 to 5.1 years.[58]

B. CASE–CONTROL AND LONGITUDINAL STUDIES IDENTIFY OTHER RISK FACTORS

With the conservative but accurate DSM-III and McKhann et al. diagnostic criteria for dementia and Alzheimer's disease,[39,48] it became feasible to select individuals with probable Alzheimer's disease with a high degree of accuracy and compare them to age- and gender-matched controls to identify other risk factors. A number of such case–control studies have been carried out during the last decade.[59] Family history, of course, has been known as a risk factor for Alzheimer's disease for decades and certainly have been confirmed in case–control studies, particularly in those dealing with subjects with onset before the age of 75. Another risk factor demonstrated to be a relatively strong risk factor in a collaborative reanalysis of 12 case studies by EURODEM was head injury associated with a loss of consciousness or a brief hospitalization.[60] Additional risk factors of interest reported by the EURODEM analysis include a history of severe depression, a history of Down's syndrome in a relative, a history of Parkinson's disease in a first-degree relative, and perhaps a history of advanced maternal age.

Another provocative finding, obtained in one longitudinal study that included cardiovascular as well as neurological workups on a yearly basis, the Bronx Aging Study, is that myocardial infarct is a risk factor in elderly women. This finding takes on added interest in view of the finding that the Apolipoprotein E4 allele is a risk factor for both heart disease and Alzheimer's disease. This finding has yet to be confirmed in other studies. However, Sparks et al.[61] have reported a very significant increase in plaques in neocortex in medical examiner cases of elderly individuals who had a 75% stenosis of a coronary vessel compared to those who did not have heart disease.

C. LACK OF EDUCATIONAL ATTAINMENT AS A RISK FACTOR FOR ALZHEIMER'S DISEASE AND OTHER PROGRESSIVE DEMENTIAS

In 1988, Mortimer[62] considered two sets of risk factors for Alzheimer's disease: social variables, such as education and occupation, and individual psychological characteristics including intelligence, personality, and stress. He argued (p. 39) that "… psychosocial factors act primarily to reduce the margin of intellectual reserve to a level where a more modest level of brain pathology results in a diagnosable dementia." He predicted that as a consequence these psychosocial risk factors would have their strongest association in late onset at a time when the aging process has reduced the normal brain reserve.

We had the opportunity to confirm these predictions. In 1987, Drs. David Salmon, Igor Grant, and Robert Katzman at UCSD were invited to participate in a survey of the prevalence of dementing disorders in a randomly selected population of 5055 elderly who lived in the Jin-An district in Shanghai, China,[63] which was carried out by Mingyuan Zhang and colleagues at the Shanghai Institute of Mental Health in collaboration with Drs. William Liu, Paul Levy, and Elena Yu at the University of Illinois in Chicago. An unexpected finding was that 27.2% of the cohort had never been to school, i.e., had no education whatsoever; 36.7% had received elementary education, many only 1 to 2 years; and 36.1% had middle school educations or higher, with doctoral degrees, thus constituting a very wide spread in the educational spectrum in this community. During the first phase it was quickly apparent that those without formal education would obtain quite low scores on the Chinese version of the Mini-Mental State Examination that we had used, so following the recommendations of Kittner and associates[64] we used education-specific cut-off scores on this examination in selecting subjects for a more intensive clinical evaluation. It was interesting that the deficits in those with no education extended beyond reading or calculation; approximately 90% of those without formal education were unable to copy the overlapping pentagons figure on the Mini-Mental State Examination. Individuals who had never held a brush or pencil early in life were not able to learn to use these tools at age 75.

In the second phase of this survey, an intensive clinical examination based on DSM-III and NINCDS–ADRDA criteria was carried out on subjects who were below the education-specific cutoff scores on the Chinese version of the Mini-Mental Status Examination plus 5% of the remaining subjects from phase 1. The work-up included a major illness history, physical examination, neurological examination, psychiatric interview, depression scales, and neuropsychological tests. Functional change was measured by dementia symptom lists, the Pfeffer functional scale and the Instrumental Activities of Daily Living and Activities of Daily Living scales. Clinical diagnoses made by the examining physicians were subsequently reviewed by experienced neurologists and psychiatrists. There was a very dramatic effect of education on the prevalence of dementia and of Alzheimer's disease, particularly among the women. For example, among 75- to 84-year-old women, the prevalence of dementia was 3.9% in those with middle school or more education, 12.6% in those with elementary school, and 18% in those with no education. Even though we used education-specific cut-off points, we were concerned that the known relationship of mental status test to education might have confounded the diagnostic process. We therefore carried out a further analysis of the data using computer algorithms to determine the diagnosis. Reanalysis of data using computer diagnoses based only on impairment of instrumental activities of daily living and dementia symptoms reported by informant shows an almost identical effect of low education. Moreover, the finding in this analysis and in the original analysis that the noneducated individuals under the age of 75 seldom have an increased risk of dementia whereas this risk is present over the age of 75 again suggests that the education effect in this cohort is real and is consistent with the Mortimer prediction.

A similar effect of education was observed in studies of the prevalence of dementia carried out in France, Sweden, Italy, Finland, and Israel as well as in studies of incident cases of dementia carried out in North Manhattan. An exception has been the Framingham study which did not show an education effect. Additional supportive evidence in regard to the education effect is found in studies of longevity without functional impairment in an order of Catholic sisters as well as from studies of incident cases of cognitive impairment in the EPESE studies (White).[65] With regard to the strength of the education effect, this must be determined in a multivariate analysis taking age into account because age is such a powerful determinant, and lack of education is much more common in older individuals. With such multivariate analysis in the Shanghai study, the relative risk for those with middle school education vs. noneducation was 2.04 and in the Bordeaux study it was 1.94.

Still, it must be remembered that while education is a risk factor, that Alzheimer's disease is a democratic disease. Individuals in any occupation or of any intellectual ability may be afflicted. An example is George Beadle, a Nobel laureate who was, in large part, personally responsible for opening up the area of biochemical genetics and who also served as the President of the University of Chicago for 7 years, who died in the 1980s at age 86 of Alzheimer's disease. However, in many community studies, lack of education is an important risk factor.

IX. FROM "FAMILIAL PREDISPOSITION" TO MULTIPLE GENOTYPES

A critical aspect of the etiology of Alzheimer's disease that is now being resolved is the role of specific genes and genetic mutations in predisposing individuals to the disorder. As far back as the mid-1920s familial cases of Alzheimer's disease were reported, but more extensive studies began decades later (see Jarvik[66] for a succinct summary of the work to be described). In 1952 Sjögren[67] reported a markedly increased risk of Alzheimer's disease in the parents of 36 patients with the presenile onset of dementia. Larsson and co-workers[68] subsequently carried out a study of senile dementia in Sweden and found a threefold increase in risk in parents and siblings. Indeed numerous case–control studies have subsequently confirmed an approximately threefold risk of developing Alzheimer's disease if one has a first-degree relative with the disorder. Of particular interest is the Kallman[69] study of 108 twin pairs among which only 8.0% of dizygotic twin pairs were concordant but 42.5% of monozygotic twin pairs were concordant. These various investigators were split between an autosomal dominant gene with incomplete penetrance and a polygenic inheritance. Jarvik[66] (p. 274) stated that her "own bias is in favor of genetic heterogeneity … It is likely, I think, that even if one day we will be able to define clinically a relatively homogeneous entity we will still have a group of genetically distinct, even if clinically indistinguishable, disorders."

Jarvik's prediction has proven correct. Mutations that cause or predispose to Alzheimer's disease have been identified at three loci and likely exist at others. These mutations include single- or double-point mutations bracketing the β-amyloid sequence of the APP gene on chromosome 21 responsible for a well-studied handful of cases of presenile onset that are truly autosomal dominant, a still-to-be-sequenced, probably dominant, genetic mutation at a well-defined locus on chromosome 14 also involved in subjects with onset before age 65 and the ε4 allele of the Apolipoprotein E gene on chromosome 19 which is co-dominant for Alzheimer's disease with onset later in life and which in the heterozygous state predisposes toward Alzheimer's disease but with less than a 50% expression at age 85. Moreover, genetic data indicate that still other genes important in the etiology of Alzheimer's disease are yet to be defined. These advances are described in more detail in chapters 12, 14, and 16.

An interesting prediction in regard to gene–age–education interaction can be made. If the majority of those individuals with an Apolipoprotein ε4 allele who will develop Alzheimer's disease have already contracted the disorder, then the exponential rate of increase in the incidence and prevalence of dementia that occurs between ages 65 and 85 might be markedly reduced at still more advanced ages. Moreover, if the education effect is due to earlier onset of dementia in those with low education, then at still more advanced ages (e.g., over age 90), there should be a greater increase in the number of new cases of dementia in those with higher education and perhaps a fall-off in the incidence of dementia in those with no education. Testing this prediction will require following a large cohort into their 10th decade of life.

REFERENCES

1. Bick, K. L., The early story of Alzheimer's disease, in *Alzheimer's Disease*, Terry, R. D., Katzman, R., and Bick, K. L., Eds., Raven Press, New York, 1994, 1.
2. Newton, R. D., The identity of Alzheimer's disease and senile dementia and their relationship in senility, *J. Mental Sci.*, 94, 225, 1948.
3. Neumann, M. A. and Cohn, R., Incidence of Alzheimer's disease in a large mental hospital: relation to senile psychosis and psychosis with cerebral arteriosclerosis, *Arch. Neurol. Psychiatr.*, 69, 615, 1953.
4. Terry, R. D., Neurofibrillary tangles in Alzheimer's disease, *J. Neuropathol. Exp. Neurol.*, 22, 629, 1963.
5. Kidd, M., Paired helical filaments in electron microscopy in Alzheimer's disease, *Nature*, 197, 192, 1963.
6. Divry, P., Cerebral ageing, *J. Belge Neurol. Psychiatry*, 47, 65, 1947.
7. Terry, R. D., Gonatas, N. K., and Weiss, M., Ultrastructural studies in Alzheimer's presenile dementia, *Am. J. Pathol.*, 44, 269, 1964.
8. Glenner, G. G. and Wong, C. W., Alzheimer's disease: Initial report of the purification and characterization of a novel cerebrovascular amyloid protein, *Biochem. Biophys. Res. Commun.*, 120, 885, 1984.
9. Glenner, G. G. and Wong, C. W., Alzheimer's disease and Down's syndrome: sharing of a unique cerebrovascular amyloid fibril protein, *Biochem. Biophys. Res. Commun.*, 122, 1131, 1984.
10. Goldgaber, D., Lerman, M. I., McBride, O. W., Saffiotti, U., and Gajdusek, D. C., Characterization and chromosomal localization of a cDNA encoding brain amyloid of Alzheimer's disease, *Science*, 235, 877, 1987.
11. Robakis, N., Wisniewski, H. M., Jenkins, E. C., Devine-Gage, E. A., Houck, E., Yao, X.-L., Ramakrishna, N., Wolfe, G., Silverman, W. P., and Brown, W. T., Chromosome 21q21 sublocalization of gene encoding β-amyloid peptide in cerebral vessels and neuritic (senile) plaques of people with Alzheimer's disease and Down syndrome, *Lancet*, 2, 384, 1987.
12. St. George-Hyslop, P. H., Tanzi, R. E., Polinsky, R. J., Haines, J. L., Nee, L., Watkins, P. C., Myers, R. H., Feldman, R. G., Pollen, D., Drachman, D., Growdon, J., Bruni, A., Foncin, J.-F., Salmon, D., Frommelt, P., Amaducci, L., Sorbi, S., Placentini, S., Stewart, G. D., Hobbs, W. J., Conneally, P. M., and Gusella, J. F., The genetic defect causing familial Alzheimer's disease maps on chromosome 21, *Science*, 235, 885, 1987.
13. Kang, J., Lemaire, H.-G., Unterbeck, A., Salbaum, M. J., Masters, C. L., Grzeschik, K.-H., Multhaup, G., Beyreuther, K., and Müller-Hill, B., The precursor of Alzheimer's disease amyloid A4 protein resembles a cell-surface receptor, *Nature*, 325, 733, 1987.
14. Iqbal, K., Grundke-Iqbal, I., Smith, A. J., George, L., Tung, Y.-C., and Zaidi, T., Identification and localization of a τ peptide to paired helical filaments of Alzheimer's disease, *Proc. Natl. Acad. Sci. U.S.A.*, 86, 5646, 1989.

15. Selkoe, D. J., Ihara, Y., and Salazar, F. J., Alzheimer's disease: insolubility of partially-purified paired helical filaments in sodium dodecyl sulfate and urea, *Science*, 215, 1243, 1982.
16. Brion, J. P., Passareiro, H., Nunez, J., and Flament-Durand, J., Mise en evidence immunologique de la proteine tau au niveau des lesions de degenerescence neurofibrillaire de la maladie d'Alzheimer, *Arch. Biol.*, 95, 229, 1985.
17. Suzuki, K. and Terry, R. D., Fine structural localization of acid phosphatase in senile plaques in Alzheimer's presenile dementia, *Acta Neuropathol.*, 8, 276, 1967.
18. Wisniewski, H. M., Narang, H. K., and Terry, R. D., Neurofibrillary tangles of paired helical filaments, *J. Neurol. Sci.*, 27, 173, 1976.
19. Blessed, G., Tomlinson, B. E., and Roth, M., The association between quantitative measures of dementia and of senile change in the cerebral grey matter of elderly subjects, *Br. J. Psychiatry*, 114, 797, 1968.
20. Hamos, J. E., DeGennaro, L. J., and Drachman, D. A., Synaptic loss in Alzheimer's disease and other dementias, *Neurology*, 39, 355, 1989.
21. Masliah, E., Terry, R. D., Alford, M., DeTeresa, R., and Hansen, L. A., Cortical and subcortical patterns of synaptophysin-like immunoreactivity in Alzheimer's disease, *Am. J. Pathol.*, 138, 235, 1991.
22. Terry, R. D. and Katzman, R., Alzheimer's disease and cognitive loss, in *Principles of Geriatric Neurology*, Katzman, R. and Rowe, J., Eds., F. A. Davis, Philadelphia, 1992, 207.
23. Terry, R. D., Masliah, E., Salmon, D. P., Butters, N., DeTeresa, R., Hill, L. R., Hansen, L. A., and Katzman, R., Physical basis of cognitive alterations in Alzheimer's disease: synapse loss is the major correlate of cognitive impairment, *Ann. Neurol.*, 30, 572, 1991.
24. Bowen, D. M., Smith, C. B., White, P., and Davison, A. N., Neurotransmitter–related enzymes and indices of hypoxia in senile dementia and other abiotrophies, *Brain*, 99, 459, 1976.
25. Davies, P. and Maloney, A. J. R., Selective loss of central cholinergic neurons in Alzheimer's disease, *Lancet*, 2, 1403, 1976.
26. Drachman, D. A. and Leavitt, J., Human memory and the cholinergic system, *Arch. Neurol.*, 30, 113, 1974.
27. Johnston, M. V., McKinney, M., and Coyle, J. R., Evidence for a cholinergic projection to neocortex from neurons in the basal forebrain, *Proc. Natl. Acad. Sci. U.S.A.*, 76, 5392, 1979.
28. Whitehouse, P. J., Price, D. L., Struble, R. G., Clark, A. W., Coyle, J. T., and DeLong, M. R., Alzheimer's disease and senile dementia: loss of neurons in the basal forebrain, *Science*, 215, 1237, 1982.
29. Rossor, M. and Iversen, L. L., Non-cholinergic neurotransmitter abnormalities in Alzheimer's disease, *Br. Med. Bull.*, 42, 70, 1986.
30. Katzman, R., The prevalence and malignancy of Alzheimer's disease; A major killer, *Arch. Neurol.*, 33, 217, 1976.
31. Gruenberg, E. M., A Mental Health Survey of Older Persons, in *Comparative Epidemiology of the Mental Disorders*, Hoch, P. C. and Zubin, J., Eds., Grune & Stratton, New York, 1961, 13.
32. Jellinger, K., Neuropathological aspects of dementias resulting from abnormal blood and cerebrospinal fluid dynamics, *Acta Neurol.*, 76, 83, 1976.
33. Fox, P., From senility to Alzheimer's disease: the rise of the Alzheimer's disease movement, *Milbank Fund. Q.*, 67, 58, 1989.
34. Lombardo, N. E., Alzheimer's disease and related disorders association: birth and evolution of a major voluntary health association, in *Understanding Alzheimer's Disease*, Aronson, M. K., Eds., Scribners and Sons, New York, 1988, 323.
35. Ron, M. A., Toone, B. K., Garralda, M. E., and Lishman, W. A., Diagnostic accuracy in presenile dementia, *Br. J. Psychiatry*, 134, 161, 1979.
36. Kiloh, L. G., Pseudodementia, *Acta Psychiatr. Scand.*, 37, 336, 1961.
37. Folstein, M. F. and McHugh, P. R., Dementia syndrome of depression, in *Alzheimer's Disease*, Katzman, R., Terry, R. D., and Bick, K. L., Eds., Raven Press, New York, 1978, 87.
38. Wells, C. E., Pseudodementia, *Am. J. Psychiatry*, 136, 895, 1979.
39. American Psychiatric Association Task Force on Nomenclature and Statistics, Ed., *Diagnostic and Statistical Manual of Mental Disorders (DSM-III)*, American Psychiatric Association, Washington, DC, 1980.
40. Larson, E. B., Reifler, B. V., Sumi, S. M., Canfield, C. G., and Chinn, N. M., Diagnostic evaluation of 200 elderly outpatients with suspected dementia, *J. Gerontol.*, 40, 536, 1985.
41. Katzman, R., Brown, T., Fuld, P., Peck, A., Schechter, R., and Schimmel, H., Validation of a short orientation-memory-concentration test of cognitive impairment, *Am. J. Psychiatry*, 140, 734, 1983.
42. Roth, M., The natural history of mental disorder in old age, *Br. J. Psychiatry*, 101, 281, 1955.
43. Shapiro, M. B., Post, F., Lofbing, B., and Inglis, J., Memory function in psychiatric patients over 60: Some methodological and diagnostic implications, *J. Mental Sci.*, 102, 233, 1956.
44. Folstein, M. F., Folstein, S. E., and McHugh, P. R., "Mini-Mental State". A practical method for grading the cognitive state of patients for the clinician, *J. Psychiatr. Res.*, 12, 189, 1975.
45. Lawton, M. P. and Brody, E. M., Assessment of older people: self-maintaining and instrumental activities of daily living, *Gerontologist*, 9, 179, 1969.
46. Katz, S., Ford, A. B., Moskowitz, R. W., Jackson, B. A., and Jaffe, M. W., Studies of illness in the aged. The index of ADL: a standardized measure of biological and psychosocial function, *JAMA*, 185, 914, 1963.
47. Pfeffer, R. I., Kurosaki, T. T., Harrah, C. H., Jr., Chance, J. M., Bates, D., Detels, R., Filos, S., and Butzke, C., A survey diagnostic tool for senile dementia, *Am. J. Epidemiol.*, 114, 515, 1981.

48. McKhann, G., Drachman, D., Folstein, M., Katzman, R., Proce, D., and Stadlan, E. M., Clinical diagnosis of Alzheimer's disease: report of the NINCDS–ADRDA Work Groups under the auspices of Department of Health and Human Services Task Force on Alzheimer's Disease, *Neurology*, 34, 939, 1984.
49. Tomlinson, B. E., Blessed, G., and Roth, M., Observations on the brains of demented old people, *J. Neurol. Sci.*, 11, 205, 1970.
50. Tatemichi, T. K., Desmond, D. W., Paik, M., Figueroa, M., Gropen, T. I., Stern, Y., Sano, M., Remien, R., Williams, J. B., Mohr, J. P., et al., Clinical determinants of dementia related to stroke, *Ann. Neurol.*, 33, 568, 1993.
51. Olichney, J. M., Hansen, L., Hofstetter, C. R., Grundman, M., Katzman, R., and Thal, L. J., Cerebral infarction in Alzheimer's disease is associated with severe amyloid angiopathy and hypertension, *Arch. Neurol.*, 92, 702, 1995.
52. Hachinski, V., Cerebral blood flow: differentiation of Alzheimer's disease from multi-infarct dementia, in *Aging*, Katzman, R., and Terry, R. D., and Bick, K. L., Eds., Raven Press, New York, 1978, 97.
53. Rosen, W. G., Terry, R. D., Fuld, P. A., Katzman, R., and Peck, A., Pathological verification of ischemic score in differentiation of dementias, *Ann. Neurol.*, 7, 486, 1980.
54. Chui, H. C., Teng, E. L., Henderson, V. W., and Moy, A. C., Clinical subtypes of dementia of the Alzheimer type, *Neurology*, 35, 1544, 1985.
55. Erkinjuntti, T., Differential diagnosis between Alzheimer's disease and vascular dementia: evaluation of common clinical methods, *Acta Neurol. Scand.*, 76, 433, 1987.
56. Román, G. C., Tatemichi, T. K., Erkinjuntti, T., Cummings, J. L., Masdeu, J. C., Garcia, J. H., Amaducci, L., Orgogozo, J. M., Brun, A., Hofman, A., Moody, D. M., O'Brien, M. D., Yamaguchi, T., Grafman, J., Drayer, B. P., Bennet, D. A., Fisher, M., Ogata, J., Kokmen, E., Bermejo, F., Wolf, P. A., Gorelick, P. B., Bick, K. L., Pajeau, A. K., Bell, M. A., DeCarli, C., Culebras, A., Korczyn, A. D., Bogousslavsky, J., Hartmann, A., and Scheinberg, P., Vascular dementia: diagnostic criteria for research studies. Report of the NINDS–AIREN International Workshop [see comments], *Neurology*, 43, 250, 1993.
57. Evans, D. A., Funkenstein, H., Albert, M. S., Scherr, P. A., Cook, N. R., Chown, M. J., Hebert, L. E., Hennekens, C. H., and Taylor, J. O., Prevalence of Alzheimer's disease in a community population of older persons, *JAMA*, 262, 2551, 1989.
58. Jorm, A. F., Korten, A. E., and Henderson, A. S., The prevalence of dementia: a quantitative integration of the literature, *Acta Psychiatr. Scand.*, 76, 464, 1987.
59. Katzman, R. and Kawas, C., The epidemiology of dementia and alzheimer disease, in *Alzheimer Disease*, Terry, R. D., Katzman, R., and Bick, K. L., Eds., Raven Press, New York, 1994, 105.
60. Mortimer, J. A., van Duijn, C. M., Chandra, V., Fratiglioni, L., Graves, A. B., Heyman, A., Jorm, A. F., Kokmen, E., Kondo, K., Rocca, W. A., Shalat, S. L., Soininen, H., and Hofman, A., Head trauma as a risk factor for Alzheimer's disease: a collaborative re-analysis of case–control studies, *Int. J. Epidemiol.*, 20(Suppl. 2), 28, 1991.
61. Sparks, D. L., Hunsaker, J. C., Scheff, S. W., Kryscic, R. F., Henson, J. L., and Markesbery, W. R., Cortical senile plaques in coronary artery disease, aging and Alzheimer's disease, *Neurobiol. Aging*, 11, 601, 1990.
62. Mortimer, J. A., Do psychosocial risk factors contribute to Alzheimer's disease?, in *Etiology of Dementia of Alzheimer's Type*, Henderson, A. S. and Henderson, J. H., Eds., John Wiley & Sons, New York, 1988, 39.
63. Zhang, M., Katzman, R., Jin, H., Cai, G., Wang, Z., Qu, G., Grant, I., Yu, E., Levy, P., and Liu, W. T., The prevalence of dementia and Alzheimer's disease (AD) in Shanghai, China: impact of age, gender and education, *Ann. Neurol.*, 27, 428, 1990.
64. Kittner, S. J., White, L. R., Farmer, M. E., Wolz, M., Kaplan, E., Moes, E., Brody, J. A., and Feinleib, M., Methodological issues in screening for dementia: The problem of education adjustment, *J. Chron. Dis.*, 39, 163, 1985.
65. White, L., Katzman, R., Losonczy, K., Salive, M., Wallace, R., Berkman, L., Taylor, J., Fillenbaum, G., Evans, D., and Havlik, R., Association of education with incidence of cognitive impairment in three established populations for epidemiologic studies of the elderly, *J. Clin. Epidemiol.*, 47, 363, 1994.
66. Jarvik, L. F., Genetic Factors and Chromosomal Aberrations in Alzheimer's Disease, Senile Dementia, and Related Disorders, in *Alzheimer's Disease: Senile Dementia and Related Disorders*, Katzman, R., Terry, R. D., and Bick, K. L., Eds., Raven Press, New York, 1978, 273.
67. Sjögren, T., Sjögren, H., and Lingren, G. H., Morbus Alzheimer and morbus Pick., *Acta Psychiatr. Neurol. Scand.*, Suppl. 52, 1952.
68. Larsson, T., Sjogren, T., and Jacobson, G., Senile dementia: a clinical, sociomedical and genetic study, *Acta Psychiatr. Scand.*, 39(Suppl. 167), 1, 1963.
69. Kallmann, F. J., Genetic aspects of mental disorders in later life, in *Mental Disorders in Later Life*, Vol. II, Kaplan, O. J., Eds., Stanford University Press, Stanford, 1956, 26; 1956.

RECOMMENDED READINGS

Katzman, R., Alzheimer's disease, *N. Engl. J. Med.*, 314, 964, 1986.
Terry, R. D., Katzman, R., and Bick, K. L., Eds., *Alzheimer Disease*, Raven Press, New York, 1993.

Chapter 3

A HISTORY OF THE MORPHOLOGY OF ALZHEIMER'S DISEASE

_____ Robert D. Terry

In 1906 the pathologist/psychiatrist Alois Alzheimer reported to a group of German psychiatrists the story of a 55-year-old woman who died after several years of progressive dementia, and in whose brain he had found both senile plaques and neurofibrillary tangles.[1] Alzheimer had applied newly discovered silver stains to the tissue in order to better delineate these microscopic lesions. Plaques had been previously seen, presumably with aniline stains, but not in association with dementia, while cortical tangles had not been previously described. The head of Alzheimer's department in Munich was Emil Kraepelin, who at the time was a dominant figure in European psychiatry, and who eagerly promoted the notion of psychiatric disease being based on organic brain changes. Kraepelin applied Alzheimer's name to the newly described syndrome of dementia-plaques-tangles in the eighth edition of his important text _Psychiatrie_ in 1910.

The two lesions, i.e., the intraneuronal neurofibrillary tangle and the neuropil plaque, are still regarded as the most important diagnostic markers and by most investigators as being the most important elements in the pathogenesis of dementia. The components of these lesions were not ascertained until the application of electron microscopy in the early 1960s, more than 50 years subsequent to Alzheimer's first light microscopic description.

During that half century, however, several important findings were added to the picture and to our understanding. In 1911, Simchowicz reported the presence of granulovacuolar bodies in hippocampal pyramidal neurons and occasionally in neurons of the basal nucleus of Meynert.[2] They are very rare elsewhere, and their significance is still unknown. In 1927, the Belgian Divry recognized that the more or less amorphous material in the core of the plaque is amyloid.[3] This abnormal fibrillar protein, which is now known to be derived from a normal large precursor protein,[4] is currently believed by many investigators to be the major pathogenetic factor. Scholtz recognized amyloid in the cortical and meningeal blood vessels in 1938,[5] and it was the latter location which gave Glenner the opportunity to isolate and sequence the amyloid peptide some 45 years later.[6]

At the time of my first interest in Alzheimer's disease in 1959, there was very little current epidemiologic, clinical, or investigative activity in the field. That most cases of senile dementia were due to Alzheimer's disease was not recognized prior to Corsellis' 1962 book.[7] In 1959 Saul Korey, who was Chief of Neurology and a well-trained neurochemist at the Einstein College of Medicine, and Robert Terry decided to study the disease utilizing brain biopsy tissue, not because the clinical importance of the disorder was known to us, but rather because the problem seemed to be accessible to our technology. That was the case in the sense that the disease was fatal and thus the biopsy procedure could do relatively little harm even at worst. Second, the changes were diffuse so that the neurosurgeon could remove a small portion (less than 1 gram) from any "silent" region of the neocortex and could expect it to contain lesions. Third, it had distinctive histologic changes such that a histopathologic diagnosis could be made. A great neurosurgeon, Leo M. Davidoff, performed about a half dozen cortical biopsies at Einstein within the first few years, and none of these patients had any post-operative difficulties.

The tangles were easily found with the electron microscope, and were revealed to be made up curious, twisted fibers which Kidd, working simultaneously at Maida Vale Hospital with McMenemy in London, reported correctly as paired helical filaments (PHF),[8] but which we in New York thought were twisted tubules.[9] In any case, they did not appear to be identical to normal neurofilaments although the dimensions were about the same. Similarly, they appeared not to have the same electron density as neurotubules, which, in fact, were rather poorly preserved in the fixatives available at the time. PHF are now known to be made up largely of hyperphosphorylated tau protein,[10] and this process of abnormal phosphorylation undoubtedly plays a major role in the overall pathogenesis of AD. The twisted structures of the tangle are not universally accepted as PHF. A flat twisted ribbon has been recently suggested by atomic force microscopy.[11]

The senile plaques were much more difficult to identify and delineate in those early days. We ultimately determined[12] that at the center of these spherical lesions were more or less compact bundles of filaments representing amyloid fibers. Surrounding them were groups of unmyelinated neuronal processes, many of which were distended and contained PHF identical to those of the tangle. Many of these neurites terminated in presynaptic boutons which were also enlarged and contained many degenerating mitochondria and dense bodies, as well as clusters of synaptic vesicles. The synaptic gap and the postsynaptic terminal were usually normal. Most of the dystrophic neurites were, therefore, axonal. Astrocytic perikarya are often found on the periphery of the plaque with their filament-filled processes infiltrating the lesion. Microglia are also frequently present in and around the plaque. These cells are often deeply indented by finger-like projections of amyloid bundles. It was subsequently determined by others that in normal aging the neurites of the plaque, although dystrophic, did not contain PHF. In the normal elderly there may be large numbers of plaques, but few or no perikaryal tangles in the cortex; in the absence of tangles, PHF are not to be found in the plaques. These lesions in normal aging contain the same amyloid (β-protein) as do the plaques of the disease.

Most current investigators have not been able to find a significant correlation between the concentration of plaques and the severity of the dementia, in contrast to the earlier, very influential report of Blessed, Tomlinson and Roth.[13] The amyloid burden does not seem to be the cause of dementia.

To add further confusion, some cases of clinically typical Alzheimer's disease are found to have plaques in a concentration consistent with disease but without tangles in the neocortex.[14] PHF are present, however, in entorhinal and hippocampal regions. About two thirds of these plaque-only cases display Lewy bodies in the neocortex, and this latter situation has come to be called the "Lewy body variant".[15] However, there are still significant numbers of elderly demented patients who have many plaques in the neocortex, without neocortical tangles, or Lewy bodies.

A few years after the original electron microscopy, plaques very similar to those of the human were found in aged primates[16] of several species and in old dogs.[17] These lesions differed from human only in that the dystrophic neurites did not contain paired helical filaments. Neuronal tangles are absent. The amyloid in the plaque cores reacted with antibodies prepared from human amyloid.

The dog and monkey thus became the first available animal models of the disease, but they are not entirely satisfactory in that they are not convenient for laboratory work and that they both lack the neurofibrillary tangles. Aluminum came up in this regard when we found that rabbits treated intracisternally with aluminum salts developed fibrillar masses in certain neuronal groups.[18,19] Ultrastructural studies, however, revealed that these fibers were identical to normal neurofilaments, and subsequent chemical analyses bore this out. PHF are quite different. Nevertheless, this finding stimulated research on the relationship of aluminum to Alzheimer's disease, and this issue has not yet been settled.

Cell counting was greatly facilitated by the development of computerized image analysis. The image requires considerable manual editing because of the frequent crowding of cells, and the necessary elimination of vascular cells and artifacts. The technique demonstrated the expected major loss of large neurons in the Alzheimer neocortex amounting to about 35%.[20] The difference between neuron counts in early onset Alzheimer's disease and age-matched normals is highly significant and very obvious. In the more common late-onset cases, there is a smaller but still significant difference from age-matched normals.[21] Not all morphometrists agree with this position. It was a few years later that the same instruments were used for analysis of neuron numbers as a function of normal aging.[22] There it was found that the number of large neurons progressively decreased, but the number of small neurons increased about equally. It was therefore concluded that the large neurons were shrinking, rather than being lost as in AD. All these data are still debated, with at least one group even stating that there is no neuron loss in Alzheimer's disease.[23] Simple microscopic examination of cortex, even without counts, would seem to belie this last position.

In 1976 and early 1977, three neuropharmacologic papers[24-26] were published almost simultaneously in Britain which together enormously increased investigative interest in AD. All demonstrated a highly significant diminution of choline acetyltransferase, thereby proving that the cholinergic system was particularly vulnerable in the disease. Soon thereafter, Whitehouse et al. showed that neurons of the basal nucleus of Meynert, the major source of cortical and hippocampal cholinergic projections, were markedly diminished in number and were frequently affected by tangles.[27] It was not long before other neurotransmitter deficiencies were found, and corresponding neuronal losses demonstrated, as, for example, the locus ceruleus in regard to norepinephrine[28] and the dorsal raphe associated with diminished serotonin.[29] Transmitter deficiencies in the disease are probably caused by the loss of the neurons in which the particular molecule is synthesized.

Silver stains of the Alzheimer neocortex display apparently broken neuritic processes, and this has been recognized for several decades. It was in 1987 that Kowall and Kosik recognized that these fragments are abnormal dendritic processes.[30] These are called neuropil threads, and they have been found to contain the same hyperphosphorylated tau which is the major component of paired helical filaments.

It has long been known that the hippocampal pyramids are very susceptible to tangle formation. The significance of these lesions in the entorhinal cortex was relatively recently emphasized, first by the findings of Hyman et al.[31], and more recently by those of Braak.[32] Hyman showed that the death of entorhinal layer 2 neurons by way of tangle formation leads to loss of the perforant pathway into the hippocampus. Disease in deeper layers of the entorhinal cortex diminishes the efferent target from the hippocampus, which itself is thus isolated. Braak established six stages in the progression of Alzheimer's disease, based largely on the presence of tangles. Most observers agree that the earliest stage involves a few such lesions in the transentorhinal region extending in the second stage into entorhinal cortex and then increasing in hippocampal and neocortical areas through stage six. These stages can be correlated with clinical severity.

Synaptic terminals are only about a micron in diameter and therefore have been enumerated only since the advent of electron microscopy.[33] More recently, immunocytochemistry and its quantitative evaluation by densitometry[34] or by confocal microscopy[35] have made this enumeration more convenient. These latter techniques depend largely on the presence of synaptophysin, which is an antigenic protein integral to the membrane of the synaptic vesicles. In fact, even electron microscopy has been largely dependent on the presence of these vesicles for recognition of the presynaptic bouton, although an older ultrastructural method utilized the phosphotungstic acid reaction on the postsynaptic thickening. All methods agree that there is a significant loss of synaptic terminals in the AD cortex. This change correlates more strongly with the ante-mortem psychometric data than does any other morphologic or biochemical finding.[36] The loss of synapses is proportionally greater than the loss of neuronal cell bodies, and so one can infer that the synapses are lost before the cell body. Such a sequence might well be the result of deficient axoplasmic flow, as was first suggested on other grounds in 1967.[37] There is evidence indicating that neuronal microtubules are destabilized because apolipoprotein E-4 instead of E-3 leaves the tau protein normally bound to microtubules accessible to abnormal phosphorylation.[38] The inadequacy of the microtubule transport mechanism would lead to diminished axoplasmic flow whether the phosphorylated tau is formed into paired helical filaments or is simply present in solution rather than bound to tubules. Diminished axoplasmic flow would lead to dystrophic changes in neurites and to loss of the synaptic terminals. That destruction of synapses is tantamount to a loss of the normal connectivity upon which cognition is based.[39]

The changes undergone by the brain in the process of normal aging explain, at least in major part, the differences between early-onset AD and the late-onset form. The older normal brain has lost synapses and has shrunken or lost pyramidal neurons. This still normal older brain is, therefore, closer to a threshold of minimal connectivity where signs of dementia would appear with only relatively little further loss due to disease.

Since the mid 1980s and the isolation and sequencing of β-amyloid by Glenner,[6] the majority of laboratory research on Alzheimer's disease has centered on this peptide and its precursor protein APP. This large protein has both trophic and toxic epitopes leaving the possibility that filamentous amyloid is but a bystander or marker. Another still unproven possibility is that intraneuronal amyloid or the amyloid gathered almost invisibly at the synapse leads to destruction of the latter and ultimately the cell body itself. Transgenic mouse models utilizing mutations of the amyloid gene with a variety of promotors are at this time becoming somewhat closer in their resemblance to the human disease.[40]

Modeling experiments, be they spontaneous in the subhuman primate or transgenic manipulations of mice, are almost always attempts to mimic the morphologic changes of the human disease. Since it is now accepted that loss of synapses in the neuropil is the ultimate cause of dementia, a useful model must present this change. Morphology and morphometry remain important techniques in this regard as well as to further general understanding of the pathophysiology of Alzheimer's disease.

REFERENCES

1. Alzheimer, A. Uber eine eigenartige Erkrankung der Hirnrinde, *Algemeine Zeitschrift fur Psychiatrie*, 64, 146, 1097.
2. Simchowicz, T., Histopathologische Studien uber die senile demenz, in *Histologie und Histopathologische Arbeiten uber die Grosshirnrinde*, Nissl, F., Alzheimer, A., Eds., Fisher, Jena, Germany, 1911, 1.
3. Divry, P., Etude histo-chimique des plaques senile, *J. Belge. Neurol. Psychiat.,* 27, 643, 1927.
4. Kang J., Lemaire, H.-G., Unterbeck, A., Salbaum, J. M., Master, C. L., et al. The precursor of Alzheimer's disease amyloid A4 protein resembles a cell-surface receptor, *Nature*, 325, 733, 1987.
5. Scholtz, W., Studien zur Pathologie der Hirngefasse. II. Die drusige Entartung de Hirnarterien und Capillaren, *Z. Gesamte Neurol Psychiatr.*, 162, 694, 1938.
6. Glenner, G. G. and Wong, C. W., Alzheimer's disease and Down's syndrome: sharing of a unique cerebrovascular amyloid fibril protein, *Biochem. Biophys. Res. Commun.*, 122, 1131, 1984.
7. Corsellis, J. A. N., *Mental Illness and the Aging Brain*, Oxford University Press, 1962, 1.
8. Kidd, M., Paired helical filaments in electron microscopy in Alzheimer's disease, *Nature*, 197, 192, 1963.
9. Terry, R. D., The fine structure of neurofibrillary tangles in Alzheimer's disease, *J. Neuropathol. Exp. Neurol.*, 22, 629, 1963.
10. Brion, J. P., Passariro, H., Nunez, J., and Flament-Durand, J., Immunologic detection of tau protein in neurofibrillary tangles of Alzheimer's disease, *Arch. Biol.*, 26, 229, 1985.
11. Pollanen, M. S., Markiewicz, P., Bergeron, C., and Goh, M. C., Twisted ribbon structure of paired helical filaments revealed by atomic force microscopy, *Am. J. Pathol.*, 144, 869, 1994.
12. Terry, R. D., Gonatas, N. K., and Weiss, M., Ultrastructural studies in Alzheimer's presenile dementia, *Am. J. Pathol.,* 44, 269, 1964.
13. Blessed, G., Tomlinson, B. E., and Roth, M., The association between quantitative measures of dementia and of senile changes in the cerebral grey matter of elderly subjects, *Br. J. Psych.*, 114, 797, 1968
14. Terry, R. D., Hansen, L. A., DeTeresa, R., Davies, P., Tobias, H., and Katzman, R., Senile dementia of the Alzheimer type without neocortical neurofibrillary tangles, *J. Neuropathol. Exp. Neurol.*, 146, 262, 1987.
15. Hansen, L. A., Masliah, E., Terry, R. D., and Mirra, S. S., A neuropathological subset of Alzheimer's disease with concomitant Lewy body disease and spongiform change, *Acta. Neuropath.*, 78, 194, 1989.
16. Wisniewski, H. M., Ghetti, B., and Terry, R. D. Neuritic (senile) plaques and filamentous changes in aged Rhesus monkeys, *J. Neuropathol. Exp. Neurol.,* 32, 566, 1973.
17. Wisniewski, H. M., Johnson, A. B., Raine, C. D., Kay, W. J., and Terry, R. D., Senile plaques and cerebral amyloidosis in aged dogs. A histochemical and ultrastructural study, *Lab. Invest.*, 23, 287, 1970.
18. Klatzo, I., Wisniewski, H., and Streicher, E., Experimental production of neurofibrillary degeneration I. Light microscopic observations, *J. Neuropathol. Exp. Neurol.*, 24 187, 1965.

19. Terry, R. D. and Pena, C., Experimental production of neurofibrillary degeneration. 2. Electron microscopy, phosphatase histochemistry and electron probe analysis, *J. Neuropathol. Exp. Neurol.,* 24, 200, 1965.
20. Terry, R. D., Peck, A., DeTeresa, R., Schechter, R., and Horoupian, D. S., Some morphometric aspects of the brain in senile dementia of the Alzheimer type, *Ann. Neurol.,* 10, 184, 1981.
21. Hansen, L. A., DeTeresa, R., Davies, P., and Terry, R. Neocortical morphometry, lesion counts, and choline acetyltransferase levels in the age spectrum of Alzheimer's disease, *Neurology,* 38, 48, 1988.
22. Terry, R. D., DeTeresa, R., and Hansen, L. A., Neocortical cell counts in normal human adult aging, *Ann. Neurol.,* 21, 530, 1987.
23. Regeur, L., Badsberg-Jensen, G., Pakkenberg, H., Evans, S. M., and Pakkenberg, B., No global neocortical nerve cell loss in brains from patients with senile dementia of Alzheimer's type, *Neurobiol. Aging,* 15, 347, 1994.
24. Davies, P. and Maloney, A. J. R., Selective loss of central cholinergic neurons in Alzheimer's disease, *Lancet,* II, 1403, 1976.
25. Bowen, D. M., Smith, C. B., White, P., Flack, R. H. A., Carrasco, L., et al. Chemical pathology of the organic dementias. II. Quantitative estimation of cellular changes in post-mortem brains, *Brain,* 100, 427, 1977.
26. Perry, E. K., Gibson, P. H., Blessed, G., Perry, R. H., and Tomlinson, B. E. Neurotransmitter enzyme abnormalities in senile dementia. Choline acetyltransferase and glutamic acid decarboxylase activities in necropsy brain tissue, *J. Neurol. Sci.,* 34, 247, 1977.
27. Whitehouse, P. J., Price, D. L., Clark, A. W., Coyle, J. T., and Delong, M. R. Alzheimer's disease: evidence for selective loss of cholinergic neurons in the nucleus basalis, *Ann. Neurol.,* 10, 122, 1981.
28. Bondareff, W., Mountjoy, C. Q., and Roth, M., Selective loss of neurones of origin of adrenergic projection to cerebral cortex (nucleus locus coeruleus) in senile dementia, *Lancet,* I, 783, 1981.
29. Yamamoto, T. and Hirano, A., Nucleus raphe dorsalis in Alzheimer's disease: neurofibrillary tangles and loss of large neurons, *Ann. Neurol.,* 17, 573, 1985.
30. Kowall, N. W. and Kosik, K. S., Axonal disruption and aberrant localization of tau protein characterize the neuropil pathology of Alzheimer's disease, *Ann. Neurol.,* 22, 639, 1987.
31. Hyman, B. T., Van, H. G. W., Damasio, A. R., and Barnes, C. L., Alzheimer's disease: cell-specific pathology isolates the hippocampal formation, *Science,* 225, 1168, 1984.
32. Braak, H. and Braak, E., Neuropathological staging of Alzheimer-related changes, *Acta Neuropathol.,* 82, 239, 1991.
33. Scheff, S. W., DeKosky, S. T., and Price, D. A., Quantitative assessment of cortical synaptic density in Alzheimer's disease, *Neurobiol. Aging,* 11, 29, 1990.
34. Masliah, E., Terry, R. D., Alford, M., and DeTeresa, R., Quantitative immunohistochemistry of synaptophysin in human neocortex: an alternative method to estimate density of presynaptic terminals in paraffin sections, *J. Histochem. Cytochem.,* 6, 837, 1990.
35. Masliah, E., Terry, R. D., Mallory, M., Alford, M., and Hansen, L. A., Diffuse plaques do not accentuate synapse loss in Alzheimer's disease, *Am. J. Pathol.* 137, 1293, 1990.
36. Terry, R. D., Masliah, E., Salmon, D. P., et al., Physical basis of cognitive alterations in Alzheimer's disease: synapse loss is the major correlate of cognitive impairment, *Ann. Neurol.,* 30, 572, 1991.
37. Suzuki, K. and Terry, R. D. Fine structural localization of acid phosphatase in senile plaques in Alzheimer's presenile dementia, *Acta. Neuropathol.,* 8, 276, 1967.
38. Strittmatter, W. J., Weisgraber, K. H., Goedert, M., et al. Hypothesis: microtubule instability and paired helical filament formation in the Alzheimer's disease brain as a function of apolipoprotein E genotype, *Exp. Neurol.,* 125, 163, 1994.
39. Hof, P. R. and Morrison, J. H., The cellular basis of cortical disconnection in Alzheimer's disease and related dementing conditions, in *Alzheimer Disease,* Terry, R. D., Katzman, R., and Bick, K. L., Eds., Raven Press, New York, 1994, 1.
40. LaFerla, F. M., Tinkle, B. T., Bieberich, C. J., Haudenscheld, C. C., and Jay, G., The Alzheimer's Aβ peptide induces neurodegeneration and apoptotic cell death in transgenic mice, *Nature Gen.,* 9, 21, 1995.

EPIDEMIOLOGY

Chapter 4

PUTATIVE RISK FACTORS FOR ALZHEIMER'S DISEASE

Richard Mayeux

CONTENTS

I. INTRODUCTION

Alzheimer's disease as a disorder of later life or occurring during the presenium has been considered an example of a "complex " disorder.[1] By definition, complex disorders result from the variable contributions of one or more genes and from environmental influences. No single gene or risk factor is "necessary or sufficient" to cause the disease. Thus, the risk of developing Alzheimer's disease probably depends on the number and impact of the contributing genes and risk factors rather than on the presence or absence of any single mutation, polymorphism, or risk factor. Individuals with different combinations of genes or risk factors would be expected to have variable degrees of risks for Alzheimer's disease. The complex genetics of Alzheimer's disease are discussed elsewhere in this book, but we will discuss the extent to which certain genes and risk factors may increase the risk of Alzheimer's disease either directly or through interactions.

II. RISK FACTORS AND CAUSAL INFERENCE

Risk factors are antecedents that are considered to be a component of the disease pathway. Cause and causal inference are the subject of great philosphical debate among scientists.[2-4] The "cause" of a disease has been defined "as an event, condition or characteristic that plays an essential role in producing an occurrence of the disease." Rothman[4] argues that cause is a relative concept. For example, he cites that while smoking causes lung cancer, it does not do so in everyone. Smoking probably causes lung cancer only in those individuals susceptible to those effects of smoking. Nonetheless, risk factors, both genetic and enviromental, may be considered causal by researchers if they are found in a higher proportion of individuals with than without the disease or if the risk of developing the disease over a specified time is greater for those individuals with, than those without, a particular risk factor. However, it is often very difficult to distinguish between a causal and noncausal association for any given factor and a disease. Epidemiologists often rely on a set of principles first described by Hill,[2] and further developed and refined over the last few decades by Susser[3,5] and Rothman[4] (Table 1). In brief, associations should be strong on the argument that weak associations may be due to condounding or bias. Consistency and specificity of the relationship between the putative risk factor and disease are also important criteria. Temporal relationship is the most difficult to establish in cross-sectional or case-control studies of Alzheimer's disease. This criterion requires that the risk factor be present before the disease. Because ascertainment of cases and information regarding risk factors is often obtained at the same time, it is often difficult to confirm the timing of the exposure with regard to disease onset. Biological gradient or "dose–response" implies that as the degree of exposure increased to a putative risk factor or as the number of genes or "gene dose" increases, the risk of disease will be greater. Biologic plausibility is also an important criterion, demanding a biological reason for any causal association.

TABLE 1   Causal Inference

1. Strength of association
2. Consistency
3. Specificity[a]
4. Temporality or direction of association
5. Biologic gradient or "dose response"
6. Plausibility (biological)
7. Coherence (cause-effect relationship is biologically possible)
8. Experimental evidence (not always available)[a]
9. Analogy (similar effects of related exposures)[a]

   [a]   Note that these principles of causal inference remain controversial, while the others are generally well accepted.

III. BIAS

In epidemiological studies two or more groups are usually compared for the frequency of exposure to putative risk factor or factors. Procedures in the selection of either cases or controls can lead to a biased or invalid study. Methods used for the selection of both cases and controls are the subject of intense discussion.[6] Selection bias can result from any known or unknown influence motivating the way in which the selection of subjects for the study occurred. For example, if an individual is convinced that exposure to certain toxic fumes leads to Alzheimer's disease, then individuals with a history of such an exposure might seek to participate in a study of toxic fumes and Alzheimer's disease. The *self-selection* bias in this type of study might lead to the conclusion that toxic fumes are related to the cause of Alzheimer's disease.

Diagnostic bias can also be a problem. Berkson's bias refers to the probability of a hospitalization among patients with one or more conditions compared with that among patients with only one of the conditions. Thus, individuals drawn from hospital populations are likely to be different and most likely "sicker" than a group of cases drawn from a general population. This type of bias extends to the use of cases in tertiary centers or specialized centers. It is quite likely that the patients in a specialized center are also self-selected, and the motivation for coming to the clinic is immeasurable. Thus, any set of risk factors, environmental or genetic, might be unique to such a group of individuals.

The use of prevalent vs. incident cases in observational, correlative or case-control studies can also be a source of bias. Because prevalence is the product of incidence times duration, prevalent cases may acknowledge factors that promote longer and better survival than incident cases. Thus, one is obtaining risk factors potentially related to survival rather than disease risk. As with the other forms of bias, *prevalent case* bias or Neyman's fallacy promotes the underlying concern that the relationship between a risk factor and disease is different for those who participate (self-selected, specialty clinical hospital cases, or prevalent cases) than for individuals who would have been eligible to participate but were otherwise aware of the study.[6]

Information bias primarily concerns the collection of information from participants in a study. For case-control studies of risk factors the potential for one type of information bias, *recall* bias, is always present. Cases and controls differ in that one has the disease the other does not. This difference, while obvious, may affect recall of exposure in different for cases than for controls. This is futher complicated in studies of Alzheimer's disease where the individual is not capable of describing previous exposures. A spouse or family member may be called upon to provide such information. Alzheimer's disease may have affected the ability of a family member or spouse to remain objective in recalling past exposures in their affected family member. Differential missclassification (usually in cases) of exposure in a study has disasterous effects on validity. A highly motivated spouse as an informant for a patient with Alzheimer's disease might have strong opinions about a potential risk factor-disease relationship, whereas a control or his or her spouse may not have such opinions. This leads to differential missclassification of exposures and could promote an association where none existed. Nondifferential missclassification of exposure is less severe, favoring a null effect of no association. Nondifferential exposure often occurs when the ability to remember an exposure (e.g., early life event) is equal for both cases and controls. Differential recall bias can be overcome by using a prospective cohort design in which exposure to risk factors is obtained before individuals develop disease.

IV. CONFOUNDING

Confounders are, by definition, extraneous factors that are related to the disease and to a risk factor or exposure related to the disease.[4] The confounder ususally predicts disease in the absence of any risk factor. Perhaps the best known confounder is age. Advancing age is associated not only with Alzheimer's disease, but with a large number of disorders. Thus, age is not a cause, but represents a confounder because it is involved in the relationship between any putative risk factor (environmental or genetic) and disease.

It is often difficult to be certain that a risk factor is a confounder and not a component of the disease pathway. Scientific judgment, experience, and investigation can help to clarify these relationships. In fact, the relationship between a confounder and disease may be stronger than that between a specific risk factor and disease. Finally, potential confounders must be accounted for by statistical adjustment or stratification in order to fully appreciate the relationship between a risk factor and disease. Nonetheless, the effects of strong confounders such as age may not be fully eliminated.

V. DISEASE PATHWAY

The model of the classical disease pathway offers a way of conceptualizing how and when risk factors act in the process of disease. *Etiology* is a term used to refer to a specific cause, while *pathogenesis* defines the mechanism by which the etiology results in disease. The period between exposure to the cause and the initiation of the disease process is referred to as the *induction period*. This period of time is dependent on the etiology or cause; no specific time period can be defined. The period between the induction of disease and its detection has been termed by Rothman[4] as the *latency period*.

In a chronic disease such as Alzheimer's disease both the latency and induction periods may be lengthy. By considering each type of antecedent risk factor, their potential impact on the disease pathway can be determined. Risk factors that are likely to act during the induction period will, most likely, have direct effects on risk. Traumatic head injury is an example of a risk factor that is considered by some to increase the risk of Alzheimer's disease by promoting the extracellular release of β-amyloid in brain.[7] Thus, by acting as an inducer of disease, head injury might be expected to increase the risk of Alzheimer's disease.

Queries concerning exposures during the latency period, however, might actually indentify risk factors that modify (increase or decrease) the risk associated with the true etiology or, alternatively, factors that might result from the disease. For example, several case-control investigations had suggested that cigarette smoking is associated with a decreased risk of Alzheimer's disease.[8,9] These observations have been made in living patients and controls. While it is possible that smoking decreases the risk of disease, it is also possible that smoking behavior diminishes as a result of the disease. Thus, a reduction in smoking during the latency period might actually reflect a manifestation of disease not a true modifier of disease risk. As clinicians continue to improve their ability to identify the disease at its first manifestations, this type of problem may diminish in analytic studies of Alzheimer's disease.

VI. TYPES OF ANALYTIC STUDIES OF RISK FACTORS

The *case–control* study estimates the "odds" of being exposed to a risk factor, given disease. An estimation of relative risks, under the rare disease assumption, is possible, but Alzheimer's disease may not be a rare disease in the age group over 65. The case–control design has limitations in that patient status and risk factors are determined at the same time. Therefore, the temporal sequence is often difficult to establish and one cannot measure incidence rates of disease in those exposed and unexposed to a risk factor. Thus, it is difficult to establish attributable risks (risk differences) between those exposed and unexposed. The advantage of a case-control study is its relatively low cost.

The *cohort study* allows calculation of incidence rates in the exposed and unexposed, but requires follow-up of a large number of individuals because risk factor data are collected prior to disease onset. It is costly, and investigators are not always able to control confounding variables and maintain high follow-up rates. The risk factors under observation may change during the period of observation. An alternative, but less often used method, is the *case–base* method in which a random (stratified) sample of the base or referent population is interviewed for the putative risk factors. Then all incident cases are identified from the entire base population over a specified time period and the frequencies of risk factors in these cases are similarly determined. Because the sampled base yields essentially complete information on the base population, the investigator is able to estimate rates of disease in those exposed and unexposed to the risk factors of interest, assess attributable risk, and establish risk profiles with considerable economy over the cohort method. The problem of temporal direction is difficult to establish in this type of investigation because the same issues that limit the usefulness of case-control studies apply here as well: ascertainment of patient status and risk factors occurs at the same time.

Thus, while case–control and case–base studies are economical, they may only be useful for deriving hypotheses in the investigation of Alzheimer's disease. Definitive analytic studies need to rely on prospective, cohort studies of risk factors.

VII. SPECIFIC RISK FACTORS FOR ALZHEIMER'S DISEASE

A. GENETIC RISK FACTORS AND SPECIFIC GENE LOCI IN ALZHEIMER'S DISEASE

The evidence suggesting that Alzheimer's disease is related to genetic factors is compelling.[10-16] A family history of dementia has been found to be far more likely in patients with Alzheimer's disease than among controls in numerous case-control studies. Familial aggregation of a dementia resembling Alzheimer's disease in first-degree relatives of patients known to have Alzheimer's diease has also been consistently observed. In at least one investigation, the authors observed that the cumulative risk of Alzheimer's disease among first-degree relatives approached 50% by the 8th decade compared with 20% among relatives of controls and suggested that this might imply that Alzheimer's disease represents an age-dependent autosomal dominant disease.[10] There are a large number of multigenerational families in which cases of Alzheimer's disease are distributed in an autosomal dominant pattern,[10-21] and there is also higher concordance of Alzheimer's disease among monozygotic twins compared with dizygotic twins.[17-21]

Some forms of familial Alzheimer's disease are due to mutations in three distinct genes: the amyloid precursor protein (APP) on chromosome 21, presenilin I on chromosome 14 and presenilin II gene on chromosome 1. Together, these three loci may account for a large number of familial cases with onset of Alzheimer's disease beginning after the third decade of life.

Several rare point mutations at codons in the APP gene on chromosome 21 mutations are associated with familial AD with onset of symptoms between ages 50 and 60.[22-26] The mutation results in an over expression of the β amyloid protein and the accumulation of amyloid deposits in the brain, but how this causes Alzheimer's disease is unknown. The presenilin genes on chromosome 14 (presenilin I) and chromosome 1 (presenilin II) encode similar transmembrane proteins also of uncertain function.[27-29] Because both genes encode intracellular membrane proteins,[30] that are likely to be involved in intercellular signalling that specify cell fate.[31] However, the phenotypes differ in that presenilin I is associated with a rapidly progressive form of disease beginning between the ages of 30 and 40 years and complete penetrance, while the presenilin II mutation has a more variable age-at-onset with incomplete penetrance. Table 2, below outlines the genes associated with early-onset familial Alzheimer's disease. These three genes are considered deterministic, in that individuals with these mutations almost always develop the disease phenotype.

In 1991, Pericak-Vance and associates.[32] reported linkage to a region on chromosome 19 among relatives of families with the most common form of late-onset Alzheimer's disease. This was followed by the discovery of an association between late-onset Alzheimer's disease and the gene for apolipoprotein-E (*APOE*), which is also located on chromosome 19.[33] In numerous cross-sectional

TABLE 2   Genes Related to Alzheimer's Disease

Location	Gene	Early-Onset	Late-Onset	Penetrance
Ch21pter-q21	Amyloid precursor protein	Ages 40–60	No	Complete
Ch14q24.3	Presenilin I	Ages 30–50	No	Complete
Ch 1q	Presenilin II	Ages 30–65	Rare	Incomplete
Ch19q13.2	Apolipoprotein-E	Rare	Ages 60–75	Incomplete

and case-control studies patients with Alzheimer's disease are found to be significantly more likely than their peers to have one or more copies of the ε4-type allele of Apo-E.[34-40] Roses and co-workers found the *APOE* gene, in particular the ε4 allelic variant, to be associated with both sporadic and familial Alzheimer's disease of both late onset.[41,42] However, early onset Alzheimer's disease may also be associated.[38,43] In both cross-sectional and case-control studies, *APOE*ε4 homozygosity is associated with a nearly tenfold increase in risk, while *APOE*ε4 heterozygosity is associated on average with an approximate fourfold increase in risk. The attributable risk related to the presence of one or more *APOE*ε4 gene may be as high as 40 to 50% in some populations. The association between *APOE*ε4 and Alzheimer's disease has been investigated mostly in North American and European Caucasian populations and to a lesser extent in other populations including Finnish[45] and African-Americans.[44,46] In one community-based study of African-Americans the association between *APOE*ε4 heterozygosity and Alzheimer's disease was attenuated in African-Americans relative to Caucasians,[46] suggesting both similarities and differences in the genetic factors related to Alzheimer's disease among individuals of distinct ethnic groups. Interactions between the *APOE* genotype and various environmental factors is now the subject of numerous investigations.[47,48]

B. DOWN'S SYNDROME AND ALZHEIMER'S DISEASE

Because adults with Down's syndrome invariably develop the neuropathological changes of Alzheimer's disease by age 40, many investigators have examined the frequency of this disorder among families of patients with Alzheimer's disease. Indeed, in case-control studies, the risk of Alzheimer's disease associated with a family history of Down's syndrome was increased two- to threefold.[49] However, Schupf et al.[50] used a unique approach to investigate the familial risk of Alzheimer's disease among the familes of adults with Down's syndrome. She and her associates proposed that because most of the nondisjunction events in Down's syndrome are of maternal origin, there might be an increased frequency of Alzheimer's disease among mothers, but not among fathers. They also posited that the shared susceptibility might involve an accelerated aging process, leading to the birth of a child with Down's syndrome in relatively young mothers and to increased risk of dementia in the mother as well as her relatives. Among the family members of persons with Down's syndrome they found the risk of an AD-like dementia among mothers who were young *before age 35* when their child with DS was born was five times that of mothers who had children with other types of mental retardation, while the risks of dementia among mothers who were older *over age 35* at the proband's birth was comparable to that of mothers of children with other types of mental retardation. Risk of dementia was not increased for fathers of patients with DS. This may imply a common genetic susceptibility to Down's synrome and Alzheimer's disease.

C. PARKINSON'S DISEASE AND ALZHEIMER'S DISEASE

First-degree relatives of patients with Alzheimer's disease have about three times the risk of Parkinson's disease.[51] The effect was even more robust among families with a family history of Alzheimer's disease.[52] Conversely, Marder et al.[53] found that first-degree relatives of demented patients with Parkinson's disease had at least six times the risk of dementia than nondemented patients with Parkinson's disease. This familial aggregation of Alzheimer's disease and Parkinson's

TABLE 3   Risk Factors Most Consistently Associated with Alzheimer's Disease

Risk Factor	Direction	Presumed Mechanism
Education and occupation	Negative	"Cognitive reserve" Surrogate for unknown factor(s)
Parental age	Positive	Advanced physiologic aging
Depression	Positive	Neurotransmitter alterations
Antiinflammatories	Protective	Prevents complement activation
Estrogen	Protective	Throphic; Aβ-APP metabolism
Head injury	Positive	↑ Aβ and APP in brain
Smoking	Protective	Enhanced nicotinic receptor function

disease with and without dementia has also been interpreted as a possible indication of shared genetic etiology between these two degenerative diseases.

VIII. RISK FACTORS ASSOCIATED WITH ALZHEIMER'S DISEASE (TABLE 3)

A. DEMOGRAPHIC CHARACTERISTICS

The risk of Alzheimer's disease has been frequently related to several factors related to culture, education, and socioeconomic status. Culture has profound effects on the frequency of Alzheimer's disease.[54-59] Whether these effects are direct or mediated through other genetic or enviromental effects remains to be determined. Illiteracy and reduced years of formal education have been associated with Alzheimer's disease. In a prospective study, Stern and associates[59] found that the cumulative risk of Alzheimer's disease was significantly increased among elderly with less than 8 years of education and lesser degrees of occupational achievement compared with those of a similar age with more education and greater occupational achievement. In that prospective study, the number of years of education and subsequent occupation seemed to act synergistically in reducing or increasing the risk of Alzheimer's disease. Each of the following possible explanations have been suggested for this association: (1) a *"detection bias"*, in which fewer years of education could lead to impaired performance on neuropsychological tests, increasing the likelihood of being diagnosed with Alzheimer's disease. Under this hypothesis, higher false-positive rates would be expected among poorly educated and higher false-negative rates among better educated persons; (2) increased *"cognitive reserve"*, implying that higher education may alter brain function in some way to reduce the clinical manifestations of disease in susceptible individuals; (3) a *"confounder"*, in which low education may be associated (see definition above) with another variable that is causally related to Alzheimer's disease (e.g., occupational exposure such as glues;[60] (4) a *"direct effect"* in which low educational attainment is a very early manifestation of the pathological processes that lead to Alzheimer's disease; (5) a *"causal link"*, low education may directly result in Alzheimer's disease.

Stern et al.,[57] reported an inverse relationship between duration of formal education and degree of reduction in rCBF flow in the parietooccipital region of the brain in patients with Alzheimer's disease of comparable severity. Analogous trends are found in subjects with more complex occupations. Both are compatible with either a "detection bias" or a "cognitive reserve" hypothesis, but do not necessarily rule out other possibilities.

Parental age at the time of birth may also influence the risk of dementia, though these studies are inconsistent.[61] Late maternal and paternal age have both been identified as potential antecedents. The biological basis for the association stems from the relationship between parental age and Down's syndrome. Thus, again investigators have proposed a similar mechanism involving shared susceptibility.

B. PSYCHIATRIC AND MEDICAL ILLNESSES (AND THEIR POSSIBLE TREATMENTS)

Investigators have found that a prior history of depression may increase the risk of Alzheimer's disease.[62] A prior history of "medically treated" depression can be associated with a threefold increase in risk of Alzheimer's disease. Whether depression represents a sign of impending disease or an early manifestation remains to be determined, but even when depression occurred 10 years earlier the risk remained significant. Devanand et al.[63] found that even a persistently depressed mood might increase in parallel with cognitive failure, and that depressed mood alone was associated with increase risk of incident dementia (Table 3).

Thyroiditis has been associated with increased risk of Alzheimer's disease among women but the exposure is an infrequent one. Heyman et al.[64] suggested that thyroid hormone might influence or increase the risk of disease by altering neurotransmitter function.

Rheumatoid arthritis and its treatment, particularly the use of either sterioidal or nonsteroidal antiinflammatory agents,[60,65] are found less frequently than expected among patients with Alzheimer's disease. Moreover, case-control studies of discordant twins found a 50 to 75% reduction in the risk of Alzheimer's disease among twins consuming nonsteroidal antiinflammatory agents.[65] Because chronic inflammation has been associated with amyloid deposition and because amyloid depostion may actually activate the complement cascade, antiinflammatory agents could play an important role in disease pathogenesis.

Parkinsonism as manifest by the extrapyramidal signs, rigidity or postural change, has been observed in healthy elderly and can also be an independent predictor of incident dementia. In the 3-year follow-up of over 250 community-dwelling elderly, those with extrapyramidal signs had nearly a fivefold increase in risk of dementia.[66]

The use of estrogen may also be associated with a decreased risk of Alzheimer's disease. Estrogen co-localizes with basal forebrain cholinergic nuclei[67] and may actually act as a growth factor in promoting neuronal survival and plasticity. Women who took estrogen had about a 50% reduction in occurrence of Alzheimer's disease in a prospective study of mortality rates.[68] Further, women who began menstruation at later ages had higher risk of Alzheimer's disease compared with women who had earlier onset of menstruation.

C. ENVIRONMENTAL RISK FACTORS

Traumatic head injury satisfies many of the criteria for causality[69] and is compatible with hypotheses concerning amyloid. Autopsy studies of individuals with head injuries[70] and professional boxers[7] confirm biologic connections to Alzheimer's disease. Several case-control studies have confirmed an association between head injury and Alzheimer's disease,[71-75] but these observations have been controversial. The effect of head injury on the risk of Alzheimer's disease may be restricted to individuals with *APOE* genotypes containing one or more copies of ε4, however.[47]

Cigarette smoking has been purported to act as a protective factor.[76] Biological evidence that smoking facilitates nicotinic receptor function could mean that smoking delays some of the signs of Alzheimer's disease.[76,77] While a history of smoking was less frequent among cases than a control group, certain inconsistencies warrant further study. For example, smokers with Alzheimer's disease have a much earlier age of onset than nonsmokers, and it is difficult to exclude reporting bias in the case-control design. Furthermore, the presence of an *APOE*-ε4 allele has been related to diminished smoking behavior.[48]

Few toxins have been associated with increased risk of Alzheimer's disease. Aluminium, which has been considered a neurotoxin by some,[78] was not associated with increased risk of Alzheimer's disease when subjects were queried about antacids or antiperspirants.[60] In a large, comprehensive case-control study in Canada, an association between occupational exposure to glues, pesticides, and fertilizers was reported. The risk was greatest for subjects with lower education. This interesting observation needs further exploration.

IX. CONCLUSIONS

Analytic studies of Alzheimer's disease are critical to identifying important, potentially modifiable antecedent factors. Clearly, investigations thus far indicate that this disease is likely to be best understood as a "complex" disorder in which genetic and environmental (or nongenetic factors) each play significant roles. Moreover, the way in which genes and environmental factors interact in the pathogenesis of Alzheimer's disease will be crucial to developing effective interventions.

REFERENCES

1. Plomin, R., Owen, M. J., and Mc Guffin, P., The genetic basis of complex human behaviors, *Science,* 264, 1733, 1994.
2. Hill, A. B., The environment and disease: association or causation?, *Proc. R. Soc. Med.,* 58, 295, 1965.
3. Susser, M., *Causal Thinking in the Health Sciences Concepts and Strategies in Epidemiology,* Oxford University Press, New York, 1973.
4. Rothman, K. J., *Modern Epidemiology,* Little, Brown, Boston, 1986, 7.
5. Susser, M., What is a cause and how do we know one? A grammar for pragmatic epidemiology, *Am. J. Epidemiol.,* 133, 635, 1991.
6. Lasky, T. and Stolley, P. D., Selection of cases and controls, *Epidemiol. Rev.,* 16, 6, 1994.
7. Roberts, G. W., Allsop, D., and Bruton, C. J., The occult aftermath of boxing, *J. Neurol. Neurosurg. Psychiat.,* 53, 373, 1990.
8. van Duijn, C. M. and Hofman, A., Relation between nicotine intake and Alzheimer's disease, *BJM,* 302, 1491, 1991.
9. Graves, A. B., White, E., Koespell, T., et al., A case-control study of Alzheimer's disease, *Ann. Neurol.,* 28, 766, 1990.
10. Breitner, J. C. S., Silverman, J. M., Mohs, R. C., et al., Familial aggregation in Alzheimer's disease: comparison of risk among relatives of early- and late-onset cases, and among male and female relatives in successive generations, *Neurology,* 38, 207, 1988.
11. Huff, F. J., Auerbach, B. A., Charkravarti, A., et al., Risk of dementia in relatives of patients with Alzheimer's disease, *Neurology,* 38, 786, 1988.
12. Mayeux, R., Sano, M., Chen, J., et al., Risk of dementia in first-degree relatives of patients with Alzheimer's disease and related disorders, *Arch. Neurol.,* 48, 269, 1991.
13. Goudsmit, J., White, B. J., and Weitkamp, L. R., Familial Alzheimer's disease in two kindred of the same geographic and ethnic origin, *J. Neurol. Sci.,* 49, 79, 1981.
14. Bird, T., Lampe, T. H., Nemens, R. N., et al., Familial Alzheimer's Disease in American descendants of the Volga Germans: probable genetic founder effect, *Ann. Neurol.,* 23, 25, 1988.
15. Bird, T. D., Sumi, S. M., Nemens, E. J., et al., Phenotypic heterogeneity in familial Alzheimer's disease: a study of 24 kindred, *Ann. Neurol.,* 25, 12, 1988.
16. Farrer, L., Meyers, R. H., Cupples, L. A., et al., Transmission and age-at-onset patterns in familial Alzheimer's disease: evidence for heterogeneity, *Neurology,* 40, 395, 1990.
17. Nee, L. E., Eldridge, R., Sunderland, T., et al., Dementia of the Alzheimer type: clinical and family study of 22 twin pairs, *Neurology,* 37, 359, 1987.
18. Zubenko, G. S., and Ferrell, R. E., Monozygotic twins concordant for probable Alzheimer's disease and increased platelet membrane fluidity, *Am. J. Med. Genet.,* 29, 431, 1988.
19. Cook, R. H., Schneck, S. A., and Clark, D. B., Twins with Alzheimer's disease, *Arch. Neurol.,* 38, 300, 1981.
20. Creasey, H., Jorm, A., Longley, W., et al., Monozygotic twins discordant for Alzheimer's disease, *Neurology,* 39, 1474, 1989.
21. Renvoize, E. B., Mindhan, R. H. S., Stewart, M., et al., Identical twins discordant for presenile dementia of the Alzheimer type, *Br. J. Psychiat.,* 149, 509, 1986.
22. Goate, A., Chartier-Harlin, M.-C., Mullan, M., et al., Segregation of a missense mutation in the amyloid precursor protein gene with familial Alzheimer's disease, *Nature,* 349, 704, 1991.
23. Chartier-Harlin, M.-C., Crawford, F., Houlden, H., et al., Early-onset Alzheimer's disease caused by mutations at codon 717 of the beta-amyloid precursor protein gene, *Nature,* 353, 844, 1991.
24. Citron, M., Oltersdorf, T., Haass, C., et al., Mutation of the beta-amyloid precursor protein in familial Alzheimer's disease increases beta-protein production, *Nature,* 360, 672, 1992.
25. Murrell, J., Farlow, M., Ghetti, B., Benson, M. D., A mutation in the amyloid protein associated with hereditary Alzheimer's disease, *Science,* 254, 97, 1991.
26. Naruse, S., Igarashi, S., Kobayashi, H., et al., Mis-sense mutation Val-to-Ile in exon 17 of amyloid precursor protein gene in Japanese fimilial Alzheimer's disease, *Lancet,* 337, 1342, 1991.
27. Sherrington, R., Rogaev, E. I., Liang, Y., et al., Cloning of a gene bearing missense mutations in early-onset familial Alzheimer's disease, *Nature, 375,* 754, 1995.

28. Levy-Lahad, E., Wijsman, E. M., Nemens, E., et al., A familial Alzheimer's disease locus on chromosome 1, *Science,* 269, 970, 1995.

29. Levy-Lahad, E., Wasco, W., Poorkal, P., et al., Candidate gene for the chromosome 1 familial Alzheimer's disease locus, *Science,* 269, 973, 1995.

30. Kovacs, D. M., Fausett, H. J., Page, K. J., et al., Alzheimer-associated presenilins 1 and 2: neuronal expression in brain and localization to intracellular membranes in mammalian cells, *Nat. Medicine,* 2, 224, 1996.

31. Levitan, D., Greenwald, I., Facilitation of lin-12-mediated signalling by sel-12, a Caenorhabditis elegans S182 Alzheimer's disease gene, *Nature,* 377, 351, 1995.

32. Pericak-Vance, M. A., Bebout, J. L., Gaskell, P. C., et al., Linkage studies in familial Alzheimer's disease: evidence for chromosome 19 linkage, *Am. J. Hum. Genet.,* 48, 1034, 1991.

33. Strittmatter, W. J., Saunders, A. M., Schmechel, D., et al., Apolipoprotein E: high affinity binding to beta-amyloid and increased frequency of type 4 allele in late-onset familial Alzheimer's disease, *Proc. Natl. Acad. Sci. U.S.A.,* 90, 1977, 1993.

34. Saunders, A. M., Strittmatter, W. J., Schmechel, D., et al., Association of Apolipoprotein E allele-ε4 with late-onset familial and sporadic Alzheimer's disease, *Neurology,* 43, 1467, 1993.

35. Poirier, J., Davignon, J., Bouthillier, D., et al., Apolipoprotein E polymorphism and Alzheimer's disease, *Lancet,* 342, 697, 1993.

36. Payami, H., Kaye, J., Heston, L. L., et al., Apolipoprotein-E genotype and Alzheimer's disease, *Lancet,* 342, 738, 1993.

37. Saunders, A. M., Strittmatter, W. J., Pericak-Vance, M. A., et al. Apolipoprotein-E ε4 allele distributions in late-onset Alzheimer's disease and in other amyloid-forming diseases, *Lancet,* 342, 710, 1993.

38. Mayeux, R., Stern, Y., Ottman, R., et al., The apolipoprotein ε4 allele in patients with Alzheimer's disease, *Ann. Neurol.,* 34, 752, 1993.

39. Brogaonkar, D. S., Schmidit, L. C., Martin, S. E., et al., Linkage of late-onset Alzheimer's disease with apolipoprotein-E type 4 on chromosome 19, *Lancet,* 342, 625, 1993.

40. Corder, E. H., Saunders, A. M., Strittmatter, W. J., et al., Gene dose of apolipoprotein-E type 4 allele and the risk of Alzheimer's disease in late onset families, *Science,* 261, 921, 1993.

41. Roses, A. D., Strittmatter, W. J., Pericak-Vance, M.A., Corder, E. H., Saunders, A. M., and Schmechel, D. E., Clinical application of Apolipoprotein E genotyping to Alzheimer's disease, *Lancet,* 343, 1564, 1994.

42. Corder, E. H., Saunder, A. M., Risch, N. J., et al., Apolipoprotein E type 2 allele decreases the risk for late onset Alzheimer's disease, *Nature Genetics,* 7, 180, 1994.

43. Van Duijn, C. M., de Knijff P., Cruts, M., Wehnert, A., Havekes, L. M., Hofman, A., and Van Broeckhoven, C., Apolipoprotein E4 allele in a population-based study of early-onset Alzheimer's disease, *Nature Genet.,* 1, 74, 1994.

44. Hendrie, H. C., et al., Apolipoprotein E genotypes and Alzheimer's disease in a community study of elderly African-Americans, *Ann. Neurol.,* 37, 118, 1995.

45. Kuusisto, J., et al., Association of apolipoprotein E phenotypes with late onset Alzheimer's disease: population based study, *Br. Med. J.,* 309, 636, 1994.

46. Tang, M.-X., Maestre, G., Tsai, W.-Y., et al., Relative Risk of Alzheimer's Disease and Age-at-Onset Based on *APOE* Genotypes Among Elderly African-Americans, Caucasians and Hispanics in New York City, *Am. J. Hum. Genetics,* 58, 554, 1996.

47. Mayeux, R., Ottman, R., Maestre, G., Ngai, C., Tang, M.-X., Ginsberg, H., Chun, M., Tycko, B., and Shelanski, M. S., Synergistic effects of traumatic head injury and Apolipoprotein-ε4 in Patients with Alzheimer's disease, *Neurology,* 45, 555, 1995.

48. Van Duijn, C. M., Havekes, L. M., Van Broeckhoven, C., de Knijff, P., and Hofman, A., Apolipoprotein E genotype modifies the association between smoking and early-onset Alzheimer's disease, *Br. J. Med.,* 392, 1491, 1991.

49. Heyman, A. L., Wilkinson, W. E., Hurwitz, B. J., et al., Alzheimer's disease: genetic aspects and associated clinical disorders, *Ann. Neurol.,* 14, 507, 1983.

50. Schupf, N., Dapell, D., Lee, J., Ottman, R., and Mayeux, R., Increased risk for Alzheimer's disease in mothers of adults with Down syndrome, *Lancet,* 344, 353, 1994.

51. Hofman, A., Schulte, W., Tanja, T. A., van Duijn, C. M., Haaxma, R., Lameris, R. J., Otten, V. M., and Saan, R. J., History of dementia and Parkinson's disease in 1st-degree relatives of patients with Alzheimer's disease, *Neurology,* 39, 1589, 1989.

52. Van Duijn, C. M., Clayton, D. G., Chandra, V., Fratiglioni, L., Graves, A. B., Heyman, A, Jorm, A. F., Kokmen, E., Kondo, K., Mortimer, J. A., Rocca, W. A., Shalat, S. L., Soininen, H., and Hofman, A., Interaction between genetic and environmental risk factors of Alzheimer's disease: a reanalysis of case-control studies, *Genetic Epidemiol.,* 11, 539, 1994.

53. Marder, K., Flood, P., Cote, L., and Mayeux, R., A pilot study of risk factors for dementia in Parkinson's disease, *Movement Dis.,* 5, 156, 1990.

54. Zhang, M., Katzman, R., Salmon, D., et al., The prevalence of dementia and Alzheimer's disease in Shanghai, China: impact of age, gender and education, *Ann. Neurol.,* 27, 428, 1990.

55. Gurland, B., in *Clinical Aspects of Alzheimer's Disease and Senile Dementia,* Miller, E. and Cohen, G. D., Eds. 1981, 61.

56. Fratiglioni, L., Grut, M., and Forsell, Y., Prevalence of Alzheimer's disease and other dementias in an elderly urban population: relationship with age, sex and education, *Neurology,* 41, 1866, 1991.

57. Stern, Y, Alexander, G., Prohovnik, I., and Mayeux, R., Inverse relationship between education and parietotemporal perfusion deficit in Alzheimer's disease, *Ann. Neurol.,* 32: 371, 1992.

58. Gurland, B., Wilder, D., Cross, P., Lantigua, R., Teresi, J., Bolivar, M., Barret, V., and Mayeux, R., Relative rates of dementia by multiple case definitions, over two prevalence periods, in three cultural groups, *Am. J. Geriatr. Psych.,* 1994.

59. Stern, Y., Gurland, B., Tatemichi, T. K., Tang, M.-X., Wilder, D., and Mayeux, R., Influence of education and occupation on the incidence of dementia, *JAMA,* 271, 1004, 1994.

60. The Canadian Study of Health and Aging, Risk factors for Alzheimer's disease in Canada, *Neurology,* 44, 2073, 1994.

61. Rocca, W. A., van Duijn, C. M., Fratiglioni, L., Graves, A. B., Heyman, A., Jorm, A. F., Kokmen, E., Kondo, K., Mortimer, J. A., Shala, S.L., Soininen, H., and Hofman, A., Maternal age and Alzheimer's disease: a collaborative re-analysis of case-control studies, *Int. J. Epidemiol.,* 20(Suppl. 2), 21, 1991.

62. Jorm, A. F., van Duijn, C. M., Fratiglioni, L., Graves, A. B., Heyman, A., Kokmen, E., Kondo, K., Mortimer, J.A., Rocca, W.A., Shalat, S.L., Soininen, H., and Hofman, A., Psychiatric history and related exposures as risk factors for Alzheimer's disease: a collaborative re-analysis of case-control studies, *Int. J. Epidemiol.,* 20(Suppl. 2), 43, 1991.

63. Devanand, D. P., Sano, M., Tang, M.-X., Taylor, S., Gurland, B. J., Wilder, D., Stern, Y., and Mayeux, R., Depressed mood and the incidence of Alzheimer's disease in the community elderly, submitted.

64. Heyman, A., Wilkinson, W. E., Stafford, J. A., Helms, M.J., Sigmon, A.H., and Weinberg, T., Alzheimer's disease: A study of epidemiological aspects, *Ann. Neurol.,* 15, 335, 1984.

65. Brietner, J., Gau, B. A., Welsh, K. A., Plassman, B. L., McDonald, W. M., Helms, M. J., and Anthony, J. C., Inverse association of anti-inflammatory treatments and Alzheimer's disease: initial results of a co-twin study, *Neurology,* 44, 227, 1994.

66. Richard, S. M., Stern, Y., and Mayeux, R., Subtle extrapyramidal signs can predict the development of dementia in elderly individuals, *Neurology,* 43, 2184, 1993.

67. Toran-Allerand, C. D., Miranda, R. C., Bentham, W. D. L., Sohrabji, R., Brown, T.J., Hochberg, R. B., MacLusky, N. J., *Proc. Natl. Acad. Sci. U.S.A.,* 89, 4668, 1992.

68. Paganini-Hill, A. and Hendersen, V., Estrogen deficiency and risk of Alzheimer's disease in women, *Am. J. Epidemiol.,* 140, 256, 1994.

69. Roberts, G. W., Gentleman, S. M., Lynch, A., and Graham, D. I., Beta A4 amyloid protein deposition in brain after head trauma. *Lancet,* 338, 1422, 1991.

70. Clinton, J., Ambler, M. W., and Roberts, G. W., Post-traumatic Alzheimer's disease: preponderance of a single plague type, *Neuropathol. Appl. Neurobiol.,* 17, 69, 1991.

71. Mortimer, J. A., French, L. R., Hutton, J. T., and Schuman, L. M., Head trauma as a risk factor for Alzheimer's disease, *Neurology,* 35, 264, 1985.

72. Graves, A. B., White, E., Koepssell, T. D., et al., The association between head trauma and Alzheimer's disease, *Am. J. Epidemiol.,* 131, 491, 1990.

73. van Duijn, C. M., Tanja, T. A., Haaxma, R., et al., Head trauma and the risk of Alzheimer's disease, *Am. J. Epidemiol.,* 135, 775, 1992.

74. Mortimer, J. A., van Duijn, C. M., Chandra, V., et al. Head trauma as a risk factor for Alzheimer's disease: A collaborative re-analysis of case-control studies, *Int. J. Epidemiol.,* 20(Suppl.), 28, 1991.

75. Mayeux, R., Ottman, R., Tang, M.-X., Noboa-Bauza, L., Marder, K., Gurland, B., and Stern, Y., Genetic susceptibility and head injury as risk factors for Alzheimer's disease among community-dwelling elderly persons and their first-degree relatives, *Ann. Neurol.,* 33, 494, 1993.

76. Graves, A. B., van Duijn, C. M., Chandra, V., et al., Alcohol and tobacco consumption as risk factors for Alzheimer's disease. A collaborative re-analysis of case-control studies, 20(Suppl.), 48, 1991.

77. Hebert, L. E., Scherr, P. A., Beckett, L. A., et al., Relation of smoking and alcohol consumption to incident Alzheimer's disease, *Am. J. Epidemiol.,* 135, 347, 1992.

78. Rifat, A. L., Eastwood, M. R., Crapper McLachlan, D. R., and Corey, P. N., Effect of exposure of miners to aluminium powder, *Lancet,* 2, 1162, 1990.

Chapter 5

DESCRIPTIVE EPIDEMIOLOGY OF ALZHEIMER'S DISEASE

Denis A. Evans

CONTENTS

I. PREVALENCE AND INCIDENCE OF ALZHEIMER'S DISEASE

Alzheimer's disease is an extremely common condition among older persons. Estimates of exactly how common the disease is vary substantially, with most of the variation due to two difficulties in measuring it precisely. First, the onset of the disease is typically by minute degrees over an extended period of time, and it is difficult or impossible to establish a precise point in this course at which normality ends and disease begins. The second difficulty is the infrequency with which Alzheimer's disease is detected and recorded in the routine delivery of health care. Thus, estimates of the prevalence of the disease, i.e., the percentage of persons who have the illness at any one time, have varied widely. The higher estimates are from community-based studies in which samples of older persons in the general population undergo evaluation using specified diagnostic criteria that attempt to include disease that is mild in severity. Estimates that depend on health care systems or informant report to detect disease have typically been much lower, even for societies that provide excellent access to health care, especially if consideration is restricted to more severe disease.

Studies[1] conducted in the 1980s in East Boston, Massachusetts, a geographically defined U.S. community, estimated that 10.3% of persons 65 years of age and older living in the community met criteria for the clinical diagnosis of "probable Alzheimer's disease" as established by the Joint Work Group of the National Institute of Neurological and Communicative Disorders and Stroke and the Alzheimer's Disease and Related Disorders Association (NINCDS/ADRDA criteria).[2] These figures agree reasonably well with previous prevalence estimates from a study of a southern California retirement community[3] that also applied specified diagnostic criteria to a defined population. In contrast, prevalence estimates that depend on diagnoses made in the routine delivery of health care have been much lower. It is very likely that these difference largely reflect variation in methodological approaches rather than substantial differences in occurrence of disease in different populations.

Estimates of the incidence of Alzheimer's disease, i.e., the number of new cases of the disease arising in a defined period of time, have, in general, been in agreement with prevalence estimates and comparisons across studies have reflected similar methodological differences. Annual incidence rates for Alzheimer's disease in the East Boston population, determined independently of the prevalence estimates were 0.6% for persons 65 to 69 years old; 1.0% for persons 70 to 74 years old; 2.0% for persons 75 to 79 years old; 3.3% for persons 80 to 84 years old; and 8.4% for persons 85 years of age and older.[4] In contrast, studies[5,6] using a well-established registry in Rochester, Minnesota, a city with good access to health care, that ascertained disease through health care records resulted in incidence estimates that were much lower than those from the East Boston Studies.

The concept of prevalence, i.e., the number or proportion of persons with a condition at a point in time, includes both elements of incidence, the rate at which the condition arises over a specified time period, and duration of the disease. A disease that has a high incidence but a short duration because it is rapidly fatal will have lower prevalence than will a disease with the same incidence but of longer duration. By taking duration of disease or mortality due to a disease into account, one can therefore compare incidence and prevalence estimates. One of the major problems in measuring occurrence of Alzheimer's disease arises because the most accurate assessments for the illness include formal evaluation of subjects' cognition, typically with neuropsychological performance tests. These tests, however, do not measure cognitive performance equally among all individuals; there are large differences according to educational, social, and cultural factors. Thus, even if tests that are relatively insensitive to educational and cultural differences are used, it is easy to confuse poor performance due to these factors with mild disease. Incidence studies have a substantial methodological advantage in this situation. These studies are measuring the occurrence of new disease in a population previously determined to be free of the disease. Optimally, this means that each study participant has been seen and at least briefly evaluated at the beginning of the study to determine the absence of disease. Thus, at the evaluation for disease incidence, one can be reasonably certain that any observed cognitive impairment represents real change since the previous assessment, not merely a life-long pattern of low function or testing error. It is noteworthy that the independently determined cumulative incidence estimates for Alzheimer's disease in the East Boston population are in close agreement with the previous prevalence estimates after taking into account the increase in risk of death due the disease. This suggests that the persons identified as having mild Alzheimer's disease in the prevalence study actually had the disease rather than merely having cognitive performance that was underestimated or reflected life-long low function. If the latter were the case, one would anticipate that rather than being in agreement with the prevalence estimates, the cumulative incidence estimates would have been substantially lower. The differences between studies depending on health care systems or informants to detect Alzheimer's disease and studies using direct assessments of population samples may be even greater for incidence estimates than for prevalence estimates because the new-onset disease assessed in incidence studies is typically mild and even more likely to be undetected in the routine delivery of health care or to be inapparent to informants.

II. CRITERIA FOR DISEASE DIAGNOSIS

In the U.S., two criterion systems are commonly used for the formal clinical diagnosis of Alzheimer's disease: the Diagnostic Criteria for Dementia of the Alzheimer's Type of the fourth edition of the Diagnostic and Statistical Manual of Mental Disorders of the American Psychiatric Association[7] (DSM-IV criteria) and the NINCDS/ADRDA criteria for the diagnosis of probable Alzheimer's disease. The logic of the two criterion systems is fairly similar. Both require impairment in memory as well as in one or more additional domains of cognitive function. The introduction of the NINCDS/ADRDA criteria in 1984 represented a major advance because of the emphasis on the use of formal neuropsychological performance testing as a means of detecting and categorizing cognitive impairment. Recent revisions of the DSM criteria have also tended to reflect this emphasis.

DSM-IV criteria can be difficult to implement in epidemiological studies because of the requirement for "significant impairment in social or occupational functioning"[7] for the diagnosis. Conceptually, impairment of social function and impairment of occupational function are probably best seen as possible consequences of a condition rather than as criteria for its diagnosis. To a limited extent, the inclusion of these requirements in disease criteria may serve a useful purpose: eliminating from a diagnosis of Alzheimer's disease some situations of mild or transient impairment. The disadvantages are substantial, however. Whether or not social and occupational impairments arise or are apparent depends not only on the disease itself but on extensive considerations external to the disease. The typical age of retirement is 65 years, and the great majority of Alzheimer's disease occurs above this age; occupational impairment can only be detected among those still employed. Impairments of social functions and ability to detect them also depend strongly on factors external to the disease. In general, such dysfunction will be more obvious among persons with extensive social networks and substantial demands on their time than it will among persons who live alone with few contacts with relatives, friends, and neighbors. In epidemiological studies, these difficulties can produce nonuniform measurement of disease according to the circumstances of the individual participant; the impact of the nonuniform measurement is increased because the circumstances favoring detection of social and occupational impairment are related to other variables of substantial interest such as gender and social status. Women, for example, are less likely to be occupationally active, and, because, on average, they live longer than men and usually survive their husbands, older women are much more likely to live alone. In practice many studies attempt to meet the DSM-IV requirement for impairment of social or occupational function by utilizing brief scales of functional impairment such as activities of daily living. This solution has limited appeal, however. These scales are typically composed of items reflecting physical and cognitive function more than social or occupational function. The effect is to maintain the conceptual difficulty of introducing consequences into a disease definition while broadening the range of consequences.

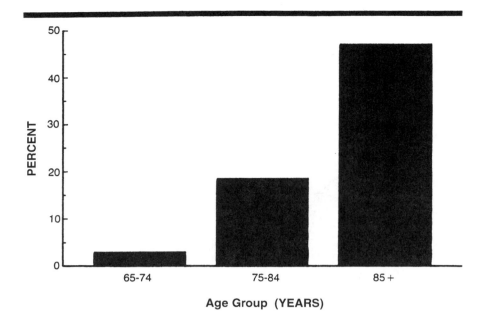

FIGURE 1   Prevalence of Alzheimer's disease among persons 65 years-of-age and older residing in a geographically defined U.S. community, East Boston Massachusetts. From Evans, D. A., Funkenstein, H. H., Albert, M. S., et al., *JAMA.,* 1989, 262:2254.

III. AGE AND ALZHEIMER'S DISEASE

One of the most distinctive features of Alzheimer's disease is its age range. Early-onset cases certainly do occur, and the neuropathology of the condition was originally described by Alzheimer in tissue from a middle-aged woman. Nonetheless, relative to its occurrence in later years, the disease is uncommon before the age of 65 years and, within the over-65 age group, the prevalence of the condition is dramatically related to age. Figure 1 summarizes age-specific prevalence estimates from the East Boston Studies. Despite wide variation in prevalence and incidence estimates, almost all studies have shown striking increases in the occurrence of the disease with age. At least one report[8] has raised the possibility that the age-specific incidence of the condition ceases to rise after age 90 based on a small number of subjects in this age group. In general, findings from other studies have not strongly supported this, however. It currently seems more likely that the age-specific incidence continues to rise with advancing age as least as far as adequate numbers of study participants permit one to estimate.

IV. THE IMPACT OF ALZHEIMER'S DISEASE ON PUBLIC HEALTH

The increase in incidence of Alzheimer's disease with increasing age has profound implications for the impact of the disease on the public health. The age group 85 years of age and older has been the fastest growing age group of the population in the United States and in many other developing countries for several decades,[9] and this trend will continue well into the next century. Because this oldest age group of the population is also the group with the highest incidence of Alzheimer's disease, the number of persons with this illness will also increase at a rapid rate if no preventive measures for the disease are found. Figure 2 shows the anticipated growth in the number of persons with Alzheimer's disease in the United States population from 1980 to 2050 both overall

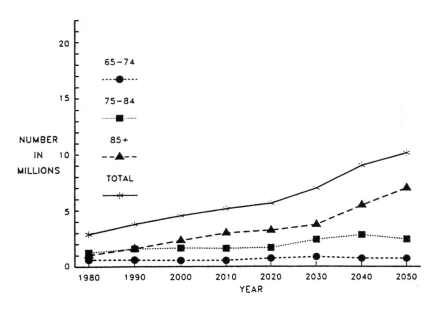

FIGURE 2 Projected number of persons 65 years-of-age and older with probable Alzheimer's disease in the U.S. population from 1980 through 2050 by three age subgroups, using U.S. Census middle projection of population growth. Disease prevalence data from studies in East Boston, Massachusetts, adjusted for years of education. From Evans, D. A., Scherr, P. A., Cook, N. R., et al., *Milbank Q,* 1990, 68:278.

and according to three age groups. In 1980, there were approximately 2.9 million persons with the illness; currently, in 1996, approximately 4 million persons in the U.S. have Alzheimer's disease, and it is estimated that by 2050, this number will have increased to over 10 million.[10] It is clear that the growth in the total number of persons with the disease is driven by the dramatic increase in the number of persons in the over-85 age group with this illness. In contrast, the number of persons 65 to 75 years of age with Alzheimer's disease is expected to remain relatively constant over this time period, and the number in the 75- to 84-year-old age group will increase only moderately.

These estimates should be interpreted with caution, however. As noted above prevalence estimates for the illness vary widely; these estimates are based on figures from the East Boston studies, one of the higher estimates of current disease prevalence, referred to the entire U.S. population. In addition, future projections of disease prevalence are subject to error in projecting population growth. The estimates in Figure 2 are based on the U.S. Census Bureau middle series projections which make intermediate assumptions. Whatever current prevalence estimates for Alzheimer's disease are selected, however, and whatever reasonable estimates of future population growth are used, it is clear that the combination of the strong relation of occurrence of the disease to age and the continued rapid growth of the oldest population age groups will result in a large increase in the number of persons with this disease in the U.S. and other developed countries. It should be emphasized that the overall pattern of this growth in number of affected persons does not depend on the exact criteria used for disease diagnosis. As previously noted, Alzheimer's disease arises by minute degrees and prevalence estimates vary substantially according to where, along a continuum between normality and severe disease, one places a cut point demarcating disease from non-disease. Where this cut point is placed, of course, affects one's estimate of the absolute number of persons in each age group who have the illness. It does not, however, affect the relation between age and disease incidence and prevalence. The large number of persons in the oldest age group with the illness represents a full range of disease severity; relative to younger age groups, it is not selectively composed of persons with mild or equivocal symptoms of disease. Although there have been few formal studies of the issue, this growth in the number of persons with Alzheimer's disease in the oldest population age groups will also likely have a strong impact on the presentation of disease to clinicians. The oldest age group is also the one in which other chronic diseases are most common, so it is likely to become less common for persons to come to the attention of health-care providers because of Alzheimer's disease. Increasingly, Alzheimer's disease will present as only one of several health problems.

Estimating the full economic impact of Alzheimer's disease has proved difficult. It doubtlessly accounts for a substantial fraction of institutional long-term care costs in the U.S., but as noted above, many persons in the oldest age groups have multiple severe health problems and, for many persons, it is difficult to attribute institutionalization to any single disease; reimbursement requirements can also affect the way in which diagnoses are listed and coded. Further, many costs of the disease are less apparent than for other conditions. Most of the people who have the illness are no longer in the work force. Most persons with the illness remain in the community for a substantial length of time with care provided by family members. It is difficult to accurately estimate the cost of these informal services or the indirect costs from loss of work time and opportunities for advancement by care providers. With these uncertainties and the substantial variation in incidence estimates of the disease, it is not surprising that estimates of its economic impact are somewhat imprecise, but estimates ranging from approximately $20 billion to over $80 billion annually depending on the costs included have been made.[11-13]

V. GENDER AND ALZHEIMER'S DISEASE

The substantial majority of persons with Alzheimer's disease are women because women, on average, live longer than men in developed societies and occurrence of the disease is strongly related to age. It is less clear whether women are at higher risk of developing the illness than are men of the same age. Studies have been divided on this issue; overall, however, more studies than not suggest that women, apart from age, are at higher risk. This conclusion should be viewed with considerable caution, however, for several methodological reasons. Thoughtful consideration of this issue requires uniform measurement of Alzheimer's disease in defined populations. It is very difficult for studies of clinical groups or population studies that use health-care systems to identify persons with the disease to address the issue because persons coming to the attention of a health-care system and identified by it as having Alzheimer's disease likely represent only a small nonrandom fraction of all persons with the illness. Further, gender substantially influences health-care utilization. Even for population studies that directly measure occurrence of the disease, the role of gender is a difficult issue. As noted above, risk of Alzheimer's disease increases strongly with age and, within the older age groups of almost all populations from developed countries, women, will on average be older than men. Thus, analyses investigating whether there is increased risk associated with female gender, apart from age, must take age into account very carefully; the effect of age is so strong that even small uncertainties can obscure the relation of gender. In addition, incidence studies are strongly preferable to prevalence studies in investigating this issue. As noted above, prevalence depends on the duration of the disease as well as its incidence. Because of their better average survival overall, women will tend to live longer after the onset of Alzheimer's disease on average even if there is no differential effect according to gender of the disease on survival because they will be less likely to die of other causes. Thus, if incidence of Alzheimer's disease among men and women were equal, one would expect slightly higher prevalence among women due only to longer duration with the illness.

Unfortunately, most population studies have been of Alzheimer's disease prevalence and have had small enough numbers of persons in the oldest age groups, in which the disease is most common, that precise adjustment for the effects of age on disease risk has been difficult. Thus, in spite of the overall tendency of population studies to report higher prevalence among women than among men of the same age, the issue of the effect of gender on risk of Alzheimer's disease is probably best regarded as an unsettled one.

VI. ALZHEIMER'S DISEASE AND MORTALITY

The effect of Alzheimer's disease on mortality can be assessed in several ways. One approach is to examine death certificates with regard to how frequently Alzheimer's disease is noted as a cause of death. This approach has several limitations, however. Many persons in the oldest age groups in which the occurrence of Alzheimer's disease is highest have several health conditions at the time of death. Assigning responsibility for death among these various conditions is a matter of somewhat uncertain judgment. Further, because Alzheimer's disease tends to be underrecognized in the routine delivery of health care, it is expected that it should be underrecognized as a cause of death as well. A more revealing approach is to measure the occurrence of Alzheimer's disease and other illnesses and compare the survival of persons with this illness to those without it. This approach has been followed in a number of settings. The greatest number of studies have been in nursing homes, other long-term-care institutions, or among persons identified as having the illness in specialized outpatient clinics. In general, these studies have suggested that Alzheimer's disease has a large adverse impact on survival. Estimates from these studies have varied widely, but at least some studies[14,15] have reported severalfold increases in risk of death associated with Alzheimer's disease. The special features of these settings limit, to some degree however, the inferences that can be drawn from these studies. The spectrum of Alzheimer's disease seen in a special clinic or in a long-term-care setting may be unusual and affected by many factors. It is difficult to select a comparison group for those with Alzheimer's disease. Nursing home patients without Alzheimer's disease, for example, will have been admitted to the facility for some other reason which may well influence their risk of death.

Studies of Alzheimer's disease and mortality in the general population have fewer limitations, but have been less common. The results of the East Boston Studies[16] suggested that the overall impact of Alzheimer's disease on risk of death is moderate rather than extreme with on average, those with the illness having a 44% increased risk of death over a period of follow-up of slightly less than 5 years. Risk of death in this study varied greatly according to severity of disease, however. Those with mild or moderate cognitive impairment had no cachexia and approximately the same risk of death as other persons of the same age and gender in the population, but those with both severe cognitive impairment and cachexia had approximately a 4.7-fold increased risk of dying. These results from a range of studies in different settings appear most compatible with a moderately increased risk of death associated with Alzheimer's disease overall; persons with mild disease have relatively little increased risk of dying, but those with advanced disease either in the community or in institutions have a substantial elevation of mortality.

VII. ALZHEIMER'S DISEASE AND NORMAL AGING

The close relation between the occurrence of Alzheimer's disease and age and its high incidence in the oldest age groups have given rise to discussions of whether what we call Alzheimer's disease is actually a part of the normal aging process. This is a complex, multifaceted issue that cannot be fully explored here; some aspects of the descriptive epidemiology of Alzheimer's disease are relevant to it, though. The word "normal" can have several connotations, and the sense of this question depends on how the word is used. In a statistical sense, the word can be defined precisely in terms of the parameters of a normal distribution. This is not usually the way in which the word "normal" is used in discussing this issue. Rather, it is more likely to be used as a synonym for "natural" or "inevitable", conveying a sense of a process that is somehow intrinsic to the human organism and not susceptible to modification.

On the basis of present knowledge, it is impossible to predict to what degree, if any, Alzheimer's disease is inevitable; our present understanding of its pathogenesis and of the basic mechanisms of aging are much too limited to permit anything but conjecture. It is probably not correct, though, to draw a conclusion that the disease is inevitable or natural from any of the three features most characteristic of descriptive epidemiology: its age distribution, its high frequency in the oldest groups of the population, or its characteristic gradual onset.

The lessons learned from other common chronic diseases are highly instructive in this regard. Gradual onset by minute degrees, so that it is difficult to separate mild disease from no disease, is recognized as characteristic of many common chronic diseases, including osteoarthritis, chronic obstructive lung disease, and hypertension. In addition such slow progressive onset is likely common in many other diseases but this gradualism tends to be obscured by later, more dramatic, disease manifestations or by the ways in which we define the disease. The gradual progression of coronary atherosclerosis underlies the apparently abrupt occurrence of a myocardial infarction and the slow process of osteoporosis underlies the abruptness of a hip fracture. This does not necessarily imply that the disease is an extension of normality or that there is an absence of modifiable risk factors. Chronic obstructive lung disease provides a cogent example.[17] In all persons, lung function, as least as measured by forced expiratory volume in one second (FEV), begins to decline early in life, before the age of 20 years, and this decline continues throughout life, accelerating slightly with age. FEV levels correlate reasonably well with symptoms of chronic obstructive lung disease, with breathlessness at rest or on minimal exertion occurring at a level of about 1.0 to 0.8 liters. Cigarette smoking, the major modifiable risk factor for the illness, accelerates this loss of FEV that occurs in all persons and people who stop smoking return to a slope of loss similar to that of nonsmokers. Thus, chronic obstructive lung disease is well characterized by a measure of function that declines in everyone, has an onset that is gradual and difficult to separate precisely from nondisease, and its occurrence is strongly related to age. Yet, it is clearly not a normal or natural occurrence. Most importantly, it has well recognized risk factors, especially smoking, and reduction in this risk factor modifies or prevents the disease.

Similarly, neither high prevalence nor a strong relation between disease occurrence and age implies inevitability. Again, the examples provided by other diseases are compelling. For many common diseases, occurrence increases strongly with age. Tuberculosis in the 18th and 19th centuries, coronary heart disease in the 20th century, and osteoporosis at this time each provide an example of extremely common conditions that have identifiable risk factors, at least some of which are potentially modifiable. For now, the most reasonable attitude seems to be to act on the assumption that modifiable risk factors will be identified for Alzheimer's disease as well.

REFERENCES

1. Evans, D. A., Funkenstein, H. H., Albert, M. S., et al., Prevalence of Alzheimer's disease in a community population higher than previously reported, *JAMA,* 262, 2251, 1989.
2. McKhann, G., Drachman, D., Folstein, M., Katzman, R., Price, D., and Stadlan, E. M., Clinical diagnosis of Alzheimer's disease: report of the NINCDS-ADRDA Work Group under the auspices of Department of Health and Human Services Task Force on Alzheimer's Disease, *Neurology,* 34, 939, 1984.
3. Pfeffer, R.I., Afifi, A. A., and Chance, J. M., Prevalence of Alzheimer's disease in a retirement community. *Am. J. Epidemiol.,* 125, 420, 1987.
4. Hebert, L. E., Scherr, P. A., Beckett. L. A., et al., Age-specific incidence of clinically diagnosed Alzheimer's disease in a community population, *JAMA,* 273, 1354, 1995.
5. Schoenberg, B. S., Kokmen, E., and Okazaki, H., Alzheimer's disease and other dementing illnesses in a defined U.S. population: incidence rates and clinical features, *Ann. Neurol.,* 22, 724, 1987.
6. Kokmen, E., Chandra, V., and Schoenberg, B. S., Trends in incidence of dementing illness in Rochester, Minnesota, in three quinquennial periods, 1960–1974. *Neurology,* 38, 975, 1988.
7. American Psychiatric Association, *Diagnostic and Statistical Manual of Mental Disorders,* 4th ed., American Psychiatric Association, Washington, DC, 1994.
8. Gruenberg, E. M., Hagnell, O., and Öjesjö, L., The rising prevalence of chronic brain syndrome in the elderly, in *Society, Stress and Disease: Aging and Old Age,* Levi, L. and Kagan A. R., Eds., Oxford University Press, London, 1987.
9. U.S. Bureau of the Census, America in Transition: An Aging Society. Current population reports, Series P-23, No. 128, U.S. Government Printing Office, Washington, D.C., 1983.

10. Evans, D. A., Scherr, P. A., Cook, N. R., et al., Estimated prevalence of Alzheimer's disease in the United States, *Milbank Q.,* 68, 267, 1990.
11. Huang, L. F., Cartwright, W.S., and Hu, T. W., The economic cost of senile dementia in the United States, 1985, *Publ. Hlth. Rep.,* 103, 3, 1988.
12. Rice, D. P., Fox, P. J., Max, W., Webber, P. A., Lindeman, D.,A., Hauck, W. W., and Segura, E., The economic burden of Alzheimer's disease care, *Hlth. Affairs,* 12, 164, 1993.
13. Ernst, R. L., and Hay, J. W., The U.S. economic and social costs of Alzheimer's disease revisited, *Am. J. Publ. Hlth.,* 84, 1261, 1994.
14. Varsamis, J., Zuchowski, T., and Maini, K. K., Survival rates and causes of death in geriatric psychiatric patients. A six-year follow-up study, *Can. Psychiat. Assoc. J.,* 17, 17, 1972.
15. Knopman, D. S., Kitto, J., Deinard, S., et al., Longitudinal study of death and institutionalization in patients with primary degenerative dementia, *J. Am. Geriatr. Soc.,* 36, 108, 1988.
16. Evans, D. A., Smith, L. A., Scherr, P. A , et al., Risk of death from Alzheimer's disease in a community population of older persons, *Am. J. Epidemiol.,* 134, 403, 1990.
17. Fletcher, C., Peto, R., Tinker, C., and Speizer, F. E., *The Natural History of Chronic Bronchitis and Emphysema,* Oxford University Press, London, 1976.

Chapter **6**

METHODS OF SCREENING FOR SURVEY RESEARCH ON ALZHEIMER'S DISEASE AND RELATED DEMENTIAS BASED ON EXPERIENCE IN THE NORTH MANHATTAN AGING PROJECT

_____ **Barry J. Gurland**

CONTENTS

0-8493-8997-6/97/$0.00+$.50
© 1996 by CRC Press, Inc.

I. INTRODUCTION

Screening will be considered only for the purposes of research, and then only epidemiological research. A system of clinical inquiry[1,2] is of a quite different nature than that designed for research. It is tempting but misleading to transfer to clinical settings the methods found successful in epidemiology, or conversely. Even within the scope of epidemiology, each study must be first conceived as a system of case finding and ascertainment before appropriate methods of screening can be properly constructed. By these tokens, it is not sound practice for choice of screening methods to be determined by the popularity of an instrument or its success in other hands.

II. PURPOSES OF SCREENING

In studies of the epidemiology of dementia, the prime purpose of screening is usually construed as improving the efficiency of case finding.[3,4] Maximum efficiency occurs when those purposes of the study that build on distinctions between cases and non-cases are achieved with the least possible expenditure of resources. Only by carefully defining the study purposes can the degree of precision and efficiency required in the separation of cases and non-cases for testing the study hypotheses be determined.

In a design that employs a screen to refer possible cases to a research diagnostic process, an ideal screen would capture all cases in a population, and refer none of the non-cases. Further, the ideal screen would, besides being reliable and valid, be brief, easily learned and administered, tactful, repeatable, culture fair, and rapidly scored in the field. No existing screen has all these features; reasoned compromises must be made. A key choice is between the virtues of referring to diagnosis the potential cases and not referring non-cases.

Many, if not all, widely used screens[5-10] can be set to capture all or almost all cases by the expedient of adjusting the threshold for designating a potential case.[11,12] In that instance, however, a high proportion of subjects referred to diagnosis will be non-cases, who will drain the expensive resources entailed in the logistics, personnel, and procedures of research diagnosis. In contrast, if a screen is set to refer only highly likely cases, many true cases will not be referred. The resolution of this conflict touches on several competing aims in the epidemiology of dementia.

Risk factors — Discovery of putative causative, aggravating, or precipitating precedents of dementia (e.g., see References 13 and 14) or its subtypes is optimized by a clean separation of cases and non-cases in a representative sample of elders. The less clean this separation, the more noise enters the analysis of relative risk, and the larger the size of samples that must be mustered for finding hidden risk factors. Since error is bound to muddy the separation, it is better to err on the side of missing cases, which will be diluted by the larger number of non-cases, than including false positives among the smaller body of cases.

Public health issues — Many studies are justified, at least initially, as a means of estimating the number of dementias in a defined population or subpopulation who constitute an actual or potential demand on services.[15] The services might be formal or informal personal care, home health aides, day centers, nursing homes, general medical attention, specialist investigation of early and ambiguous cases, and the like; or might bear upon the opportunities for specific treatment of the dementing process or its behavioral symptoms. Allocation of funds for research which might provide a basis for reducing the demand on services through prevention of the dementing condition, can be similarly advocated on the basis of numbers of actual or projected numbers and proportions of dementias. Issues of need for services and prevention can be supported with the same projections but rationalized as a need to alleviate or prevent the impact of the dementing process on the quality of life of victims and their family.

In this context, relatively rough but convincing estimates will suffice. Planning or policy decisions have never been more than loosely connected to the projected data. Rhetoric, special pleading, fiscal realities, looseness in theories that relate services to data on need, and the limits of generalizability unite to widen the gap between epidemiological projections, on the one hand, and policy and planning initiatives for services and research funding, on the other hand. Given this slippage between data and action, a reasonable strategy for generating projections would be to choose a screening procedure which keeps false-positive screen classifications at a low rate, gives prominence to validating true screen positives with rigorous research diagnoses, and extrapolates missed cases by reference to diagnosis on a proportion of screen negative subjects.

Persuasive elements in projections of dementia are often introduced through transposing the well-known needs and suffering of clinically established cases of dementia onto the numbers of cases bearing the diagnosis of dementia in a population. Nevertheless, there is a great heterogeneity of need and suffering among diagnosed cases of dementia,[16-19] which is left unexpressed in reports which translate projected rates into service needs. As detailed later, numbers of cases must be apportioned to stages, subtypes, co-morbidities, and social contexts with known impacts on quality of life of patient and family, and hence on service needs. Early or mild cases are assuming greater importance as promising interventions arise and are evaluated.[20]

III. INCIDENCE AND PREVALENCE

In preparing a cohort of elders for study of new cases arising over time, it becomes important to identify and remove from the cohort as many preexisting cases as possible. Then, during the period of continuing surveillance of the non-case initial cohort, any cases found can be deemed with high confidence to have had an onset in the interval since the last survey wave, and not be a case previously missed. Thus, a premium must be placed on screening techniques that capture and classify as many cases as possible: involving screens of high sensitivity.

Nevertheless, false negatives are bound to slip through. Contamination of incidence will be higher in the first period of follow-up than in later rounds, since missed cases will be cumulatively reduced. Thus, greater accuracy and confidence in findings can be obtained by collection of incidence figures over several successive waves of survey.[21] Large cohorts, at least over 1000 strong,[22] are desirable for this approach. As a further check on the robustness of observed incidence rates, transitions of the cohort across thresholds of screening scores or other field batteries of cognitive assessments can be documented. Within limits, incidence should be the same whether indexed by new diagnoses or new transitions across a screen threshold corresponding to a high probability of diagnosis.

Comparison of incidence and duration between groups need only have equivalent and reasonably early starting points, not necessarily the earliest starting points. For some purposes the maximum duration of dementia is salient, e.g., where there is a search for immediate precedents or precipitants, or where service needs and family burden are charted over the course of the illness, or early intervention is to be instituted or tested. Maximum duration of the disease process can be many years before the diagnosis is eventually made;[24] that duration cannot be determined from contemporary survey approaches and must instead refer to duration of manifest symptoms. Indicator symptoms can be selected to match the nature of the interest in duration.

The latitude in choosing indicators of symptoms is wider for incidence studies than for prevalence purposes. All that is required for calculation of incidence and comparison of incidence between groups is that a given indicator of onset be consistent, provided that attrition from causes related to dementia is not appreciable within the period between earliest feasible indicators of onset and the stage taken as the arbitrary point of onset. It follows that a surrogate for diagnosis, such as a neuropsychological profile, may be an acceptable method for deriving incidence data.[25]

Prevalence can be increased by more new cases, or greater survival and an extended duration of cases, or an earlier onset of cases. One approach to distinguishing between these alternatives is to follow confirmed cases over time. Unfortunately, results will be highly influenced by the stage of the illness at the time of beginning the follow-up, further confounded by the very early stages being harder or easier to recognize in some demographic groups than in others.[23] Therefore, observing duration for purposes of comparing groups should be keyed to tagging cases with a new onset, joining the methods of study of prevalence with those of incidence.

IV. COMPARISON OF SUBGROUPS

Analyses may be concentrated on differences in the distribution of rates, risk factors, symptom patterns, and co-morbidities among subgroups of dementia, such as Alzheimer's disease, vascular dementias, Parkinson's disease dementia, stroke, and other secondary dementias. This focus requires an unbiased selection from each of the segments of the spectrum of subgroups of dementia, though the overall degree of completeness of case finding may not be crucial. Some of these subgroups are quite uncommon, being more easily accessible through special clinics or reporting registries than from community surveys. For example, Parkinsonian dementias cannot be accumulated to a useful extent from surveys of customary size, but can be readily gathered from neurological clinics specializing in Parkinson's disease. Care must be then taken to ensure that subgroup characteristics do not merely mirror the selective bias of a clinic.

V. CULTURAL VARIATION

Even assuming that criterion-based research diagnosis is unbiased with respect to demographic characteristics, the screening techniques may be biased and then transmit that bias to the diagnostic process.[26] Under most circumstances, the more subjects that are referred (e.g., because they are screen positive) to the diagnostic procedures, the more will be designated as cases. These biases may particularly affect comparisons between groups who come from different ethnic, income, and educational backgrounds, with education having the most powerful effect.[11,26-35] Gender comparisons may be misleading where function enters into the classification system since certain functional tasks (e.g., shopping and cooking) are by custom more practiced by women in contemporary cohorts of elders, and others (e.g., paid occupations) by men. Tasks may also offer a greater challenge to one or other gender, such as dressing or shopping.

Statistical approaches to reducing the bias in screening instruments have been developed whereby items in scales can be selected for their relative neutrality with respect to demographic group membership.[36] Alternatively, threshold scores for case definition can be raised or lowered to provide equal probabilities of diagnosis for specific groups,[31,33] or the entire range of a scale's scores can be weighted to the same effect. These are not satisfactory solutions for several reasons: they may assume that diagnosis is not biased or that there are no real differences between demographic groups (whereas findings are conflicting, especially with respect to race and education,[37-42] or that demographic characteristics such as educational achievement are constant descriptors across geography, time, and populations). Diagnosis does not necessarily act as a fail-safe check on demographic bias. Diagnosis may be biased or overcompensated,[27,42] Moreover, to restate a caution, a screen that inclines to refer more subjects to diagnosis because of demographic bias will expose more subjects to the risk of being diagnosed as cases.

Accepting that no single scale will be found unbiased by every demographic characteristic, the robustness of findings on demographic group comparisons of rates of dementia, can, nonetheless be tested by use of multiple approaches to classification. Cross-cultural comparisons that give consistent results no matter what the scale or other classificatory system will attract greater confidence that real differences are involved. Comparisons may be made with scales of varying complexity, varying threshold scores, mathematical extrapolations from scale scores, scales emphasizing function or cognition or both, diagnoses with stringent and liberal criteria, and so on.[21]

A more fundamental approach is to relinquish the elusive pursuit of unbiased classification and instead search for classification associated with equal consequences across socio-cultural groups, as discussed later under cognitive health.

VI. COMPARISON WITH OTHER STUDIES

Identical screening techniques may be employed in geographically dispersed collaborative studies with the intention of comparing results from various locations and aggregating data across sites.[43-45] Amassing large data sets permits analysis of relatively rare conditions and contexts. However, it should be demonstrated, rather than taken for granted, that the operating characteristics of identical screening techniques are constant across sites and populations. Caution about assuming identical standards from identical instruments must be exercised where the entire interview is not identical, or the interviewers are not trained by a single source, or there may be an interaction between demographic or co-morbid features of the population and the operating characteristics of the screening instrument.

VII. OPERATING CHARACTERISTICS OF SCREENS

Performance of a screen is typically evaluated by indices that bear upon sensitivity, specificity, hit rates, true and false positive and negatives, and positive and negative predictive values.[12,46,47] Such indices convey the actual performance of a scale, with a given cut-point, in respectively identifying a high proportion of true cases in a population, a high proportion of the true non-cases in a population, a high proportion of correct classifications, the actual number of persons correctly classified as cases and non-cases, and the probability of a screen-positive subject being a true case or of a screen-negative subject being a non-case. All these indices change if the cut-point is altered. The continuum of index values progressively changes as the cut-point is serially moved up or down the scale; this is represented by a receiver operating characteristics (ROC) curve.[48] Overall performance at all cut-points in toto is represented mathematically and graphically as the area under the curve (AUC).[48] A key corollary to the general rule that indices shift with the cut-point is that the indices describe the scale only as restricted to a particular cut-point. Indices should not be taken, without nominating the cut-point, as characterizing a scale; comparison of scales by indices should not be restricted to any single cut-point on each scale.

Moreover, the indices are a property of a scale interacting with a population or subpopulation. If the latter changes, the indices may change. Thus, for example, it is not accurate to describe any scale as sensitive or more sensitive than another. Almost any scale in wide use can be made to achieve a high sensitivity by adjusting the cut-point; at issue is what standards are achieved for the other operating characteristics of the scale at a given sensitivity. To compare the efficiencies of scales the indices should be made similar on at least one dimension.[12] Furthermore, indices reflect only the performance of the scale on that population, and scales can only be compared on the same population.

VIII. BATTERIES OF TESTS

In striving to heighten sensitivity while preserving good specificity of screening results, more than one instrument may be assembled to work together as a battery of tests. The combination of instruments may be relatively brief and easily administered in the field,[23,49,50] or complex, demanding expert administration and interpretation, and aimed at a target population such as early dementia.[51-54]

IX. REPORTING VS. SURVEY REGISTRIES

Registries serve as an inventory of cases of dementia from a known denominator such as a well-defined population, usually residents in a specific community with geographic boundaries. Cases may be discovered through networks of reporters in key positions, such as in medical clinics and social services where cases of dementia are likely to be found. Alternatively, cases may be found and entered in the inventory through survey of representative samples of persons from the population. Neither method by itself is likely to exhaust the pool of existing cases. Reporting networks are typically best at collecting cases which come from sociocultural groups that gravitate to hospital-based services, institutions, public system health and social services, large-scale home care organizations, or specialized clinic services; and are severe enough to be known to the service system. The reporting network tends to miss cases which are early, which find services out of area, or which enlist private services. Survey approaches have a greater reach in finding early cases or persons who seek services beyond the reporting network. The cost per case collected, disregarding the value attached to the representativeness of the sample, is much less for the reporting network than for the survey activities. The selective biases relating to preferences for and access to services is clearly greater in the reporting network method. Biases arising from degree of cooperativeness with research interviews is likely to be greater in the survey. In the reporting network method, risk factor findings may be confounded by cases entered into the registry by clinics which have a special interest in a type of risk factor, such as stroke, HIV infection, or Parkinson's disease. Also, some groups who use services more readily may have an overrepresentation of early cases relative to groups who only come to services as a last resort.

The possibility of combining reporting and survey approaches to increase the representativeness of cases at all levels of severity, co-morbid patterns, and demographic background has not been generally explored. In some populations, survey response rates can be so high that reporting systems can add very little. However, in certain situations such as in neighborhoods where community residing elders have reason to feel fearful of strangers or authority figures, or in studies involving several sequenced steps of investigation,[56] response rates may be low enough that room is left for uncertainty about the influence on findings by selective biases arising from lack of cooperation. In that instance, reporting network case finding can help to inform the study analyses about the corrections that should be introduced into group comparisons reliant on survey data. Conversely, surveys targeted to the same geographic area as the reporting network can indicate which types of cases and demographic groups have been missed by the service-based network.

X. LONGITUDINAL ASSESSMENTS

Instruments that are used for screening at baseline may be expected also to provide data on the course of the illness by repetition at periodic intervals.[55] Brief cognitive screen scores are correlated with stages of severity of dementia[56,57] but practice and ceiling (or floor) effects may emerge over time.[58]

XI. VALIDATION

Diagnosis is the conventional validator of survey classification of dementia and its subtypes.[59] An operational set of criteria (e.g., Reference 60) is selected and the requisite information is systematically collected, independent of the screening data and blind to it. A decision tree leads to diagnosis, through steps that may be more or less codified.[61,62] At one end of the spectrum of method, clinical judgment plays a governing role in matching information to criteria, while at the other end every step is quantified and a computer generates the classification according to pro-grammed instructions.[62-64] These strategies can also be combined in sequence.[23] To the extent that the diagnostic process is systematized, it may become less convincing as a validator since it may partake of more of the nature of the screening procedures and be vulnerable to the same biases and variation across sociodemographic groups. In theory, neuroimaging, neurophysiological tests, and autopsy findings may supplement or be added to diagnosis as validators [e.g., References 65 and 66]. In practice this latter class of objective validators is not collected on a large enough, nor sufficiently unbiased, sample to act in this capacity. Follow-up and review of diagnosis at intervals may be more telling but is confounded by the possibility of a differential course of illness in different sociodemographic groups.

XII. BREADTH OF DIAGNOSTIC CONCEPT

A special case of the problem posed by uncertainty regarding constancy of diagnosis across groups is the favoring of differing concepts of diagnosis in different studies or even in analysis of data from the same study. On the one hand, narrow or conservative diagnosis has the merit of identifying relatively indisputable cases of dementia, who are likely to be quite severe as well. There is a low risk of including cases with ambiguous symptoms that might slip over the threshold for case definition only in those demographic groups whose members are not used to formal testing (e.g., of cognitive functions) or have high rates of chronic physical illness with functional impair-ments that might spuriously fit criteria for diagnosis. However, early or only moderately impaired cases will be excluded and may thus hide group differences in this respect. Broad or liberal diagnosis, on the other hand, sensitive to early and mild cases, may accrue false-positive cases who have clinical characteristics that hover around the border of meeting criteria.[67-69]

XIII. COGNITIVE HEALTH

An alternative to manufacturing benchmarks for diagnosis that reside entirely in the realm of operational criteria is to establish the constancy of the meaning of diagnosis for the various comparison groups. Meaning is gained in terms of quality of life impacts,[70-72] including complaints of difficulty with memory, impairments in activities of daily living (as measured by, for example, the Index of ADL,[73] Lawton's IADL,[74] or the SAILS[75]), depression, poor self-perceived health, reduced interpersonal relationships and satisfaction, pain and other distressing symptoms, dimin-ished expectations for the future, undermined sense of dignity, and dissatisfaction with the adequacy of care. Analogous threats to the caregiver's quality of life can be gauged[76,77] as mediated through the patient's behavioral changes.[78] These qualities of life are related to cognitive impairment but may have considerable independent variance and thus must be separately assessed.[79] The useful breadth of diagnosis to adopt can be gauged by the quality of life associations of incremental enlargements of the diagnostic scope. Equivalency of diagnostic concepts across demographic groups can be derived from the impacts of given criteria on quality of life in those groups.

XIV. SURROGATE FOR DIAGNOSIS

Specified levels of screen scores are sometimes used[66] to infer the frequency and distribution of diagnoses of dementia; validation is extrapolated from previous study. Screen scores may also be combined with other systematic information that can be gathered by non-physicians and in community settings and then processed through algorithms which match the combined information to criteria for diagnosis,[63,80] separate syndromes of depression from those of dementia,[80-82] and subtype dementias. Collection and processing of information in this way has the merit of replicability and can be applied even where expert clinical evaluation is not accessible. However, it may offer a spuriously consistent standard of diagnosis across studies and groups. The relation between screen scores, symptom patterns, and diagnosis will vary in unpredictable ways across groups. Concurrent validation by criterion-based diagnosis is required for a high degree of confidence in the achievement of a constant standard of diagnosis (e.g., Reference 62).

XV. SCREENING SYSTEMS VS. INSTRUMENTS

Any method of screening for dementia is best understood as an element in a wider system of research or clinical inquiry.[83] Choices among a range of strategies and tools must be made, but these choices should be driven by the system's purposes and will be restrained by the limits of its resources. This is said to counter a common preoccupation with the properties of individual screening instruments. A sweeping assertion that underlines the system perspective is that choosing between the many widely used screening instruments for dementia should be made without regard to differences between them in psychometric properties. These differences are not constant across populations and are small compared to differences that emanate from their system context.

In view of the fluctuating performance of screening instruments in different contexts, it is more manageable to use instruments only as part of a system, rather than in isolation. Instruments then become a device for making the system work smoothly, not a dominating standard. Whichever instruments or combination of instruments are employed, their purpose is to refer efficient proportions of true cases and non-cases to the validating component of the study. It must be implicit in any two studies which stand to be compared that the validation standards, not the screening standards, are consistent. That may be difficult and typically overlooked, but it is inescapable; otherwise, consistency in screening can neither be proved nor usually obtained. If validation, classically criterion-based diagnosis, is a reliable benchmark, then screening is part of a system comprising case finding and case ascertainment (i.e., validation). In this process, screening can only be more or less efficient, not more or less wrong. If too many false positives are discovered, then the screening rules can be tightened, or loosened if the too many false negatives are observed, without altering the standards for classification. The screen cannot assume the properties of the validator. The validator is independent of the efficiency of the screen. It is correspondingly misplaced to go to great lengths in choosing between available screens on the basis of fine differences in performance.

XVI. STYLES OF ASSESSMENT

With the latitude and redirection of emphasis emerging from the concept of screening as a system,[83] a range of options opens for styles of administering screens.[23,84] Most studies try to attain the best possible case finding and ascertainment allowed by available resources. Such resources are usually dictated by the level of government or private foundation funding granted to the study and the length of time that the investigators can wait for data collection. Other resources of finite extent include the goodwill and tolerance for testing of the population under study and the morale and determination of the field interviewers. These aspects of the system might well prevail in the assembly of a screening system for a particular epidemiological study. Within reasonable limits of efficiency, one screen may be favored over another because it is more tactful, or collects information useful in other ways as well, or is more readily conducted over the telephone or other medium, or is more objective,[85,86] or is less biased by sociocultural features.

Technology can also smooth and facilitate the style of administering the screen. Lap-top computers can be programmed to scroll the screen questions and allow ratings to be entered. Inadvertent skipping of items and contradictory ratings can be preempted by the program. Complicated contingencies directing the flow of the interview can be prescribed. Immediate scoring of a high degree of complexity can be effected and the results displayed to assist decisions in the field on referral to further steps of investigation. Downloading of data into an office-based cumulative archive can be quickly accomplished and regularly scanned for monitoring of the conduct and progress of the survey.

ACKNOWLEDGMENTS

This work was supported by the following grants: (1) "North Manhattan Aging Project" — National Institute on Aging, P.I.; Barry Gurland, M.D., Co-P.I.; David Wilder, Ph.D., Project Number: 5 P01 AG7232. (2) "Epidemiology of Dementia in an Urban Community" — National Institute on Aging, P.I.; Richard Mayeux, M.D., Co-P.I.; Barry Gurland, M.D., and Yaakov Stern, Ph.D., Project Number: P01 AG07232. (3) "Active Life Expectancy Among Urban Minority Elderly" — National Institute on Aging, P.I.; Rafael Lantigua, M.D. Co-P.I.; David Wilder, Ph.D., Co-Invest.; Barry Gurland, M.D., Sidney Katz, M.D., Project Number: 5 R01 AG10489. (4) "A Transcultural Screen for Alzheimer's Disease and Related Disorders" — New York Community Trust Foundation, P.I.; Barry Gurland, M.D., Project Number *NYCT CU 50404701. (5) "The Morris W. Stroud, III, Program on Scientific Approaches to Quality of Life in Health and Aging" — Endowment Fund, Co-Directors; Barry Gurland, M.D. and Sidney Katz, M.D.

Other staff members of the North Manhattan Aging Project: Virginia Barrett, D.P.H.; Betty Barsa, M.S.W.; Mabel Bolivar, B.A.; Dr., Harold Browne, B.A.; Peter Cross, M.Phil.; Jean Denaro, M.A.; Priscilla Encarnación, B.A.; Maria Gonzalez, B.A.; Eloise Killeffer, M.Ed.; Lucia McBee, B.A.; Carmen Polanco, B.A.; Jeanne Teresi, Ph.D.; Interviewers who have completed over 100 interviews: Dr., Raul Almanzar; Carlomagno Baldi, B.A.; Carlos Garcia; Rufina Joga; Consuelo McLaughlin, B.A.; Annie Nuñez; Argentina Peralta, B.A.; Joseph Romero; Rosanne Vargas-Moneo, B.A.; Dario Zagar, B.A.

The late Dr. W. Edwards Deming designed the sampling plan for the North Manhattan Aging Project (NMAP).

We thank the Bureau of Data Management and Strategy of the Health Care Financing Administration for providing the tape files of Medicare beneficiaries.

REFERENCES

1. Gurland, B. J., Mental health assessment; the importance of assessing mental health in the elderly, *Dan. Med. Bull.,* Kellog Foundation, Special Supplement Series, 7, 33, 1989.
2. Gurland, B. J., Cote, L. J., Cross, P. S., and Toner, J. A., The assessment of cognitive function in the elderly, *Clin. Geriat. Med.,* 3(1), 53, 1987.
3. Albert, M., Smith, L. A., Scherr, P. A., Taylor, J. O., and Evans, D. A., and Funkenstein, H. H., Use of brief cognitive tests to identify individuals in the community with clinically diagnosed Alzheimer's disease, *Int. J. Neurosci.,* 57,167, 1991.
4. Blessed, G., Black, S. E., Butler, T., and Kay, D. W. K., The diagnosis of dementia in the elderly: A comparison of CAMCOG (the cognitive section of CAMDEX), the AGECAT Program, DSM-III, the Mini-Mental State Examination and some short rating scales, *Br. J. Psychiatry,* 159, 193, 1991.

5. Brink, T. L., Curran, P., Dorr, M., Janson, E., et al., The Set Test for dementia and depression, *J. Clin. Gerontol.*, 4, 69, 1986.

6. Folstein, M. F., Folstein, S. E., and McHugh, P. R., Mini-Mental State Examination: A practical method for grading the cognitive state patients for the clinician, *J. Psychiat. Res.*, 12, 189, 1975.

7. Golden, R. R., Teresi, J. A., and Gurland, B. J., Detection of dementia and depression cases with the Comprehensive Assessment Referral Evaluation interview schedule, *Int. J. Aging Hum. Dev.*, 16, 242, 1983.

8. Kahn, R., Goldfarb, A. Pollack, M., et al., Brief objective measures of mental status in the aged, *Am. J. Psychiat.*, 117, 326, 1960.

9. Katzman, R., Brown, T., Fuld, P., et al., Validation of a short orientation-memory-concentration test of cognitive impairment, *Am. J. Psychiat.*, 140, 734, 1983.

10. Pfeiffer, E., A short portable mental status questionnaire for the assessment of organic brain deficit in elderly patients, *J. Am. Geriatr. Soc.*, 22(10), 433, 1975.

11. Gurland, B. J., Wilder, D. E., Cross, P., Teresi, J., and Barrett, V. W., Screening scales for dementia: toward reconciliation of conflicting cross-cultural findings, *Int. J. Geriat. Psychiat.*, 7, 105, 1992.

12. Wilder, D. E., Cross, P., Chen, J., et al.: The operating characteristics of brief screens for dementia in a multicultural population, *Am. J. Geriat. Psychiat.*, in press.

13. Mayeux, R., Ottman, R., Tang, M.X., Noboa-Bauza, L., Marder, K., Gurland, B., and Stern, Y., Genetic susceptibility and head injury as risk factors for Alzheimer's disease among community-dwelling elderly persons and their first-degree relatives, *Ann. Neurol.*, 33(5), 494, 1993.

14. Sluss, T. K., Gruenberg, E. M., and Kramer, M., The use of longitudinal studies in the investigation of risk factors for senile dementia-Alzheimer type, in *Epidemiology of Dementia*, Mortimer, J. A. and Schuman, L. M., Eds., Oxford University Press, New York, 1981, 132.

15. Gurland, B. J. and Cross, P.S., Public health perspectives on clinical memory testing of Alzheimer's Disease and related disorders, in *The Handbook for Clinical Memory Assessment of Older Adult*, Poon, L. W., Ed., American Psychological Association, Washington, D.C., 1986, 11.

16. Gurland, B. J., Katz, S., Lantigua, R. A., and Wilder, D., Cognitive function and the elderly, Proceedings of the 1991 International Symposium on Data on Aging, National Center for Health Statistics (NCHS), U.S. Department of Health and Human Services Series, 5(7):21, 1993.

17. Sloane, P. D. and Mathew, L. J., An assessment and care planning strategy for nursing home residents with dementia, *Gerontologist,* 31, 28, 1991.

18. Stern, Y., Hesdorffer, D., Sano, M., and Mayeux, R., Measurement and prediction of functional capacity in Alzheimer's disease, *Neurology,* 40, 8, 1990.

19. Wands, K., Merskey, H., Hachinski, V. C., and Fisman, M., A questionnaire investigation of anxiety and depression in early dementia, *J. Am. Geriat. Soc.*, 38, 535, 1990.

20. Berg, L., Miller, J. P., Baty, J., and Rubin, E. H., Mild senile dementia of the Alzheimer type: IV. Evaluation of intervention, *Ann. Neurol.*, 31, 242, 1992.

21. Gurland, B. J., Wilder, D. E., Cross, P., Lantigua, R. A., Teresi, J., Bolivar, M., Barrett, V., and Mayeux, R., Relative rates of dementia by multiple case definitions, over two prevalence periods, in three cultural groups, *Am. J. Geriat. Psychiat.*, 3, 6, 1995.

22. Fukunishi, I., Hayabara, T., and Hosokawa, K., Epidemiological surveys of senile dementia in Japan, *Int. J. Soc. Psychiat.*, 37, 51, 1991.

23. Gurland, B. J., Wilder, D. E., Chen, J., Lantigua, R., Mayeux, R., and Van Nostrand, J., A flexible system of detection for Alzheimer's disease and related dementias, *Aging: Clinical and Experimental Research on Comprehensive Geriatric Assessment,* in press.

24. La-Rue, A. and Jarvik, L. F., Cognitive function and prediction of dementia in old age, *Int. J. Aging Hum. Dev.*, 25, 79, 1987.

25. Burvill, P. W., The impact of criteria selection on prevalence rates, Fifth Congress of the International Federation of Psychiatric Epidemiology, Montreal, Canada, 1990, *Psychiat. J. Univ. Ottawa,* 15, 194, 1990.

26. Escobar, J. I., Burnham, A., Karno, M., Forsythe, A., Landsverk, J., and Golding, J. M., Use of the Mini-Mental State Examination (MMSE) in a Community Population of Mixed Ethnicity: Cultural and Linguistic Artifacts, *J. Nerv. Mental Dis.*, 174, 607, 1986.

27. Gurland, B. J., The borderlands of dementia: influence of socio-cultural characteristics on rates of dementia occurring in the senium, in *Clinical Aspects of Alzheimer's Disease*, Miller, N. E., and Cohen, G., Eds., Raven Press, New York, 1981, 61.

28. Li, G., Shen, Y. C., Chen, C. H., and Zhao, Y. W., An epidemiological survey of age-related dementia in an urban area of Beijing, *Acta Psychiat. Scand.*, 79, 557, 1989.

29. Murden, R. A., McRae, T. D., Kaner, S., and Bucknam, M. E., Mini-Mental State exam scores vary with education in Blacks and Whites. *J. Am. Geriatr. Soc.*, 39(2): 149, 1991.

30. Phanthumchinda, K., Jitapunkul, S., Sitthi-Amorn, C., and Bunnag, S. C., Prevalence of dementia in an urban slum population in Thailand: validity of screening methods, *Int. J. Geriat. Psychiat.*, 16, 639, 1991.

31. Rosen, A. M. and Fox, H. A., Tests of cognition and their relationship to psychiatric diagnosis and demographic variables, *J. Clin. Psychiat.*, 47(10), 495, 1986.

32. Salmon, D. P., Riekkinen, P. J., and Katzman, R., et al.: Cross-cultural studies of dementia: a comparison of Mini-Mental State Examination performance in Finland and China, *Arch. Neurol.*, 46(7), 769, 1989.

33. Uhlmann, R. F. and Larson, E. B., Effect of education on the Mini-Mental State Examinations a screening test for dementia, *J. Am. Geriat. Soc.*, 39, 876, 1991.

34. Yu, E. S., Liu, W. T., Levy, P., and Zhang, M., Cognitive impairment among elderly adults in Shanghai, China, *J. Gerontol.*, 44, S97, 1989.

35. Baker, F. M., Dementing illness in African American populations: evaluation and management for the primary physician, *J. Geriat. Psychiat.*, 24, 73, 1991

36. Teresi, J., Golden, R., Cross, P., Gurland, B., Kleinman, M., and Wilder, D., Item bias in cognitive screening measures: comparisons of elderly White, Afro-American, Hispanic and high and low educational subgroups, *J. Clin. Epidemiol.*, 48, 473, 1995.

37. de la Monte, S. M., Hutchins, G. M., and Moore, G. W., Racial differences in the etiology of dementia and frequency of Alzheimer lesions in the brain, *J. Natl. Med. Assoc.*, 81, 644, 1989.

38. Folstein, M. F., Bassett, S. S., Anthony, J. C., and Romanoski, A. J., Dementia: a case ascertainment in a community survey, *J. Gerontol.*, 46, 132, 1991.

39. Fratiglioni, L., Grut, M., Forsell, Y., and Viitanen, M., Prevalence of Alzheimer's disease and other dementias in an elderly urban population: Relationship with age, sex, and education, *Neurology*, 41, 1886, 1991.

40. Heyman, A., Fillenbaum, G., Prosnitz, B., and Raiford, K., Estimated prevalence of dementia among elderly Black and White community residents, *Arch. Neurol.*, 48, 594, 1991.

41. Li, G., Shen, Y. C., Chen, C. H., and Zhau, Y. W., A three-year follow-up study of age-related dementia in an urban area of Beijing, *Acta Psychiat. Scand.*, 83, 99, 1991.

42. O'Connor, D. W., Pollitt, P. A., and Treasure, F. P., The influence of education and social class on the diagnosis of dementia in a community population, *Psychol. Med.*, 21(1), 219, 1991.

43. Launer, L. J. and Hofman, A., Studies on the incidence of dementia: the European perspective, *Neuroepidemiology*, 11, 127, 1992.

44. Kua, E. H., The prevalence of dementia in elderly Chinese, *Acta Psychiat. Scand.*, 83, 5, 1991.

45. George, L. K., Landerman, R., Blazer, D. G., and Anthony, J. C., Cognitive impairment, in *Psychiatric Disorders in America, The Epidemiologic Catchment Area Study*, Robins, L. N., and Regier, D. A., Eds., The Free Press, New York, 1991, 291.

46. Fillenbaum, G., Comparison of two brief tests of organic brain impairment, MSQ and the short portable MSQ, *J. Am. Geriat. Soc.*, 28, 381, 1980.

47. Ganguli, M., Belle, S., Ratcliff, G., Seaberg, E., Huff, F.J., von der Porten, K., and Kuller, L. H., Sensitivity and specificity for dementia of population-based criteria for cognitive impairment: the MoVIES Project, *J. Gerontol. Med. Sci.*, 48, M152, 1993.

48. Metz, C. C., Basic principles of ROC analysis, *Semin. Nuclear Med.*, 8, 283, 1978.

49. Gurland, B., Golden, R., Teresi, J., and Challop, J., The SHORT-CARE: an efficient instrument for the assessment of depression, dementia and disability, *J. Gerontol.*, 39, 166, 1984.

50. Commenges, D., Gagnon, M., Letenneur, L., Dartigues, J. F., Barberger-Gateau, P., and Salamon, R., Improving screening for dementia in the elderly using Mini-Mental State Examination subscores, Benton's Visual Retention Test, and Isaac's Set Test, *Epidemiology*, 3, 185, 1992.

51. Cohn, J. B., Wilcox, C. S., and Lerer, B. E., Development of an "early" detection battery for dementia of the Alzheimer type, *Prog. Neuro Psychopharmacol. Biol. Psychiat.*, 15, 433, 1991.

52. de-Rotrou, J., Forette, F., Hervy, M. P., and Tortrat, D., The Cognitive Efficiency Profile: Description and validation in patients with Alzheimer's disease, *Int. J. Geriat. Psychiat.*, 6, 501, 1991.

53. Flicker, C., Ferris, S. H., and Reisberg, B., Mild cognitive impairment in the elderly: predictors of dementia, *Neurology*, 41, 1006, 1991.

54. Hill, R. D., Storandt, M., and LaBarge, E., Psychometric discrimination of moderate senile dementia of the Alzheimer type, *Arch. Neurol.*, 49, 377, 1992.

55. Jonker, C. and Hooyer, C., The AMSTEL project: Design and first findings: The course of mild cognitive impairment of the aged: A longitudina 14-year study, Fifth Congress of the International Federation of Psychiatric Epidemiology, Montreal, Canada, 1990, *Psychiat. J. Univ. Ottawa*, 15, 207, 1990.

56. Davis, P. B., Morris, J. C., and Grant, E., Brief screening tests vs. clinical staging in senile dementia of the Alzheimer type, *J. Am. Geriat. Soc.*, 38, 129, 1990.

57. Warren, E. J., Grek, A., Conn, D., et al.: A correlation between cognitive performance and daily functioning in elderly people, *J. Geriat. Psychiat. Neurol.*, 2(2), 96, 1989.

58. Brink, T. L., Markoff, C, Martinez, N., and Curran, P., Mental status questionnaire for senile confusion: practice effect in English and Spanish speaking subjects, Convention of the Western Psychological Association, San Jose, CA, 1985, *Clin.-Gerontol.*, 4, 29, 1986.

59. Schofield, P., Tang, M., Marder, K., et al. Reliability and consistency in the diagnosis of Alzheimer's disease and related conditions in community based studies, *Neurology*, 43, A23, 1993.

60. American Psychiatric Association, *Diagnostic and Statistical Manual of Mental Disorders (DSM-IV)*, 4th ed., American Psychiatric Association, Washington, D.C., 1994.

61. Stern, Y., Andrews, H., Pittman, J., Sano, M., Tatemichi, T., Lantigua, R., and Mayeux, R., Diagnosis of dementia in a heterogeneous population: development of a neurophysiological paradigm-based diagnosis of dementia and quantified correction for the effects of education, *Arch. Neurol.,* 49, 453, 1992.

62. Copeland, J. R., Dewey, M. E., and Griffiths-Jones, H. M., Dementia and depression in elderly persons: AGECAT compared with DSM III and pervasive illness, *Int. J. Geriat. Psychiat.,* 5, 47, 1990.

63. Copeland, J. R. M., Gurland, B. J., Dewey, M. E., Kelleher, M.J., Smith, A. M. R., and Davidson, I. A., Is there more dementia, depression and neurosis in New York? A comparative community study of the elderly in New York and London using the computer diagnosis, AGECAT, *Br. J. Psychiat.,* 151, 466, 1987.

64. Lobo, A., Saz, P., and Dia, J. L., The AGECAT "organic" section as a screening instrument for minor cognitive deficits, Fifth Congress of the International Federation of Psychiatric Epidemiology, Montreal, Canada, 1990, *Psychiat. J. Univ. Ottawa,* 15, 212, 1991.

65. Blessed. G., Tomlinson, B. E., and Roth, M., The association between qualitative measure of dementia and senile change with cerebral matter of elderly subjects. *Br. J. Psychiatry,* 114, 792, 1968

66. Morris, J. C., McKeel, D. W., Storandt, M., and Rubin, E. H., Very mild Alzheimer's disease: informant-based clinical, psychometric, and pathologic distinction from normal aging, *Neurology,* 41, 469, 1991.

67. O'Connor, D. W., Pollitt, P. A., Hyde, J. B., and Miller, N. D., Clinical issues relating to the diagnosis of mild dementia in a British community survey, *Arch. Neurol.,* 48, 530, 1991.

68. Mowry, B. J., and Burvill, P. W., A study of mild dementia in the community using a wide range of diagnostic criteria, *Br. J. Psychiat.,* 153, 328, 1988.

69. Rosenman S., The validity of the diagnosis of mild dementia, *Psychol. Med.,* 21(4), 923, 1991.

70. Katz, S. and Gurland, B. J., Science of quality of life of elders: challenges and opportunity, in *The Concept and Measurement of Quality of Life in the Frail Elderly,* Birren, J., Lubben, J. E., Rowe, J. C., Deutchman, D. E., Eds., Academic Press, Los Angeles, 1991, 16:335.

71. Gurland, B. J., Quality of life in elders with borderzone cognitive impairment, in *Quality of Life of the Elderly.* Proceedings of the Fifth Sendai International Conference. Sendai, Japan, June 28–29, 1993. WHO-Collaborating Center for Well-Being in Aging, c/o Tohoku University School of Medicine, Japan.

72. Gurland, B. and Katz, S., The outcomes of psychiatric disorder in the elderly: relevance to quality of life, in *Handbook of Mental Health and Aging,* Birren, J. E., Sloane, R. B., and Cohen, E. D., Eds., Academic Press, Los Angeles, 1992, 230.

73. Katz, S., Ford, A. B., Moskowitz, R. W., Jackson, B. A., and Jaffe, M. W., Studies of illness in the aged. The index of ADL: A standardized measure of biological and psychosocial function, *JAMA,* 185, 914, 1963.

74. Lawton, M. P. and Brody, E. M., Assessment of older people: self maintaining and instrumental activities of daily living, *Gerontologist,* 9, 179, 1969.

75. Mahurin, R. K., DeBettignies, B. H., and Pirozzolo, F. J., Structured assessment of independent living skills: preliminary report of a performance measure of functional abilities in dementia, *J. Gerontol.,* 46, P58, 1991.

76. Brodaty, H. and Hadzi, P. D., Psychosocial effects on careers of living with persons with dementia, Australian and New Zealand, *J. Psychiat.,* 24, 351, 1990.

77. O'Connor, D. W., Pollitt, P. A., Roth, M., and Brook, C. P., Problems reported by relatives in a community study of dementia, *Br. J. Psychiat.,* 156, 835, 1991.

78. Rubin, E. H., Morris, J. C., Storandt, M., and Berg, L., Behavioral changes in patients with mild senile dementia of the Alzheimer's type, *Psychiat. Res.,* 21, 55, 1987.

79. Inouye, S. K., Albert, M. S., Mohs, R., Sun, K., and Berkman, L. F., Cognitive performance in a high-functioning community-dwelling elderly population, *J. Gerontol. Med. Sci.,* 48(4), M146, 1993.

80. Copeland, J. R., Gurland, B. J., Dewey, M. E., and Kelleher, M. J., The distribution of dementia, depression and neurosis in elderly men and women in an urban community: assessed using the GMS-AGECAT package, *Int. J. Geriat. Psychiat.,* 2, 177, 1987.

81. Henderson, A. S., Co-occurrence of affective and cognitive symptoms: The epidemiological evidence, *Dementia,* 1, 119, 1990.

82. O'Connor, D. W. and Roth, M., Coexisting depression and dementia in a community survey of the elderly. *Int. Psychogeriat.,* 2, 45, 1990.

83. Gurland, B. J. and Wilder, D. E., A systems approach to the uses of brief scales of cognitive impairment and depressed mood: assessment of elders in primary medical care settings, in *Geriatric Assessment Technology: The State of the Art,* Rubenstein, L. Z., Wieland, D., and Bernabei, R., Proceedings of the International Conference: Geriatric Assessment Technology: the State of the Art, Florence, Italy, June 19–21, 1994, in Press.

84. Wilder, D. E., Gurland, B. J., Chen, J., Lantigua, R. A., Katz, S., and Killeffer, E. H. P., and Encarnacion, P., Interpreting subject and informant reports of function in screening for dementia, *Int. J. Geriat. Psychiat.,* 9(11), 827, 1994.

85. Kuriansky, J. and Gurland, B., The Performance Test of Activities of Daily Living, *Int. J. Aging Hum. Dev.,* 7, 343, 1976.

86. Gurland. B., Cross, P., Chen, J., and Wilder, D., A new performance test of adaptive cognitive functioning: the Medication Management Test (MMT), *Int. J. Geriat. Psychiat.,* 9(11), 875, 1994.

DIAGNOSIS

Chapter 7

DIAGNOSIS OF ALZHEIMER'S DISEASE

John C. Morris

CONTENTS

I. DEFINITION OF DEMENTIA

Diagnostic criteria for dementia as established by the current version of the *Diagnostic and Statistical Manual* (DSM-IV) of the American Psychiatric Association require "the development of multiple cognitive deficits that include memory impairment and at least one of the following: aphasia, apraxia, agnosia, or a disturbance in executive functioning"[1] where executive functioning is the ability to inhibit inappropriate responses and to select key information and behaviors for action. The cognitive disturbances in dementia must be sufficient to interfere with accustomed activities or relationships and represent a decline from a higher level of functioning, i.e., a demented person performs his or her usual activities less well than previously (or relinquishes them altogether) because of cognitive loss. Dementia typically has a progressive course. Particularly in the milder stages, the pattern of decline may be nonuniform such that some categories of function are impaired more than others but global dementia predominates eventually as nearly all mental function is lost in later stages.

II. DIFFERENTIATION OF DEMENTIA FROM NONDEMENTED AGING

Dementia is a syndrome of brain dysfunction and has many possible causes. Because dementia primarily is experienced by elderly persons, perhaps the most difficult issue in differential diagnosis is to determine the threshold for cognitive impairment in relation to the cognitive changes associated with "normal" aging. The clinical overlap of these two conditions creates diagnostic dilemmas and has suggested to some a continuum where dementia simply is an exaggerated form of aging.[2] The tendency for increased individual variation among elderly persons in physiological and psychological function,[3] coupled with differences in lifestyle (e.g., exercise), educational attainment, and factors such as nutrition, complicates interindividual and intergenerational comparisons and further blurs the boundaries of "normal" and "abnormal" cognitive function. The terms "usual" and "successful" aging have been introduced to correspond to elders with little or no discernible loss of function ("successful aging") from those with clinically evident changes associated with age, such as reduced mobility caused by degenerative joint disease.[4] For cognition, however, the degree to which decline may occur and still be part of "usual" or "successful" aging is yet to be determined, in part because there are few prospective cognitive studies of carefully characterized elders that are followed to post-mortem examination. The uncertainty in defining "normal" performance in the older adult population is reflected in the statement that "to draw a distinction between disease and normal aging is to attempt to separate the undefined from the undefinable".[5]

With these limitations in mind, the general consensus is that some aspects of cognition decline with age.[6] Age-associated declines are noted on measures of secondary memory, such as recalling a recently learned string of digits or list of words, although the use of cues can compensate for this deficit in nondemented elderly persons.[7] Age-associated decline also has been noted in cerebral processing resources[8] that are needed to encode and retrieve information. This decline results in decreased capacity for working memory,[9] wherein desired information (e.g., a long distance telephone number) must be maintained during performance of another cognitive activity (e.g., counting change needed for the telephone call). Terms such as "benign senescence", "mild cognitive impairment", and "age-associated memory impairment" have been coined to describe these memory changes, the implication being that they fall short of the definition of dementia. Too few longitudinal data currently exist to show whether some or all of these "benign" conditions ultimately will progress to overt dementia. For at least some individuals, these deficits are not "benign" but rather seem to presage dementia.[10] From a clinical standpoint, nondemented aging generally is assumed when memory changes are nonprogressive and do not interfere substantively with everyday functioning, although there may be increased reliance on compensatory strategies (e.g., making lists). The critical information about whether or not there is interference with accustomed activities often depends on the observations of someone who knows the individual well, such as the spouse or an adult child. Self-reported memory complaints of older adults usually are not predictive of progressive cognitive decline[11] and tend to correlate better with personality traits and depression than with dementia.[12,13] In contrast, collateral source information about how function has changed relative to past performance can be sensitive to even very mild cognitive impairment[14] that may not be detected reliably by standard cognitive tests.[15,16]

The diagnosis of early dementia thus rests on the informant-based clinical judgment that cognitive changes are sufficient to interfere with everyday performance. Documentation of impairment on quantitative cognitive measures provides diagnostic support, but because these measures may be insensitive to very mild change, dementia cannot be diagnosed simply on the basis of cut-off scores on cognitive tests. Neuropsychological measures do play an important role in monitoring cognitive performance over time, which may be necessary in some cases to confirm the diagnosis. Development of biological markers for dementing illnesses[17,18] and more sensitive neuropsychological batteries[19] eventually may improve the differentiation of dementia from nondemented aging.

III. CLINICAL DIAGNOSTIC CRITERIA FOR ALZHEIMER'S DISEASE

In 1984, the Work Group convened by the National Institute of Neurological and Communicative Disorders and Stroke (NINCDS) and the Alzheimer's Disease and Related Disorders Association (ADRDA) published criteria[20] that helped standardize the diagnosis of Alzheimer's disease (AD), by far the leading cause of dementia.[21] These criteria established three levels of diagnostic confidence. In a demented person, *probable AD* is present when dementia is characterized by gradual onset and progression and when other systemic or brain disorders that potentially could cause dementia are absent. *Possible AD* is diagnosed if there are variations in the presentation or course of dementia or when another potentially dementing disorder (e.g., stroke) is present but is believed not to be responsible for dementia. The term *definite AD* is reserved for cases of clinically diagnosed AD in which there is histopathological confirmation by cerebral biopsy or autopsy. The NINCDS-ADRDA criteria for probable AD are equivalent to other sets of criteria, such as those for *dementia of the Alzheimer type* published in DSM-IV (see Table 1). In the demented person without known cause, the salient diagnostic feature for AD is the gradual onset and progression of dementia.

The NINCDS-ADRDA criteria were adopted by the multi-center Consortium to Establish a Registry for Alzheimer's Disease (CERAD) for its standardization and reliability studies of clinical, neuropsychological, and neuropathological assessments used to characterize probable AD. Very high inter-rater reliability has been demonstrated for the CERAD neuropsychological instruments[22] and the accuracy of CERAD clinical methods for the diagnosis of AD as validated by neuropathological examination has been approximately 90%.[23] The reliability and validity of NINCDS-ADRDA criteria have been confirmed in other multicenter studies.[24,25] Use of informant-based clinical methods and standardized diagnostic criteria, such as those employed in CERAD, routinely yield diagnostic accuracy rates for AD of 85% or greater;[23,26,27] in the absence of such methods, however, accuracy rates fall to 58% or even lower.[28,29]

IV. CLINICAL COURSE AND PHENOMENOLOGY OF ALZHEIMER'S DISEASE

The clinical manifestations of AD are pleiotropic. Although core symptoms are present in nearly all cases, there often is heterogeneity in mode of presentation, rate of progression, and expression of associated features such as age at onset, family history of dementia, and behavioral and motor complications. Some clinical features may be present at one stage of the illness but not

TABLE 1   Clinical Diagnostic Criteria for Alzheimer's Disease

DSM-IV dementia of the Alzheimer type[1]	NINCDS-ADRDA Probable Alzheimer's disease[20]

Development of multiple cognitive deficits
  Memory impairment
    At least one of the following:
      Aphasia
      Apraxia
      Agnosia
      Disturbed executive functioning
      (planning, organizing, sequencing,
      abstracting)
Course characterized by continued gradual
  cognitive and functional decline
Deficits are sufficient to interfere significantly
  in social and occupational functioning and
  represent a decline from past functioning
Other causes (medical, neurologic,
  psychiatric) of dementia are excluded
	Dementia established by examination and documented by
	  objective testing
	Deficits in two or more cognitive areas
	Progressive worsening of memory and other cognitive functions
	No disturbance in consciousness
	Onset between 40 and 90 years of age
	Absence of systemic disorders or other brain diseases that could
	  account for the progressive deficits in memory and cognition
	Diagnosis is supported by
	  Progressive deficits in language (aphasia), motor skills (apraxia),
	    and perception (agnosia)
	  Impaired activities of daily living and altered patterns of
	    behavior
	  Family history of similar disorders
	  Consistent laboratory results (e.g., cerebral atrophy on
	    computed tomography)

Note: DSM-IV — Diagnostic and Statistical Manual of Mental Disorders, 4th edition; NINCDS-ADRDA — National Institute of Neurological and Communicative Disorders and Stroke/Alzheimer's Disease and Related Disorders Association.

From Morris, J. C., *Handbook of Dementing Illnesses,* Marcel Dekker, New York, 1994, 78. With permission.

another. In spite of its rich and varied phenomenology, a general picture of probable AD in mild, moderate, and severe stages can be described and is presented here.

Probable AD begins insidiously, and it is often impossible to precisely date its onset. Several years may pass before the family recognizes that everyday functioning has been sufficiently compromised to the point that medical attention is sought. Forgetfulness is the typical presenting symptom. Common examples of memory deficits in this stage are the repetition of questions or statements and the misplacement of items without independent retrieval. Impaired acquisition of new information is manifested by inability to recall recent conversations or events, whereas highly learned material from years gone by may be remembered with seeming clarity. Minor geographic and temporal disorientation also may be early symptoms; the patient may need directions to find even familiar locations or ask for frequent reminders as to the date. Poor judgment and impaired problem solving occur as part of the dysexecutive syndrome wherein patients lack insight (often being unaware of their deficits), have poor attention, and experience uncharacteristic difficulty in completing tasks that involve sequencing of information, such as operating an automatic coffee maker or balancing the checkbook. Word-finding difficulty, or dysnomia, may occur as an early feature of probable AD and is associated with hesitancy of speech and reduced verbal output. Passivity, disinterest, withdrawal, and other personality changes are common symptoms even in the mild stages of dementia and occasionally may be presenting features. The mildly demented patient usually performs self-care activities (e.g., dressing; grooming and bathing; toileting) without problem and may still be engaged in many other activities of daily living, including cooking, driving, voting, and socializing with friends and family, although function in these activities usually is impaired relative to previous levels of performance. Many patients in the mild stage of probable AD appear normal to casual observers.

Progressive decline in all cognitive domains is the rule as the patient advances to the moderate stage. Memory for recent events is severely compromised and confusion about relationships and identities of relatives may occur. Accomplishing even simple tasks, such as making change or washing dishes with acceptable cleanliness, becomes difficult. Driving and other complex activities typically are relinquished by this stage and basic care often requires at least supervision by others lest inappropriate choices in clothes, missed spots in shaving, or neglect of bathing and grooming occur. The patient becomes lost easily. Language skills deteriorate further with incomplete sentences, paraphasic errors, and impaired comprehension of both written and spoken language. The moderate stage of probable AD may be complicated by troublesome behaviors. Agitation, restlessness (including wandering), day-night disorientation, suspiciousness, verbal or occasionally physical aggression, delusions (e.g., the false belief that a misplaced item has been stolen), and hallucinations (visual or auditory) occur with increasing dementia severity.[30] These behaviors can be very disruptive for caregivers and may prompt institutionalization.[31]

The severe stage of probable AD is characterized by total or near-total dependence on caregivers for even basic functions. Only fragments of memory remain; even the spouse and children may not be recognized appropriately. Verbal output is restricted to short phrases or single words. First urinary and then fecal incontinence develop. New onset generalized tonic-clonic seizures may appear in advanced probable AD;[32] the occurrence of seizures in less severe stages, however, should prompt a thorough evaluation for other epileptogenic factors. Terminal-stage AD consists of a bedridden, uncomprehending, vegetative state. Weight loss and dysphagia are nearly universal. Death usually results from aspiration, inanition, pulmonary embolus, or infection (pneumonia; urosepsis). The total duration of the clinical course of AD can range from a few years to 20 years or longer, but the average time from onset to death is in the range of 8 to 10 years.

V. STAGING INSTRUMENTS FOR ALZHEIMER'S DISEASE

There is value in identifying the mild, moderate, and severe stages of probable AD for purposes of patient management and family counseling. As has been noted, several features of probable AD display stage dependency. For example, language disturbances,[33] behavioral pathology,[30] extrapyramidal dysfunction,[34] and falls[35] are all associated with increased dementia severity. Rates of cognitive decline also are influenced by stage of dementia such that the less severe the dementia, the slower the rate of decline.[36,37] From a practical standpoint, at least some mildly demented patients may still be capable of safe driving[38] and retain competence for decision-making (e.g., durable power of attorney), whereas more impaired patients lose capacity for these functions.[39,40]

Clinical rating scales provide a global measure of dementia severity and adjust for differential levels of impairment in separate cognitive and functional domains (e.g., a patient with compromised memory and problem-solving abilities may still be independent in self-care). Because clinical scales are less influenced by demographic factors, such as education, that affect performance on quantitative cognitive measures[41,42] and are less subject to "floor" and "ceiling" effects, they can serve as clinically meaningful measures across a wide range of dementia severity. For these reasons, global staging instruments have been incorporated into longitudinal research studies of probable AD and clinical trials of antidementia drugs, where they are sensitive indicators of cognitive change.[43,44] Several widely used global scales are shown in Table 2 with other selected cognitive and behavioral measures commonly used in the clinical study of probable AD.[45-53]

VI. CLINICAL HETEROGENEITY IN ALZHEIMER'S DISEASE

Comorbidity is frequent in patients with probable AD, who are prone to develop other common age-associated illnesses. Many of these have the potential to add to cognitive impairment; a sudden worsening of dementia in a patient with probable AD almost always is caused by a superimposed condition. Many comorbid disorders are amenable to specific therapy with at least partial improvement in cognitive function. Depression and cognitive dysfunction associated with medications are among the most frequent disorders that complicate probable AD.[54]

Although probable AD develops most often after age 65 years, earlier ages of onset are well documented. Early-onset cases are more likely to represent familial forms of AD[55] and are reported to be associated with greater language dysfunction,[56] increased frequency of seizures and myoclonus,[57] and more rapid cognitive decline.[58] It is likely that age at onset modifies the clinical expression

TABLE 2   Selected Clinical Measures in Dementia

Measure	Comment
Brief Cognitive Tests	**"Bedside" Mental Status Exams**
Dementia Scale[45]	Informant-based scale of everyday memory function, ability in activities of daily living, and personality, interests, and drive; still useful when patient no longer is testable
Information-Memory-Concentration Test[45]	27 items of memory, orientation, information, and sequencing (concentration); this test and the Dementia Scale have been validated and correlated with density of Alzheimer brain lesions
Short Blessed Test[46]	Six-item weighted version of Information-Memory-Concentration Test; usually completed within 5 min, also correlated with Alzheimer histopathology
Mini-Mental State[47]	Widely used; 19 items measuring orientation, memory, concentration, language, and praxis; requires some test materials
Clinical Rating Instruments	**Global measures of dementia severity**
Clinical Dementia Rating[48]	Five-point ordinal scale; assesses cognitive ability by structured informant interview and patient testing in six domains with individual descriptors for each level of severity in each domain
Global Deterioration Scale[49]	Seven-point ordinal scale; global descriptors for each severity level
CAMDEX[50]	Five-point ordinal scale; structured informant interview and patient testing; includes Dementia Scale and the Mini-Mental State; global descriptors for each severity level
Behavioral Scales	**Noncognitive Disturbances (affective disorders, psychosis, increased activity, personality changes) impair the functional ability of the patient and represent major management problems for the family and clinician**
Geriatric Depression Scale[51]	Thirty items (either self-rated or observer rated) of depressive symptomatology in older adults
Agitation Inventory[52]	Assesses frequency of 29 agitated behaviors by caregiver questionnaire in 3 categories: physically aggressive, physically nonaggressive (e.g., disrobing, restlessness), and verbally disruptive (e.g., repetitive questions, screaming)
CERAD Behavior Rating Scale for Dementia (BRSD)[53]	Combination of items from other instruments; informant-based evaluation of broad number of behavioral problems and psychiatric symptoms of patients with dementia

Note: These instruments represent only some of the available measures.

From Morris, J. C., *Clin. Geriatr. Med.,* 10, 262, 1994. With permission.

of probable AD, both because of environmental influences (e.g., dementia will be perceived as more disabling and "severe" in a 48 year old corporate executive than in an 88-year-old retiree) and because of genetic factors. The influence of genotype is exemplified by the ε4 allele of apolipoprotein E which confers a dose–dependent increased risk for AD.[59] Apolipoprotein E genotype is an important susceptibility factor for AD, although its risk may be modified by other factors such as female sex[60] and ethnicity.[61,62] It already is clear that AD is genetically heterogeneous, with known genetic mutations linked to familial AD on chromosomes 21,[63] 14,[64] and 1.[65] The rapid pace of genetic advances in AD likely will result in the discovery of additional mutations and polymorphisms that contribute to phenotypic heterogeneity.

As noted earlier, the usual clinical pattern of probable AD is the gradual onset and progression of memory dysfunction and other cognitive loss. On rare occasions, patients may present with an unexplained and isolated cognitive deficit. There may be focal atrophy of cerebral regions corresponding to the single cognitive deficit and the term "asymmetrical cortical degenerative syndromes" has been proposed for these presentations.[66] Specific "focal" syndromes include progressive aphasia,[67] apraxia,[68] visuoperceptual disturbances including Balint's syndrome,[69] and behavioral or "frontal lobe" disorders.[70] In many instances, the isolated deficit may gradually dissolve into more widespread cognitive impairment consistent with probable AD; pathologically confirmed AD is known to be associated with each of the focally presenting syndromes.[68,71-73] The probability of non-AD disorders is increased, however, when language or behavioral changes are prominent early features.[25] The rare non-AD disorders associated with asymmetric cortical degenerative syndromes occasionally may even mimic probable AD. Included in this group of disorders are corticobasal ganglionic degeneration,[74] Pick's disease,[75] hippocampal sclerosis,[25] motor neuron disease,[76] and "nonspecific" dementia.[77]

There is firm evidence that Parkinson's disease and AD coexist more frequently than would be expected by chance alone,[78,79] suggesting shared risk factors or pathogenetic mechanisms. Parkinson's disease independently can cause dementia[80] and the presence of parkinsonism in probable AD is associated with more rapid cognitive decline,[81] as would be expected with the combination of two dementing disorders. The basis for the cognitive dysfunction associated with Parkinson's disease is not fully understood. The frequent presence of Lewy bodies in neocortical neurons in demented patients with Parkinson's disease provides a potential morphological correlate for dementia. However, the significance of cortical Lewy bodies has yet to be established as they are very commonly detected in patients with Parkinson's disease regardless of whether dementia is present.[82,83] Cortical Lewy bodies also are found in many patients with AD where they are associated with substantia nigral pathology and extrapyramidal dysfunction.[84] Psychosis occurring in relatively early stages of dementia has been postulated as a diagnostic feature for "diffuse Lewy body disease"[85] or the "Lewy body variant of AD"[86] but large-scale prospective studies with clinicopathological correlation will be needed to fully determine the interrelationships among Lewy body disease, Parkinson's disease, and AD.

REFERENCES

1. American Psychiatric Association, *Diagnostic and Statistical Manual of Mental Disorders,* 4th ed., American Psychiatric Association, Washington, DC, 1994.
2. Drachman, D. A., If we live long enough, will we all be demented?, *Neurology,* 44, 1563, 1994.
3. Morse, C. K., Does variability increase with age? An archival study of cognitive measures, *Psychol. Aging,* 8, 156, 1993.
4. Rowe, J. W. and Kahn, R. L., Human aging: usual and successful, *Science,* 237, 143, 1987.
5. Evans, J. G., Aging and disease, in *Research and the Aging Population. Ciba Foundation Symposium,* 134th ed., Evered, D. and Whalen, J. Eds., John Wiley & Sons, Chichester, 1988, 38.
6. Craik, F. I. M., Memory functions in normal aging, in *Memory Disorders, Research and Clinical Practice,* Yanagihara, T. and Petersen, R. C., Eds., Marcel Dekker, New York, 1991, 347.
7. Petersen, R. C., Smith, G., Kokmen, E., Ivnik, R. J., and Tangalos, E. G., Memory function in normal aging, *Neurology,* 42, 396, 1992.
8. Baltes, M. M., Kuhl, K., and Sowarka, D. Testing for limits of cognitive reserve capacity: a promising strategy for early diagnosis of dementia, *J. Gerontol.,* 47(3), P165, 1992.
9. Salthouse, T. A. and Skovronek, E. Within-context assessment of age differences in working memory, *J. Gerontol.,* 47, P110, 1992.
10. Linn, R. T., Wolf, P. A., Bachman, D. L., Knoefel, J. E., Cobb, J. L., Belanger, A. J., Kaplan, E. F., and D'Agostino, R. B. The "preclinical phase" of probable Alzheimer's disease, *Arch. Neurol.,* 52, 485, 1995.
11. Flicker, C., Ferris, S. H. and Reisberg, B., A longitudinal study of cognitive function in elderly persons with subjective memory complaints, *J. Am. Geriatr. Soc.,* 41, 1029, 1993.
12. Bolla, K. I., Lindgren, K. N., Bonaccorsy, C. and Bleecker, M. L. Memory complaints in older adults: fact or fiction? *Arch. Neurol.,* 48, 61, 1991.
13. Hänninen, T., Reinikainen, K. J., Helkala, E. L., Koivisto, K., Mykkänen, L., Laakso, M., Pyörälä, K. and Riekkinen, P., Subjective memory complaints and personality traits in normal elderly subjects, *J. Am. Geriat. Soc.,* 42, 1, 1994.
14. Koss, E., Patterson, M. B., Ownby, R., Stuckey, J. C. and Whitehouse, P. J., Memory evaluation in Alzheimer's disease: caregivers' appraisals and objective testing, *Arch. Neurol.,* 50, 92, 1993.
15. Hansen, L. A., DeTeresa, R., Davies, P., and Terry, R. D. Neocortical morphometry, lesion counts, and choline acetyltransferase levels in the age spectrum of Alzheimer's disease, *Neurology,* 38, 48, 1988.
16. Morris, J. C., McKeel, D. W., Jr., Storandt, M., Rubin, E. H., Price, J. L., Grant, E. A., Ball, M. J., and Berg, L., Very mild Alzheimer's disease: informant-based clinical, psychometric, and pathologic distinction from normal aging, *Neurology,* 41, 469, 1991.

17. Small, G. W., Mazziota, J. C., Collins, M. T., Baxter, L. R., Phelps, M. E., Mandelkern, M. A., Kaplan, A., Rue, A. L., Adamson, C. F., Chang, L., Guze, B. H., Corder, E. H., Saunders, A. M., Haines, J. L., Pericak-Vance, M. A., and Roses, A. D., Apolipoprotein E type 4 allelle and cerebral glucose metabolism in relatives at risk for familial Alzheimer's disease, *JAMA,* 273, 942, 1995.

18. Petersen, R. C., Smith, G. E., Ivnik, R. J., Tangalos, E. G., Schaid, D. J., Thobodeau, S. N., Kokmen, E., Waring, S. C., and Kurland, L. T. Apolipoprotein E status as a predictor of the development of Alzheimer's disease in memory-impaired individuals, *JAMA,* 273, 1274, 1995.

19. Masur, D. M., Sliwinski, M., Lipton, R. B., Blau, A. D., and Crystal, H. A., Neuropsychological prediction of dementia and the absence of dementia in healthy elderly persons, *Neurology,* 44, 1427, 1994.

20. McKhann, G., Drachman, D., Folstein, M., Katzman, R., Price, D. and Stadlan, E. M. Clinical diagnosis of Alzheimer's disease: report of the NINCDS-ADRDA Work Group under the auspices of Department of Health and Human Services Task Force on Alzheimer's disease, *Neurology,* 34, 939, 1984.

21. Jellinger, K., Danielczyk, W., Fischer, P., and Gabriel, E., Clinicopathological analysis of dementia disorders in the elderly, *J. Neurol. Sci.,* 95, 239, 1990.

22. Morris, J. C., Heyman, A., Mohs, R. C., Hughes, J. P., van Belle, G., Fillenbaum, G., Mellits, E. D., Clark, C., and and the CERAD investigators, The Consortium to Establish a Registry for Alzheimer's Disease (CERAD). I. Clinical and neuropsychological assessment of Alzheimer's disease, *Neurology,* 39, 1159, 1989.

23. Mirra, S. S., Heyman, A., McKeel, D. W., Sumi, S. M., Crain, B. J., Brownlee, L. M., Vogel, F. S., Hughes, J. P., van Belle, G., Berg, L., and participating CERAD neuropathologists, The Consortium to Establish a Registry for Alzheimer's Disease (CERAD). II. Standardization of the neuropathologic assessment of Alzheimer's disease, *Neurology,* 41, 479, 1991.

24. Victoroff, J., Mack, W. J., Lyness, S. A., and Chui, H. C., Multicenter clinico-pathological correlation in dementia, *Am. J. Psychiat.,* 152, 1476, 1995.

25. Blacker, D., Albert, M. S., Bassett, S. S., Go, R. C. P., Harrell, L. E., and Folstein, M. F., Reliability and validity of NINCDS-ADRDA criteria for Alzheimer's disease, *Arch. Neurol.,* 51, 1198, 1995.

26. Mendez, M. F., Mastri, A. R., Sung, J. H., and Frey, W. H., II, Clinically diagnosed Alzheimer's disease: neuropathologic findings in 650 cases, *Alzheimer Dis. Assoc. Disord.,* 6, 35, 1992.

27. Becker, J. T., Boller, F., Lopez, O. L., Saxton, J., McGonigle, K. L., and Alzheimer Research Program, The natural history of Alzheimer's disease: description of study cohort and accuracy of diagnosis, *Arch. Neurol.,* 51, 585, 1994.

28. Alafuzoff, I., Iqbal, K., Friden, H., Adolfsson, R., and Winblad, B. Histopathological criteria for progressive dementia disorders: clinical-pathological correlation and classification by multivariate data analysis, *Acta Neuropathol.,* 74, 209, 1987.

29. Homer, A. C., Honavar, M., Lantos, P. L., Hastie, I. R., Kellett, J. M. and Millard, P. H. Diagnosing dementia: do we get it right?, *Br. Med. J.,* 297, 894, 1988.

30. Drevets, W. C. and Rubin, E. H., Psychotic symptoms and the longitudinal course of senile dementia of the Alzheimer type, *Biol. Psychiat.,* 25, 39, 1989.

31. Lachs, M. S., Becker, M., Siegal, A. P., Miller, R. L., and Tinetti, M. E. Delusions and behavioral distributions in cognitively impaired elderly persons, *J. Am. Geriat. Soc.,* 40, 768, 1992.

32. Romanelli, M. F., Morris, J. C., Ashkin, K., and Coben, L. A., Advanced Alzheimer's disease is a risk factor for late-onset seizures, *Arch. Neurol.,* 47, 847, 1990.

33. Faber-Langendoen, K., Morris, J. C., Knesevich, J. W., LaBarge, E., Miller, J. P. and Berg, L., Aphasia in senile dementia of the Alzheimer type, *Arch. Neurol.,* 23, 365, 1988.

34. Morris, J. C., Drazner, M., Fulling, K., Grant, E. A., and Goldring, J., Clinical and pathological aspects of parkinsonism in Alzheimer's disease: a role for extranigral factors?, *Arch. Neurol.,* 46, 651, 1989.

35. Morris, J. C., Rubin, E. H., Morris, E. J., and Mandel, S. A. Senile dementia of the Alzheimer type: an important risk factor for serious falls, *J Gerontol.,* 42, 412, 1987.

36. Drachman, D. A., O'Donnell, B. F., Lew, R. A., and Swearer, J. M., The prognosis in Alzheimer's disease. 'How far' rather than 'how fast' best predicts the course, *Arch. Neurol.,* 47, 851, 1990.

37. Morris, J. C., Edland, S., Clark, C., Galasko, D., Koss, E., Mohs, R., van Belle, G., Fillenbaum, G., and Heyman, A., The Consortium to Establish a Registry for Alzheimer's Disease (CERAD). IV. Rates of cognitive change in the longitudinal assessment of probable Alzheimer's disease, *Neurology,* 43, 2457, 1993.

38. Hunt, L., Morris, J. C., Edwards, D., and Wilson, B. S. Driving performance in persons with mild senile dementia of the Alzheimer type, *J. Am. Geriat. Soc.,* 41, 747, 1993.

39. Drachman, D. A., Swearer, J. M., and the Collaborative Study Group, Driving and Alzheimer's disease: the risk of crashes, *Neurology,* 43, 2448, 1993.

40. Marson, D., Ingram, K., Cody, H. A., and Harrell, L. E., Assessing the competency of patients with Alzheimer's disease under different legal standards, *Arch. Neurol.,* 52, 949, 1995.

41. Tombaugh, T. N. and McIntyre, N. J. The Mini-Mental State Examination: a comprehensive review, *J. Am. Geriat. Soc.,* 40, 922, 1992.

42. Doraiswamy, P. M., Krishen, A., Stallone, F., Martin, W. L., Potts, N. L., Metz, A., and DeVeaugh-Geiss, J., Cognitive performance on the Alzheimer's disease assessment scale: effect of education, *Neurology,* 45, 1980, 1995.

43. Berg, L., Miller, J. P., Baty, J., Rubin, E. H., Morris, J. C., and Figiel, G. Mild senile dementia of the Alzheimer type. IV. Evaluation of intervention, *Ann. Neurol.*, 31, 242, 1992.

44. Knopman, D. S., Knapp, M. J., Gracon, S. I., and Davis, C. S., The clinician interview-based impression (CIBI): a clinician's global change rating scale in Alzheimer's disease, *Neurology*, 44, 2315, 1994.

45. Blessed, G., Tomlinson, B. E., and Roth, M., The association between quantitative measures of dementia and of senile change in the cerebral grey matter of the elderly subjects, *Br. J. Psychiat.*, 114, 797, 1968.

46. Katzman, R., Brown, T., Fuld, P., Peck, A., Schechter, R., and Schimmel, H., Validation of a short orientation-memory-concentration test of cognitive impairment, *Am. J. Psychiat.*, 140, 734, 1983.

47. Folstein, M. F., Folstein, S. E., and McHugh, P. R. Mini-mental State: a practical method for grading the cognitive state of patients for the clinicians, *J. Psychiatr. Res.*, 12, 189, 1975.

48. Morris, J. C., The Clinical Dementia Rating (CDR): current version and scoring rules, *Neurology*, 43, 2412, 1993.

49. Reisberg, B., Ferris, S. H., and deLeon, M. J., The Global Deterioration Scale for assessment of primary degenerative dementia, *Am. J. Psychiat.*, 139, 1136, 1982.

50. Roth, M., Tym, E., Mountjoy, C. Q., Huppert, F. A., Hendrie, H., Verma, S., and Goddard, R., CAMDEX: a standardized instrument for the diagnosis of mental disorders in the elderly with special reference to the early detection of dementia, *Br. J. Psychiat.*, 149, 698, 1986.

51. Yesavage, J. A., Geriatric Depression Scale, *Psychopharmacol. Bull.*, 24, 709, 1988.

52. Cohen-Mansfield, J. and Billig, N. Agitated behaviors in the elderly. I. A conceptual review, *J. Am. Geriat. Soc.*, 34, 711, 1986.

53. Tariot, P. N., Mack, J. L., Patterson, M. B., Edland, S. D., Weiner, M. F., Fillenbaum, G., Blazina, L., Teri, L., Rubin, E., Mortimer, J. A., and Stern, Y., The behavior rating scale for dementia of the Consortium to Establish a Registry for Alzheimer's Disease, *Am. J. Psychiat.*, 152, 1349, 1995.

54. Clarfield, A. M., The reversible dementias: do they reverse?, *Ann. Int. Med.*, 109, 476, 1988.

55. Farrer, L. A., Myers, R. H., Cupples, L. A., St.George-Hyslop, P. H., Bird, T. D., Rossor, M. N., Mullan, M. J., Polinsky, R., Nee, L., Heston, L., Van Broeckhoven, C., Martin, J. J., Crapper McLachlan, D. R., and Growdon, J. H., Transmission and age-at-onset patterns in familial Alzheimer's disease: evidence for heterogeneity, *Neurology*, 40, 395, 1990.

56. Selnes, O. A., Carson, K., Rovner, B., and Gordon, B., Language dysfunction in early- and late-onset possible Alzheimer's disease, *Neurology*, 38, 1053, 1988.

57. Bird, T. D., Sumi, S. M., Nemens, E. J., Nochlin, D., Schellenberg, G., Lampe, T. H., Sadovnick, A., Chui, H., Miner, W., and Tinklenberg, J., Phentypic heterogeneity in familial Alzheimer's disease: a study of 24 kindreds, *Ann. Neurol.*, 25, 12, 1989.

58. Huff, F. J., Growdon, J. H., Corkin, S., and Rosen, T. J., Age at onset and rate of progression of Alzheimer's disease, *J. Am. Geriat. Soc.*, 35, 27, 1987.

59. Saunders, A. M., Strittmatter, W. J., Schmechel, D., St.George-Hyslop, P. H., Pericak-Vance, M., Joo, S. H., Rosi, B. L., Gusella, J. F., Crapper McLachlan, D. R., Alberts, M. J., Hulette, C., Crain, B., Goldgaber, D., and Roses, A. D., Association of apolipoprotein E allele Î 4 with late-onset familial and sporadic Alzheimer's disease, *Neurology*, 43, 1467, 1993.

60. Farrer, L. A., Cupples, L. A., van Duijn, C. M., Kurz, A., Zimmer, R., Müller, U., Green, R. C., Clarke, V., Shoffner, J., Wallace, D. C., Chui, H., Flanagan, S. D., Duara, R., St.George-Hyslop, P., Auerbach, S. A., Volicer, L., Wells, J. M., Van Broeckhoven, C., Growdon, J. H., and Haines, J. L., Apolipoprotein E genotype in patients with Alzheimer's disease: implications for the risk of dementia among relatives, *Ann. Neurol.*, 38, 797, 1995.

61. Maestre, G., Ottman, R., Stern, Y., Gurland, B., Chun, M., Tang, M.-X., Shelanski, M., Tycko, B., and Mayeux, R., Apolipoprotein E and Alzheimer's disease: ethnic variation in genotypic risks, *Ann. Neurol.*, 37, 254, 1995.

62. Osuntokun, B. O., Sahota, A., Ogunniyi, A. O., Gureje, O., Baiyewu, O., Adeyinka, A., Oluwole, S. O., Komolafe, O., Hall, K. S., Unverzagt, F. W., Hui, S. L., Yang, M., and Hendrie, H. C., Lack of an association between apolipoprotein E Î4 and Alzheimer's disease in elderly Nigerians, *Ann. Neurol.*, 38, 463, 1995.

63. Goate, A., Chartier-Harlin, M. C., Mullan, M., Brown, J., Crawford, F., Fidani, L., Giuffra, L., Haynes, A., Irving, N., and James, L., Segregation of a missense mutation in the amyloid precursor protein gene with familial Alzheimer's disease, *Nature*, 349, 704, 1991.

64. Sherrington, R., Rogaev, E. I., Liang, Y., Rogaeva, E. A., Levesque, G., Ikeda, M., Chi, H., Lin, C., Holman, K., Tsuda, T., Mar, L., Foncin, J.-F., Bruni, A. C., Montesi, M. P., Sorbi, S., Rainero, I., Pinessi, L., Nee, L., Chumakov, I., Pollen, D., Brookes, A., Sanseau, P., Polinsky, R. J., Wasco, W., Da Silva, H. A. R., Haines, J. L., Pericak-Vance, M. A., Tanzi, R. E., Roses, A. D., Fraser, P. E., Rommens, J. M., and St.George-Hyslop, P. H., Cloning of a gene bearing missense mutations in early-onset familial Alzheimer's disease, *Nature*, 375, 754, 1995.

65. Levy-Lahad, E., Wasco, W., Poorkaj, P., Romano, D. M., Oshima, J., Pettingell, W. H., Yu, C., Jondro, P. D., Schmidt, S. D., Wang, K., Crowley, A. C., Fu, Y.-H., Guenette, S. Y., Galas, D., Nemens, E., Wijsman, E. M., Bird, T. D., Schellenberg, G. D., and Tanzi, R. E., Candidate gene for the chromosome 1 familial Alzheimer's disease locus, *Science*, 269, 973, 1995.

66. Caselli, R. J., Jack, C. R., Petersen, R. C., Wahner, H. W., and Yanagihara, T., Asymmetric cortical degenerative syndromes: clinical and radiologic correlations, *Neurology*, 42, 1462, 1992.

67. Mesulam, M. M. and Weintraub, S., Primary progressive aphasia: Sharpening the focus on a clinical syndrome, in *Heterogeneity of Alzheimer's Disease,* Boller, F., Forette, F., Khachaturian, Z. S., Poncet, M., and Christen, Y., Eds., Springer-Verlag, Berlin, 1992, 43.

68. Crystal, H. A., Horoupian, D. S., Katzman, R., and Jotkowitz, S., Biopsy-proved Alzheimer's disease presenting as a right parietal lobe syndrome, *Ann. Neurol.,* 12, 186, 1982.

69. Mendez, M. F., Mendez, M. A., Martin, R., and Smyth, K. A., Complex visual disturbances in Alzheimer's disease, *Neurology,* 40, 439, 1990.

70. Kumar, A. and Gottlieb, G., Frontotemporal dementias: a new clinical syndrome?, *Am. J. Geriat. Psychiat.,* 1, 95, 1993.

71. Green, J., Morris, J. C., Sandson, J., McKeel, D. W., and Miller, J. W., Progressive aphasia: a precursor of global dementia? *Neurology,* 40, 423, 1990.

72. Victoroff, J., Ross, G. W., Benson, D. F., Verity, M. A. and Vinters, H. V. Posterior cortical atrophy. Neuropathologic correlations, *Arch. Neurol.,* 51, 269, 1994.

73. Brun, A., Frontal lobe degeneration of non-Alzheimer type. I. Neuropathology, *Arch. Gerontol. Geriatr.,* 6, 193, 1987.

74. Arima, K., Uesugi, H., Fujita, I., Sakurai, Y., Oyanagi, S., and Andoh, S., Corticonigral degeneration with neuronal achromasia presenting with primary progressive aphasia: ultrastructural and immunocytochemical studies, *J. Neurol. Sci.,* 127, 186, 1994.

75. Graff-Radford, N. R., Damasio, A. R., Hyman, B. T., Hart, M. N., Trane, L. D., Damasio, H., VanHoesen, G. W., and Rezai, K., Progressive aphasia in a patient with Pick's disease: a neuropsychological, radiologic, and anatomic study, *Neurology,* 40, 620, 1990.

76. Cooper, P. N., Jackson, M., Lennox, G., Lowe, J., and Mann, M. A., t, Ubiquitin, and aB-crystallin immunohistochemistry define the principal causes of degenerative frontotemporal dementia, *Arch. Neurol.,* 52, 1011, 1995.

77. Knopman, D. S., Mastri, A. R., Frey, W. H., II, Sung, J. H., and Rustan, T., Dementia lacking distinctive histologic features: a common non-Alzheimer degenerative dementia, *Neurology,* 40, 251, 1990.

78. Hulette, C., Mirra, S., Wilkinson, W., Heyman, A., Fillenbaum, G. and Clark, C., The Consortium to Establish a Registry for Alzheimer's Disease (CERAD). IX. A prospective cliniconeuropathologic study of Parkinson's features in Alzheimer's disease, *Neurology,* 45, 1991, 1995.

79. Kazee, A. M., Cox, C., and Richfield, E. K., Substantia nigra lesions in Alzheimer's disease and normal aging, *Alzheimer Dis. Assoc. Disord.,* 9, 61, 1995.

80. Mayeux, R., Chen, J., Mirabello, E., Marder, K., Bell, K., Dooneief, G., Cote, L., and Stern, Y., An estimate of the incidence of dementia in idiopathic Parkinson's disease, *Neurology,* 40, 1513, 1990.

81. Storandt, M., Morris, J. C., Rubin, E. H., Coben, L. A., and Berg, L., Progression of senile dementia of the Alzheimer type on a battery of psychometric tests, in *Memory Functioning in Dementia,* Bäckman, L. Ed., Elsevier, Amsterdam, North-Holland, 1992, 10, 207.

82. Hughes, A. J., Daniel, S. E., Blankson, S., and Lees, A. J., A clinicopathologic study of 100 cases of Parkinson's disease, *Arch. Neurol.,* 50, 140, 1993.

83. de Vos, R. A. I., Jansen, E. N. H., Stam, F. C., Ravid, R., and Swaab, D. F., 'Lewy body disease': clinico-pathological correlations in 18 consecutive cases of Parkinson's disease with and without dementia, *Clin. Neurol. Neurosurg.,* 97, 13, 1995.

84. Kazee, A. M. and Han, L. Y. Cortical Lewy bodies in Alzheimer's disease, *Arch. Pathol. Lab. Med.,* 119, 448, 1995.

85. Crystal, H. A., Dickson, D. W., and Lizardi, J. E., Antemortem diagnosis of diffuse Lewy body disease, *Neurology,* 40, 1523, 1990.

86. Mirra, S. S., Hart, M. N., and Terry, R. D., Making the diagnosis of Alzheimer's disease. A primer for practicing pathologists, *Arch. Pathol. Lab. Med.,* 117, 132, 1993.

Chapter **8**

CLINICAL ASSESSMENT OF PATIENTS WITH DEMENTIA

_____ Sid Gilman

CONTENTS

0-8493-8997-6/97/$0.00+$.50
© 1996 by CRC Press, Inc.

I. INTRODUCTION

Evaluation of people who might have a dementing illness requires a carefully taken history, a thorough physical and neurological examination, and several screening laboratory tests. The initial assessment requires at least two visits to a physician's office and is usually undertaken in the outpatient setting. Depending upon the outcome of the initial assessment, additional tests may be required. For people in the early stages of dementia, follow-up examination in several months may be important to determine whether any cognitive disorders initially observed have progressed with time. Detecting the presence of dementia can be difficult and challenging, particularly in the early stages of the disorder.[1] Interviews with family members and others closely associated with the person requiring evaluation are frequently essential in detecting cognitive decline, especially with people who deny their dysfunctions. Historical information from multiple sources coupled with performance on tests of cognitive function provides the most effective means of completing the initial evaluation.[2-4]

II. HISTORY

A. PRESENTING COMPLAINT

The initial phase of the history should begin with documentation of the patient's age, sex, occupation, and identification of the patient's presenting complaints or, if the patient is asymptomatic, with any concerns expressed by family members or others capable of providing reliable historical information. Concerns expressed by the family, friends, or associates about cognitive decline in the patient should be taken as a compelling rationale for initiating an evaluation. The history should be obtained from the patient and also from a person or persons closely familiar with the patient, preferably family members or friends in frequent or constant contact with the patient.[5-7] Many people with dementing illnesses lack insight into their disabilities and may deny symptoms.[8] Often it is preferable to obtain the history from the patient alone and to examine the patient without others present to preserve the patient's dignity and to foster a trusting patient-physician relationship.[9] If the evaluation is performed without family members or friends participating, it is essential to obtain further history from these people interviewed separately, since these informants may be reluctant to discuss the patient's symptoms in the patient's presence.[10] It is important to inform the patient that a collateral history is being obtained from others to preserve a trusting relationship.

B. HISTORY OF THE PRESENT ILLNESS

After the presenting complaint has been established, a chronologically based medical history should be acquired focused upon the presenting complaint obtained from the patient, family member, or friend. The history should include the initial symptoms or signs of cognitive decline, a description of the onset, whether abrupt or gradual, and the subsequent course, also whether gradually progressive or punctuated by episodic worsening or improvement. Specific inquiries should be directed toward the common symptoms of cognitive decline, including forgetting the names of people, places, and objects; mismanaging financial affairs at work or at home; getting lost in familiar places; losing track of time; having difficulty learning and retaining new information; experiencing problems in handling complex motor skills; and becoming unable to reason logically. Specific examples of these problems are helpful. The inquiry should be directed to the patient's capabilities in the activities of daily living, including household chores, preparing meals, dressing appropriately, and managing personal hygiene. The history should include attention to other neurological complaints, including headache; loss of awareness; difficulty speaking or swallowing; incontinence of urine or stool; visual disorders; trouble hearing; and problems with walking, rising from a chair, and turning over in bed. Alterations in emotional state occur commonly in dementia and can include numerous disturbances, including depression, anxiety, change in personality, and unusual passivity or irritability.[11,12] Many patients develop delusions, commonly the notion that someone is stealing from them.[13] Hallucinations occur in dementia, but often late in the course. Other psychiatric disorders may be expressed early in the course of the disorder, including restlessness, agitation, disturbances of sleeping, wandering, and compulsive motor acts.

C. PAST HISTORY

Once the history of the present illness has been obtained, the past medical history should be documented, focusing inquiries upon relevant systemic diseases, psychiatric disorders, craniocerebral trauma, and medications. Specific questions should be posed concerning cerebrovascular disorders (transient ischemic attacks and strokes), seizures, head injury, systemic infections (including pneumonia and urinary tract infections), diabetes, risk factors for AIDS and syphilis, anemia, vitamin deficiency, cancers, drug abuse, alcohol intake, disorders of cardiac, hepatic and renal function, and nutrition. A detailed list of each medication currently used should be obtained, including prescribed drugs, particularly sedatives, anxiolytics, and antidepressants, and also over-the-counter medications, especially sedatives and analgesics. The importance of medications in evaluating cognitive decline, especially in the elderly, cannot be overly emphasized. The most common causes of reversible dementia are those associated with ingestion of medication. Many drugs have been implicated, including benzodiazepines, anticholinergics, antihypertensives, cardiac medications (digitalis preparations, calcium channel blockers, and antiarrhythmic agents), corticosteroids, nonsteroidal antiinflammatory drugs, antibiotics, antineoplastic agents, anticonvulsants, and medications for Parkinson's disease.[14]

D. FAMILY HISTORY

A history of cognitive and movement disorders in parents and siblings is an important aspect of the evaluation since many dementias are either clearly hereditary or strongly influenced by genetic factors. Many kindreds of Alzheimer's disease with autosomal dominant inheritance have been described, with loci on chromosomes 14, 19, and 21.[15-20] Many of these clearly inherited cases develop cognitive disorders at a relatively young age. Moreover, family studies of older-onset Alzheimer's disease indicate that by age 90 years, approximately 50% of the first-degree relatives of people with dementia will become demented themselves.[21,22] Recent studies indicate an association between the E4 allele of apolipoprotein E (APOE) and both familial and sporadic forms of late-onset Alzheimer's disease.[23]

In addition to Alzheimer's disease, several other progressive dementing illnesses have strong genetic influences. Huntington's disease, a degenerative disease with involuntary movement disorders and dementia, is inherited as an autosomal dominant trait. Other disorders with genetic influences are Gerstmann-Straussler syndrome, Pick's disease, and Creutzfeldt-Jakob disease. Consequently, the family history should include specific inquiry about the patient's parents, including their ages of death; disorders of the parents' siblings and parents; and disorders of the patient's siblings. The ages of death of first-degree relatives should be included in the history, particularly when there is a history of cognitive decline in one or more of these relatives.

E. SOCIAL HISTORY

If insufficiently covered in the history of the present illness or past history, a detailed inquiry should be made concerning the patient's social history. This should include the patient's educational history, military service, previous occupations, current occupation, functional status at work if still employed, hobbies, marital history, sexual history, and relationships with family and friends. Assessment of cultural and language factors is important, particularly if the patient is not primarily English-speaking, since these factors must be considered in evaluating cognitive performance.

III. PHYSICAL EXAMINATION

A general physical examination should be undertaken to assess the patient's general appearance as well as the blood pressure, pulse, and respiratory rate. If the history suggests any symptoms provoked by rising from the lying or sitting position, the blood pressure should be obtained with the patient recumbent and then standing. The examination should include attention to the heart, lungs, abdomen, and extremities, seeking evidence of arrhythmias, cardiomegaly, congestive heart failure, enlargement of the liver and spleen, and clubbing of the digits. A neurovascular examination should be undertaken to evaluate the pulses and seek bruits over the carotid arteries.

IV. NEUROLOGICAL EXAMINATION

A. INTRODUCTION

The neurological examination includes evaluation of mental status, cranial nerves, motor system, reflexes, and sensation. Experienced neurological clinicians commonly detect motor system abnormalities upon initially encountering the patient in the waiting room, including a masked face, stooped posture, tremor of the head, trunk or limbs, slowness in standing, and difficulty in beginning to walk. The patient's stance and gait may be wide based, and extrapyramidal disturbances, apraxia, and ataxia of gait can be seen as the patient walks forward or when attempting to turn. These disturbances can indicate disorders of cerebral cortical, basal ganglia, cerebellar, or posterior column function. Often evaluation of these disturbances as the patient moves from the waiting room to the examination room reveals disturbances that patients, aware that they are being scrutinized, are able to conceal during the formal neurological examination later. Scrutiny of the patient's cleanliness, dress, and mannerisms often discloses evidence of inattention to personal hygiene, neglect of personal and extrapersonal space, and subtle hemiparesis.

B. MENTAL STATUS

The mental status examination should include tests of level of consciousness, ability to concentrate, orientation, existing fund of information, registration of new information, short-term memory, long-term memory, calculations, language, praxis, judgment, and insight. The patient's level of consciousness should be characterized along a continuum from alert through drowsy, extending to stupor and coma. The ability to concentrate can be assessed from the patient's responses to each of the questions posed during the entire mental status examination and is best evaluated by the patient's ability to complete each task promptly without repeated explanations of the responses required. Tests of orientation include questions about the patient's name, age, and occupation, and identification of the year, season, date, day, and month, and the state, county, town, hospital, and floor. The patient's fund of information can be evaluated by asking for the names of the United States President, Vice-President, and the State Governor. Further inquiries should be made about current events and the significance of these events as assessed from current information in newspapers and other media sources such as television. These questions should be based upon the topics of the day. Typical questions concern the activities of the President, upcoming or immediately completed elections, and well-described conflicts in various parts of the world. Registration of information is assessed by giving the patient the names of three common objects (such as golf ball, sailboat, and automobile), naming each object one second apart, and asking the patient to repeat all three objects immediately. Details of the patient's difficulty in completing this task should be described. Short-term memory is tested by repeating the test of registration until the patient is able to name all three objects, then waiting 5 minutes and asking the patient again to name all three objects. If the patient cannot recall one or more of these items, clues to their identity should be provided (e.g., do you use one for a sport?) to determine whether the patient can recall the object with this intervention. Long-term memory can be evaluated by asking for the patient's birthday, date of marriage, date of military service if appropriate, and the dates of major events such as world wars and the dates of Christmas and other holidays. Testing the ability to calculate requires asking the patient to subtract 7 from 100 serially and to perform simple addition, subtraction, multiplication, and division. Language function should be evaluated by noting the patient's capacity to form full sentences, understand and follow three-step commands, identify right and left sides, name fingers correctly, read simple sentences, and write sentences. Difficulty in completing these tasks indicates that additional specific tests should be employed. Praxis is evaluated by assessing the patient's ability to draw and to copy diagrams of simple objects (a rectangle, square, cube, flower, clock face, and house). Difficulty with these functions requires assessment with additional tests of motor function. Judgment can be determined with the letter (what would you do if you found a stamped, addressed, sealed envelope on the street?) and fire (what would you do if you were in a crowded theater and you saw a fire?) tests. Other means of evaluating judgment and intellectual function include tests of similarity (how is a bicycle similar to an automobile?) and interpretation of proverbs (what is the meaning of the proverb, "people who live in glass houses should not throw stones"?).

Several quantitative tests of mental status function are available and can be used in the initial clinical evaluation. These include the Mini-Mental State Examination; Blessed Information, Memory, Concentration Test; Blessed Orientation, Memory, Concentration Test; Short Portable Mental Status Questionnaire; Mental Status Questionnaire; and Short Test of Mental Status.

C. CRANIAL NERVES

The cranial nerve examination should include special attention to visual acuity and fields, extraocular movements, facial mobility, disturbances of hearing, speech, and movements of the tongue, palate, and lips. Disturbances of cranial nerve function occur with normal aging.[24-27] Normal elderly persons often have sluggish pupillary responses, decreased smooth pursuit movements, and diminished saccadic frequency.[28,29] Medications for glaucoma lead to pupillary constriction and impair pupillary responses. Upward gaze can be limited in the normal elderly, but downward gaze should be intact.[30] Although taste and smell may be diminished in the normal elderly, decreased recognition of odors can be an early sign of both Alzheimer's disease and Parkinson's disease.[30] Facial immobility and hypokinetic speech can indicate extrapyramidal disorders and are common in Parkinson's disease, Alzheimer's disease with extrapyramidal symptoms, progressive supranuclear palsy, and multiple system atrophy. Spasticity of speech can be seen in disorders affecting cerebral cortical or cerebral white matter function bilaterally, including vascular diseases and neurodegenerative disorders such as olivopontocerebellar atrophy, multiple system atrophy, and amyotrophic lateral sclerosis. Ataxia of speech is common in olivopontocerebellar atrophy and in vascular and other types of pathology affecting the brainstem and cerebellum.

D. MOTOR SYSTEM

Evaluation of motor function should include descriptions of posture, gait, strength, resistance to passive manipulation of the limbs, and coordinated limb and trunk movements. Aging is often associated with osteoarthritis, which may alter posture and gait. Walking also can be slowed in the normal elderly, and difficulty with tandem walking can occur.[31] Nevertheless, a stooped position and shuffling with walking commonly occur in Parkinson's disease, Alzheimer's disease with extrapyramidal symptoms, progressive supranuclear palsy, and multiple system atrophy. Ataxia of gait can occur with cerebellar disorders and disturbances of peripheral nerve or dorsal column function. Apraxia of gait can indicate normal pressure hydrocephalus, frontal lobe degeneration of various types, and Alzheimer's disease. Muscle bulk and strength are commonly decreased in the elderly, but these changes should be general and not focal. Abnormalities of resistance to passive manipulation should not occur if the patient can relax the limbs fully. Tests of resistance to passive manipulation can reveal spasticity, indicating disturbances of corticospinal function, rigidity, suggesting extrapyramidal dysfunction, and hypotonia, which can be seen in disorders of cerebellar and sensory systems. Tests of coordination should be administered, including the finger-nose-finger, heel-knee-shin tests, and rapidly alternating movements of the hands and feet. These tests can reveal abnormalities of corticospinal, extrapyramidal, and cerebellar function.

E. REFLEXES

Examination of the reflexes should include the muscle stretch reflexes, certain cutaneous reflexes, and tests for primitive "release" reflexes. In the normal elderly, stretch reflexes can be difficult to detect, but should remain symmetrical, and the plantar responses should be flexor bilaterally. Some normal elderly can show glabellar and snout reflexes, but rooting and sucking reflexes usually indicate disorders of the cerebral cortex, primarily the frontal lobes. Similarly, grasp reflexes of the hands and feet can be detected in some normals, but commonly suggest disorders of frontal lobe function.[30]

F. SENSATION

Sensory testing in patients under evaluation for cognitive disorders should include evaluation of cold sensation, pinprick, position sense, and vibratory sense. Elderly persons commonly have reduced vibration sense in the toes and at times in the feet,[33] but this disorder should be bilateral, and cold, pinprick, light touch, and position sense should be preserved. Abnormalities of sensation suggest a neuropathy, myelopathy, or higher-level disorder and should trigger a full investigation as to cause.

V. FACTORS CONFOUNDING EVALUATION OF COGNITIVE FUNCTION

Assessment of cognitive function can be complicated by factors that interfere with patients' capacity to respond fully and appropriately to the examination. These include age, educational attainment, cultural background, psychiatric disorders, impairment of consciousness, sensory disorders, and physical disability. Both age and education influence performance on most mental status tests.[33] In recognition of the influence of age, norms that are age-specific have been developed for Mini-Mental State Examination.[34,35] Education is another important variable in test performance, and correlations have been found between Mini-Mental State Examination scores and years of education.[35] Low educational attainment can increase the likelihood of falsely positive tests,[36,37] and high education levels can introduce falsely negative scores.[38] Cultural background can affect performance on cognitive tests, particularly when language barriers are involved.[39] Social class and socioeconomic status can also influence performance on tests of mental status.[33]

Psychiatric disorders, particularly depression, can influence cognitive performance. Indeed, depression is often misidentified as dementia, and dementia can be mistaken for depression.[40] The possibility that a seemingly demented person might be depressed is important to consider, particularly since many people in the early stages of dementia are themselves depressed.[41] Depression presenting as dementia has been labeled "pseudodementia" and, more recently, "depression-related cognitive dysfunction".[42] Persons suspected of dementia should be evaluated for depression in both the medical history and in appropriate neuropsychological batteries. In addition to depression, many other psychiatric disorders can be mistaken for dementia, particularly psychotic paranoid states and schizophrenia.

Patients with disturbances of the state of consciousness, particularly delirium, can be mistakenly diagnosed as having dementia. Delirium is characterized by disturbances in attention, concentration, and consciousness, along with fluctuations in the intensity of cognitive dysfunction. Delirium results from a variety of disorders, including craniocerebral trauma, metabolic disturbances, dehydration with alterations in electrolyte levels and acid-base balance, and medication effects. Delirium can also occur in people with dementia. The sudden onset of delirium in a person with previously normal cognition or even preexistent dementia should trigger an urgent evaluation for the cause of the disorder.

As noted earlier, visual and auditory impairment can result in defective performance on mental status examinations.[43] Accordingly, correction of visual and auditory impairment prior to mental status testing is an important component of the evaluation. Physical impairments can adversely affect performance on tests requiring manual dexterity such as the Mini-Mental State Examination and require care in interpretation of the results. Alternately, tests can be utilized that do not require motor function except speech such as the Blessed Information, Memory, Concentration test.

VI. LABORATORY TESTS

A. INTRODUCTION

The clinical history, physical examination, and neurological examination provide important information indicating that the patient under evaluation may be at risk for cognitive disturbances secondary to fluid and electrolyte disorders, metabolic disturbances, and traumatic or medication-related etiologies. In addition, several blood tests along with a brain imaging examination should be made in screening for correctable causes of cognitive dysfunction.

B. SCREENING BLOOD AND URINE TESTS

A consensus conference sponsored by the National Institutes of Health recommended a battery of laboratory tests to screen for correctable causes of dementia.[44] These include a complete blood count, electrolyte panel, screening metabolic panel, thyroid function tests, levels of vitamin B_{12} and folate, tests for syphilis and, if suggested by the history, human immunodeficiency virus, urinalysis, electrocardiogram, and chest X-ray. Contradicting this view are two reports demonstrating that most of these studies are normal and suggesting that a more cost-effective panel of tests should be employed, limited to a complete blood count, thyroid function tests, and a metabolic panel.[45,46] The debate concerning the need for an extensive as opposed to a more focused screening evaluation has not been resolved, but clearly the initial history and examination conducted by an experienced clinician is the principal guide to the need for further laboratory studies. Currently we recommend following the battery recommended by the NIH Consensus Conference.[44] Although the frequency of detecting a reversible dementia is between 3 and 10% of large series of patients screened,[47,48] the need to detect patients whose cognitive disorder can be reversed cannot be overly emphasized.

C. BRAIN IMAGING

It is essential to include a brain imaging study in the evaluation of people with cognitive disorders, since this type of examination can demonstrate focal or generalized pathological changes responsible for these disorders, and the changes may not be detectable through the history and examination. The studies suitable for this evaluation include anatomical imaging with computed tomography (CT) and magnetic resonance (MR) and physiological (functional) imaging with positron emission tomography (PET) and single photon emission computed tomography (SPECT).

1. Anatomical Imaging

CT scans provide images of the brain that allow visualization of many focal and general neuropathological changes associated with cognitive disorders, including hemorrhage, infarction, tumor, and abscess.[49] CT scanning requires ionizing radiation with its attendant long-term hazards, but the dose is tolerable. In most hospitals CT scans can be performed quickly and relatively inexpensively. CT scans do not permit detection of recent infarction of the brain, and, although these scans are sensitive to recent subdural hematomas, they may fail to allow detection of bilateral chronic subdural hematomas. In addition, because of beam hardening artifacts, CT is less sensitive than MR for disorders affecting the posterior fossa.

MR imaging is the most sensitive brain imaging technique available to visualize recent infarction, small lacunar lesions, the plaques of multiple sclerosis, changes suggesting normal pressure hydrocephalus, and focal pathology in sites poorly visualized by CT, particularly the posterior fossa.[50] MR imaging presents the disadvantage of requiring placement of patients in a confined space, and a small percentage of patients cannot tolerate the examination because of claustrophobia. Inaccessibility of the patient during MR scanning also makes it difficult to use in distracted or demented people who cannot remain still. Thus far, no consensus has been achieved concerning the relative merits of CT and MR scanning in the evaluation of patients with cognitive disorders, but clearly one or the other should be used in the evaluation process.

D. FUNCTIONAL IMAGING

Information concerning brain function can be obtained through newer approaches to MR imaging and with pharmacological agents that serve as the source of radiation to produce a brain image. Currently utilized modalities are functional MRI, which currently allows visualization and measurement of cerebral blood flow, and radionuclide imaging with PET and SPECT. Functional imaging provides information that can be extremely helpful in differentiating among certain types of cognitive disorders. Although these studies are not used routinely, they are assuming increasing prominence because of their utility. PET studies of cerebral metabolism with [^{18}F]fluorodeoxyglucose have revealed hypometabolism in a characteristic distribution in Alzheimer's disease, with involvement predominantly in the posterior temporoparietal regions.[51] The pattern of hypometabolism is different in progressive supranuclear palsy than in Alzheimer's disease, involving in the former disorder chiefly the frontal cortex, basal ganglia, and brainstem, and, in Pick's disease, affecting principally the anterior portions of the frontal and temporal lobes.[51,52] In Huntington's disease the caudate nucleus and putamen are hypometabolic, and, in multiple system atrophy the cerebral cortex, basal ganglia and cerebellum are involved.[52] Regional cerebral blood flow can also be imaged, both with PET (utilizing [0^{15}]H$_2$0) and SPECT (with ^{99m}Tc-HMPAO, ^{123}I-IMP, ^{123}I-HIPDM, or ^{133}Xenon), and the distribution of changes in blood flow closely parallels that seen in studies of cerebral metabolism. Thus, the regions of the brain that are hypometabolic in Alzheimer's disease, progressive supranuclear palsy, Huntington's disease, olivopontocerebellar atrophy, and multiple system atrophy are also hypoperfused.[51-53] Both SPECT and PET studies of cerebral blood flow have proven helpful in differentiating between Alzheimer's disease, multiple infarct dementia, and normal aging.[51] Currently, a variety of ligands are under development that permit visualization of neurotransmitters and neurotransmitter receptors with PET. Among the substances under development are [^{18}F]fluorodopa and [^{11}C]dihydrotetrabenazine for examination of monoaminergic presynaptic terminals, [^{11}C]raclopride for D$_2$ dopaminergic neurotransmitter receptors, and [^{11}C]flumazenil for gamma-aminobutyric type A/benzodiazepine receptors.

VII. OTHER STUDIES

Several other investigations are indicated in the evaluation of selected patients with cognitive disorders, depending upon the results of the history and examination. Lumbar puncture is an important test when the history and examination suggest an infectious process such as bacterial, fungal, or viral meningitis or a neoplastic process such as carcinomatous meningitis. Studies are currently in process to determine whether cerebrospinal fluid immunoreactivity with a monoclonal antibody, Alz-50, might be helpful in the diagnosis of Alzheimer's disease.[54] Electroencephalography can be diagnostic in patients suspected of having Creutzfeldt-Jakob disease and seizure disorders. The finding that abnormalities in the EEG correlate with the severity of the dementia in

Alzheimer's disease[55] is interesting but does not justify the use of EEG in the regular evaluation of persons with cognitive disorder. Evoked potential studies have some promise of assisting in the diagnosis of early Alzheimer's disease, since changes in the P300 wave are associated with dementia.[56] The specificity and sensitivity of these changes, however, are inadequate to allow this test to be regarded as a definitive diagnostic tool. Roentgenograms of the skull are not helpful in the evaluation of cognitive disorders except after recent craniocerebral trauma, and cerebral arteriography is indicated only in patients with cognitive changes under evaluation for vasculitis or arteriosclerotic cerebrovascular disease.

REFERENCES

1. Lanska, D. J. and Schoenberg, B. S., The epidemiology of dementia: methodologic issues and approaches, in *Dementia*, Whitehouse, P. J., Ed., F. A. Davis, Philadelphia, 3, 1993.
2. Jorm, A. F. and Korten, A. E., Assessment of cognitive decline in the elderly by informant interview, *Br. J. Psychiatr.*, 152, 209, 1988.
3. van der Cammen, T. J. M., van Harskamp, F., Stronks, D. L., Passchier, J., and Schudel, W. J., Value of the Mini-Mental State Examination and informants' data for the detection of dementia in geriatric outpatients, *Psychol. Rep.*, 71, 1003, 1992.
4. Chaves, M. L. F. and Izquierdo, I., Differential diagnosis between dementia and depression: a study of efficiency increment, *Acta Neurol. Scand.*, 85, 378, 1992.
5. Henderson, A. S. and Huppert, F. A. The problem of mild dementia, *Psychol. Med.*, 14, 5, 1984.
6. LaRue, A., Watson, J., and Plotkin, D. A., Retrospective accounts of dementia symptoms: are they reliable?, *Gerontologist,* 32, 240, 1992.
7. Bayles, K. A. and Tomoeda, C. K., Caregiver report of prevalence and appearance order of linguistic symptoms in Alzheimer's patients, *Gerontologist,* 31, 210, 1991.
8. Grut, M., Jorm, A. F., Fratiglioni, L., Forsell, Y., Viitanen, M., and Winblad, B., Memory complaints of elderly people in a population survey: variation according to dementia stage and depression, *J. Am. Geriatr. Soc.*, 41, 1295, 1993.
9. Greene, M. G., Majerovitz, S. D., Adelman, R. D., and Rizzo, C., The effects of the presence of a third person on the physician-older patient medical interview, *J. Am. Geriatr. Soc.*, 42, 413, 1994.
10. Butler, R. N., Finkel, S. I., Lewis, M. I., Sherman, F. T., and Sunderland, T., Aging and mental health: diagnosis of dementia and depression, *Geriatrics*, 47, 49 and 55, 1992.
11. Breen, A. R., Larson, B., Reiffler, B. U., Vitaliano, P. P., and Lawrence, G. L., Cognitive performance and functional competence in co-existing dementia and depression, *J. Am. Geriatr. Soc.*, 32, 132, 1984.
12. Krishnan, K. R. R., Heyman, A., Ritchie, J. C., Utley, C. M., Dawson, D. V., and Rogers, H., Depression in early-onset Alzheimer's disease: clinical and neuroendocrine correlates, *Biol. Psychiatr.*, 24, 937, 1988.
13. Patterson, M. B., Schnell, A., Martin, R. J., Mendez, M. F., Smyth, K., and Whitehouse, P. J., Assessment of behavioral and affective symptoms in Alzheimer's disease, *J. Geriatr. Psychiatr. Neurol.*, 3, 21, 1990.
14. Morrison, R. and Katz, I. Drug-related cognitive impairment: current progress and recurrent problems, *Annu. Rev. Gerontol. Geriatr.*, 9, 233, 1989.
15. Bird, T. D., Lampe, T. H., Nemens, E. J., Miner, G. W., Sumi, S. M., and Schellenberg, G. D., Familial Alzheimer's disease in American descendents of the Volga Germans: probable genetic founder effect, *Ann. Neurol.*, 23, 25, 1988.
16. Bird, T. D., Sumi, S. M., Nemens, E. J., Nochlin, D., Schellenberg, G., Campe, T., Sadovnick, A., Chui, H., Miner, G. W., and Tinklenberg, J., Phenotypic heterogeneity in familial Alzheimer's disease: a study of 24 kindreds, *Ann. Neurol.*, 25, 12, 1989.
17. Foncin, J. F., Salmon, D., Supino-Viterbo, V., Feldman, R., Macchi, G., Mariotti, P., Scoppetta, C., Caruso, G., and Bruni, A. C., Démence présénile d'Alzheimer transmise dans une familie étendue, *Rev. Neurol.,* 141, 194, 1985.
18. Goudsmit, J., White, B. J., Weitkamp, L. R., Keats, B., Morrow, C., and Gajdusek, C., Familial Alzheimer's disease in two kindreds of the same geographic and ethnic origin, *J. Neurol. Sci.*, 49, 79, 1981.
19. Nee, L. E., Eldridge, R., Sunderland, T., Thomas, C. B., Katz, D., Thompson, K.I., Weingartner, H., Weiss, H., Julian, C., and Cohen, R., Dementia of the Alzheimer's type: clinical and family study of 22 twin pairs, *Neurology,* 37, 359, 1987.
20. St. George-Hyslop, P. H., Tanzi, R. E., Polinsky, R. J., Haines, J. L., Nee, L., Watkins, P. C., Myers, R. H., Feldman, R. H., Pollen, D., and Drachman, D., The genetic defect causing familial Alzheimer's disease maps on chromosome 21, *Science*, 235, 885, 1987.
21. Breitner, J. C. S., Silverman, J. M., Mohs, R. C., and Davis, K. L., Familial aggregation in Alzheimer's disease: comparison of risk among relatives of early- and late-onset cases, and among male and female relatives in successive generations, *Neurology,* 38, 207, 1988.

22. Mohs, R. C., Breitner, J. C. S., Silverman, J. M., and Davis, K. L., Alzheimer's disease: morbid risk among first degree relatives approximates 50% by 90 years of age, *Arch. Gen. Psychiatr.*, 44, 405, 1987.

23. Corder, E. H., Saunders, A. M., Strittmater, W. J., Schmechel, D. E., Gaskell, P. C., Small, G. W., Roses, A. D., and Pericak-Vance, M. A., Gene dose of apolipoprotein E type 4 allele and the risk of Alzheimer's disease in late onset families, *Science,* 261, 921, 1993.

24. Baloh, R. W., Neurotology of aging: vestibular system, in *Clinical Neurology of Aging*, Albert, M. L., Ed., Oxford University Press, New York, 1984, 345.

25. Cohen, M. M. and Lessell, S., Neuro-ophthalmology of aging, in *Clinical Neurology of Aging*, Albert, M. L., Ed., Oxford University Press, New York, 1984, 313.

26. Hayes, D. and Jerger, J., Neurotology of aging: auditory system, in *Clinical Neurology of Aging*, Albert, M. L., Ed., Oxford University Press, New York, 1984, 362.

27. Pizzarello, C. D., The dimensions of the problem of eye disease among the elderly, *Ophthalmology*, 94, 1191, 1987.

28. Fletcher, W. A. and Sharpe, J. A., Saccadic eye movement dysfunction in Alzheimer's disease, *Ann. Neurol.*, 20, 464, 1986.

29. Lawton, M. P. and Brody, E. M., Assessment of older people: self-maintaining and instrumental activities of daily living, *Gerontologist*, 9, 179, 1969.

30. Mayeux, R., Foster, N. L., Rossor, M., and Whitehouse, P. J., The clinical evaluation of patients with dementia, in *Dementia*, Whitehouse, P. J., Ed., F.A. Davis, Philadelphia, 1993, 92.

31. Wolfson, L. I. and Katzman, R., The neurologic consultation at age 80, in *The Neurology of Aging*, Katzman, R. and Terry, R. D., Eds., F. A. Davis, Philadelphia, 1983, 221.

32. Schaumberg, H. H., Spencer, P. S., and Ochoa, J., The aging human peripheral nervous system, in *The Neurology of Aging*, Katzman, R. and Terry, R. D., Eds., F. A. Davis, Philadelphia, 1983, 111.

33. Tombaugh, T. N., and McIntyre, N. J., The Mini-Mental State Examination: a comprehensive review, *J. Am. Geriatr. Soc.*, 40, 922, 1992.

34. Bleeker, M. L., Bolla-Wilson, K., Kawas, C., and Agnew, J., Age-specific norms for the Mini-Mental State Exam, *Neurology*, 38, 1565, 1988.

35. Crum, R. M., Anthony, J. C., Bassett, S. S., and Folstein, M. F., Population-based norms for the Mini-Mental State Examination by age and educational level, JAMA, 269, 2386, 1993.

36. Anthony, J. C., LaResche, L., Niaz, U., Korff, M. R., and Folstein, M. F., Limits of the "Mini-Mental State" as a screening test for dementia and delirium among hospital patients, *Psychol. Med.*, 12, 397, 1982.

37. Murden, R. A., McRae, T. D., Kaner, S., and Buckman, M., Mini-Mental State Exam scores vary with education in blacks and whites, *J. Amer. Geriatr. Soc.*, 39, 149, 1991.

38. O'Connor, D. W., Pollitt, P. A., Hyde, J. B., Fellows, J. L., Miller, N. D., Brook, C. P. B., and Russ, B., The reliability and validity of the Mini-Mental State in a British community survey, *J. Psychiatr. Res.*, 23, 87, 1989.

39. Loewenstein, D. A., Arguelles, T., Barker, W. W., and Duara, R., A comparative analysis of neuropsychological test performance of Spanish-speaking and English-speaking patients with Alzheimer's disease, J. Gerontol., 48, 142, 1993.

40. Office of Medical Applications of Research, NIH Consensus Development Panel on Depression in Late Life, Diagnosis and treatment of depression in late life, *JAMA*, 268, 1018, 1992.

41. Reding, M., Haycox, J., and Blass, J., Depression in patients referred to a dementia clinic: a three-year prospective study, *Arch. Neurol.*, 42, 894, 1985.

42. Stoudemire, A., Hill, C., Gulley, L. R., and Morris, R., Neuropsychological and biomedical assessment of depression-dementia syndromes, *J. Neuropsychiatr. Clin. Neurosci.*, 1, 347, 1989.

43. Peters, C. A., Potter, J. F., and Scholer, S. G., Hearing impairment as a predictor of cognitive decline in dementia, *J. Am. Geriatr. Soc.*, 36, 981, 1988.

44. Office of Medical Applications of Research, Consensus Conference on Dementia, National Institutes of Health, Differential diagnosis of dementing diseases, *JAMA*, 258, 3411, 1987.

45. Larson, E. B., Reifler, B. V., Sumi, S. M., Canfield, C. G., and Chinn, N. M., Diagnostic tests in the evaluation of dementia: a prospective study of 200 elderly outpatients, *Arch. Intern. Med.*, 146, 1917, 1986.

46. Lindenbaum, J., Healton, E. B., Savage, D. G., Brust, J., Garrett, T., Podell, E., Marcell, P., Stabler, S., and Allen, R., Neuropsychiatric disorders caused by cobalamin deficiency in the absence of anemia of macrocytosis, *N. Engl. J. Med.*, 318, 1720, 1988.

47. Barry, P. P. and Moskowitz, M. A., The diagnosis of reversible dementia in the elderly: a critical review, *Arch. Intern. Med.*, 148, 1914, 1988.

48. McIntyre, L. and Frank, J., Evaluation of the demented patient, *J. Fam. Pract.*, 24, 399, 1987.

49. Gibby, W. A. and Zimmerman, R. A., X-ray computed tomography, in *Clinical Brain Imaging: Principles and Applications*, Mazziotta, J. C. and Gilman, S., Eds., F. A. Davis, Philadelphia, 1992, p. 2.

50. Lufkin, R.B., Magnetic resonance imaging, in *Clinical Brain Imaging: Principles and Applications*, Mazziotta, J. C. and Gilman, S., Eds., F. A. Davis, Philadelphia, 1992, 39.

51. Duara, R., Dementia, in *Clinical Brain Imaging: Principles and Applications*, Mazziotta, J. C. and Gilman, S., Eds., F. A. Davis, Philadelphia, 1992, 300.

52. Mazziotta, J. C., Movement disorders, in *Clinical Brain Imaging: Principles and Applications*, Mazziotta, J. C. and Gilman, S., Eds., F. A. Davis, Philadelphia, 1992, 244.

53. Gilman, S. and Gebarski S. S., Cerebellar disorders, in *Clinical Brain Imaging: Principles and Applications*, Mazziotta, J. C. and Gilman, S., Eds., F. A. Davis, Philadelphia, 1992, 370.

54. Wolozin, B. L. and Davies, P., Alzheimer-related neuronal protein A68: specificity and distribution, *Ann. Neurol.*, 22, 521, 1987.

55. Helkala, E. L., Laulumaa, V., Soininen, H., Partenen, J., and Riekkinen, P. J., Different patterns of cognitive decline related to normal or deteriorating EEG in 3-year follow-up study of patients with Alzheimer's disease, *Neurology*, 41, 528, 1991.

56. Patterson, J. V., Michalewski, H. J., and Starr, A., Latency variability of the components of auditory event-related potentials to infrequent stimuli in aging, Alzheimer-type dementia, and depression, *Electroencephalogr. Clin. Neurophysiol.*, 71, 450, 1988.

Chapter **9**

THE USE OF TESTS AND INSTRUMENTS IN THE EVALUATION OF PATIENTS WITH DEMENTIA

Richard C. Mohs

CONTENTS

0-8493-8997-6/97/$0.00+$.50

I. ROLE OF TESTING IN DIAGNOSIS

This section is concerned with the use of structured neuropsychological and behavioral tests in the diagnosis and evaluation of persons who may have a dementing illness. As described in previous sections dementia is defined as a clinical syndrome in which the patient has deficits in more than one cognitive domain, usually including memory loss, and those deficits must be great enough to have produced some impairment in that patient's ability to function in everyday life.[1,2] The evaluation of a person with suspected dementia usually includes a clinical history, physical, and neurological examination, and often, the use of biochemical screening tests and a brain imaging study. In most cases it will also include one or more neuropsychological tests in which the patient is asked to perform highly structured tasks. The tasks are designed so that they place significant demands on the patient's memory, attention, language, judgment, control of movement, and other cognitive abilities that are impaired by brain disease. There are several reasons why such tests are given. Most important is that for the vast majority of dementing conditions, including Alzheimer's disease (AD), there is no laboratory test that directly measures the degree of brain impairment. The presence of brain impairment must be inferred from the fact that the patient is no longer able to do some of the things that he could do previously. Evidence of impaired cognitive functioning may not be evident from casual observation of the patient. For example, a patient's loss of language function may only be noticable when the patient is asked to use words that are relatively rare, or the patient's loss of movement control may be noticeable only when asked to reproduce a drawing of a complex geometric shape. Structured neuropsychological testing ensures that the patient has been observed while trying to use the cognitive abilities that are most often impaired by dementing illnesses.

Another reason to use a standard testing procedure is that it is often difficult to tell whether a patient's current cognitive ability is less than it was previously or less than it should be given the patient's age and educational background. Most structured neuropsychological tests have been given to many different people in a standardized way so that normative data for specific groups defined by age, educational background, and disease state are available. These data tell how other persons of a certain age, educational background, and disease state usually perform on those tests, and allow comparison of the new patient's results with appropriate norms.

A. TESTING IN CLINICAL PRACTICE

In clinical practice neuropsychological testing is useful when there is some reason to believe that a patient is having some problems with cognition. The patient may present with a complaint of a problem with memory or of an episode of confusion. In other cases a family member may report that the patient seems to be having difficulty with memory or has made errors in judgment or problem solving that seem out of line with previous ability. In either case a more detailed examination of the patient, including a neuropsychological examination, is warranted. The main purpose of the neuropsychological examination in these cases is to help determine whether or not the patient's current level of cognitive performance is sufficiently poor to suggest that the patient has a dementing illness. For this purpose even a very brief mental status examination such as the Mini-Mental State Exam (MMSE)[3] may be helpful, although more detailed and challenging examinations will provide a more precise picture of which aspects of the patient's cognitive functioning are preserved and which are spared. Several studies have now demonstrated that neuropsychological tests are quite sensitive for distinguishing mildly demented patients from nondemented persons of the same age, education, and racial background.[4,5]

If it is determined that the patient is impaired in one or more cognitive areas it is also important to determine the type of dementing illness. In trying to discern the most likely cause for the patient's cognitive difficulties, the clinician will again use a variety of information including clinical history, physical, neurologic, and psychiatric exams, laboratory test results, and possibly brain imaging studies. In a few instances one or more of these pieces of information will point to a specific cause for the dementia such as a tumor or stroke. However, for most of the common dementias, including AD, the cause is inferred based on the fact that all information is consistent with a certain diagnosis. Neuropsychological test results should be examined to determine the extent to which they are consistent with the pattern of impairment observed in patients with AD.

Neuropsychological tests are also useful for keeping track of changes in a patient's cognitive status over time. It is well established that cognitive function in AD patients worsens over time and data are available on the usual rate at which scores on several neuropsychological tests deteriorate in AD patients.[6,7] For some patients and their families it may be of value to know whether the patient's cognitive changes are faster, slower, or the same as the typical patient. If a patient presents with very mild cognitive impairment, it may be difficult to determine whether that patient has AD or if the symptoms are simply a reflection of age-related changes that will not progress. For those patients a follow-up neuropsychological examination in 6 to 12 months will often help to determine which possibility is correct.[8] Finally, if a patient is placed on a medication either to treat the dementia itself or to treat a comorbid condition such as depression, neuropsychological tests are useful for measuring the effect of that medication on cognitive function.[6]

B. TESTING IN COMMUNITY SCREENING PROGRAMS

Neuropsychological tests are also of some value in screening persons in the community who have not yet been brought to medical attention. The prevalence of undiagnosed AD in the community is not precisely known, but some studies suggest that it is quite high, particularly in persons over age 75.[9,10] Other studies have shown that elderly persons who show slightly impaired performance on mental status screening tests are more likely to progress to frank dementia in the near future than are elderly persons who perform very well on such screening tests.[8,11] Tests used for community screening studies are very brief in an effort to minimize the amount of time required to screen each person. Most commonly used are the Mini-Mental State Examination,[3] the test of Blessed and colleagues,[12,13] or some brief memory assessment.[10] These tests do not enable a diagnosis of AD or other dementing condition to be made. Poor scores on one of these tests simply indicates that a person has a higher probability of being demented than does a person who scores in the normal range and, therefore, that the person with the low score may need a more complete clinical evaluation. No matter what cut-off score one uses on these tests there will be both false positives (i.e., people who have a low score but are not actually demented) and false negatives (i.e., people who do not score below the cut-off score on the test but who do have a dementing illness) and the proportion of each will depend upon the cut-off score that is picked.[14]

Up to the present time these brief screening tests have been used primarily as an aid in epidemiological studies where the purpose is to get a count of the number of AD cases that is as accurate as possible. Screening programs designed to refer cases for treatment have not been instituted because the treatments available for patients with AD are only modestly effective in improving some symptoms and are not effective in modifying disease course. When treatments are available that are more effective and safer, it is likely that community screening programs with referral to clinical diagnostic and treatment centers will be quite valuable. Such programs would target people who, because of their age or relationship to an AD patient, are at increased risk of developing AD. Brief neuropsychological screening tests would play an important role in the process of deciding which persons to refer for more thorough evaluation and, possibly, for treatment.

II. WHAT TESTS SHOULD BE GIVEN?

A. COGNITIVE DOMAINS TO BE EVALUATED

Clinical descriptions of patients with AD and studies using structured neuropsychological tests have documented in some detail the areas of cognitive function that are impaired in these patients. Memory should be tested both by asking the patient to learn something new like a list of words and by asking the patient to recall previously learned information such as the names of the current and past presidents. It is also important to assess the patient's ability to remember new information such as the list of words after a delay of several minutes.[4,5] Acquisition and recall after a delay are thought to depend upon structures in the medial temporal regions of the brain including the hippocampus that are impaired early in the course of AD. Orientation, an ability heavily dependent upon memory, is tested by asking the patient questions about where he is (orientation to place), the current date and time (orientation to time), and about himself (orientation to person). Language should be tested by evaluating both expressive and receptive aspects. Expressive speech can be assessed by asking the patient to name specific objects, repeat a phrase such as "No ifs, ands or buts" and by asking the patient to use certain words in a sentence. Receptive language can be assessed by having the patient follow commands given verbally or in writing (e.g., "Point to the ceiling and then to the floor."). Praxis, the ability to perform learned motor activities at will, can be tested in several ways. In early AD there may be little impairment in praxis except in the ability to reproduce geometric drawings, a skill referred to as constructional praxis. Tests of constructional praxis usually require the patient to draw complex figures such as a clock face[15] or a three-dimensional cube.[16] Apraxia may be evident in everyday activities later in the disease when the patient will be unable even to organize the movements required for dressing or grooming.

Some tests of attention and concentration should also be included in the evaluation of patients with suspected dementia although standardization of these tests is difficult. Attention can be assessed by having the patient concentrate on some mental activity such as doing calculations or spelling a word backwards. Concentration over longer periods of time is difficult to assess simply, but can be measured to some extent by having patients do timed tests such as Trailmaking.[17]

B. COMMONLY USED TESTS

Tests for the evaluation of patients with AD can be grouped according to their length and the detail with which they probe different cognitive domains. Brief screening tests are those which can be administered in 10 to 15 minutes or less. Tests in this group include the Mini-Mental State Exam (MMSE),[3] which includes items to assess verbal memory, orientation, language, constructional praxis, and attention. The test is scored from 0, indicating severe impairment, to 30 if the patient makes no errors. Patients with AD generally score 26 or less although performance is clearly influenced by age and education as well as disease state.[14] Another widely used screening test is the Short Blessed Test,[12,13] which is even briefer than the MMSE. It includes items to assess memory, orientation, and concentration, but does not have specific probes for language or praxis impairment. Scores on the Short Blessed range from 0, for a subject who makes no errors, to 28; AD patients usually score 6 or more. Other brief screening tests such as the Mental Status Questionnaire[18] and the Short Portable Mental Status Questionnaire[19] have items that overlap to a large extent with the MMSE and the Short Blessed Test.

Longer instruments for use in clinical settings usually cover the same cognitive domains but in greater detail. One very useful battery which takes approximately 45 to 50 minutes to administer was developed by the Consortium to Establish a Registry for Alzheimer's Disease (CERAD), a group composed of investigators from AD research programs in the United States funded by the U.S. National Institute on Aging.[20] The CERAD battery contains tests of verbal memory, including immediate and delayed recall, language tests of naming and verbal fluency, drawings to test constructional praxis, as well as the MMSE. Recently, the CERAD battery has been supplemented with a brief measure of verbal intelligence, a portion of the Trailmaking test to assess psychomotor speed and concentration and additional verbal memory tests with delay for detecting very mild dementia.

Another widely used test which can be administered in about 30 to 40 minutes is the Alzheimer's Disease Assessment Scale (ADAS).[16] Some of the items included in the ADAS, which also assesses memory, language, praxis, orientation, and attention, are similar to items in the CERAD battery. The ADAS is slightly shorter, however, and also includes a set of clinician-rated items to assess the severity of noncognitive disturbances such as agitation, psychosis, and depressed mood. Because the ADAS was designed as an outcome measure for drug treatment trials, it provides specific rules for calculating overall severity scores for both cognitive and noncognitive symptoms. Both the CERAD battery and the ADAS are more comprehensive than the brief screening tests, particularly in their assessment of memory functions. Other instruments designed to evaluate the cognitive symptoms of dementia include the Mattis Dementia Rating Scale (DRS)[21] and the Syndrome Kurtztest (SKT).[22] Fewer normative data are available on these tests, but they clearly have face validity in that they test many of the appropriate cognitive domains. The SKT is the only one of the tests that is timed and therefore places heavy demands on concentration and attention; it is probably not appropriate for evaluating moderate to severely demented patients.

C. DESIRABLE TEST CHARACTERISTICS
1. Reliability
Neuropsychological test results can be more or less useful depending upon the question that is being asked and the characteristics of the test itself. Several tests have been shown to be useful in evaluating patients with suspected AD, but clinicians will probably use only one or two tests with which they are quite familiar. To compare a patient's score with published normative data or to assess change over time accurately requires that the test have a high degree of reliability. Many of the tests used most commonly to evaluate patients with AD, including the tests described above, have been shown to have a high degree of inter-rater and test-retest reliability. Assuming that these tests are given according to the published instructions, it should be possible to compare a patient's data with published norms and to conclude that measured changes over time actually reflect changes in the patient's cognitive state.

2. Validity
a. Content
Validity of any neuropsychological test refers to the ability of that test to measure what it is supposed to measure. For tests used to evaluate patients with AD, validity can be assessed by examining the content of the test and, more importantly, by examining the data obtained when relevant patient groups are tested. The content of all of the tests described in this chapter are appropriate for evaluating patients with AD since they are all selected to assess deficits in areas such as memory, language, and attention that are clearly impaired in AD. It is worth noting that many tests of intellectual function are not particularly useful for evaluating patients with dementia. Intelligence tests, aptitude tests, and neuropsychological batteries developed to identify localized brain damage are usually not appropriate for evaluating patients with suspected dementia because poor scores on these tests probably do not indicate deficits in the areas the tests were designed to assess. For many of these tests the instructions to the subjects are quite complex and would be difficult for a patient with dementia to follow because of their memory and language difficulties. As an example, patients with AD often perform poorly on IQ tests, not because they have low intelligence, but simply because they cannot comprehend or remember the instructions for many components of an IQ test.

b. Distinguishing AD from Age-Related Memory Loss
Normative data from nondemented persons are available for several of the widely used tests, including the MMSE, the CERAD battery, the ADAS, and the Blessed Test. Normative data from population studies are most comprehensive for the MMSE, and these include norms indicating how scores are affected by age and eduction.[14] Substantial normative data are also available for the CERAD battery. These data indicate that performance in nondemented persons is most influenced by education, with less-educated persons scoring lower on the CERAD measures of language and praxis but not on the memory tests.[23] There are also small but significant race differences in performance on the CERAD language and praxis measures with African Americans scoring slightly

lower than age and education-matched Caucasian Americans.[24] These normative data are particularly important if test scores are used to distinguish patients with early AD from elderly persons who have benign age-related memory problems. A test for which the effects of age and education are not known will be less useful in early diagnosis.

Several studies have demonstrated that the most prominent difference between early AD and age-related memory loss is a deficit in acquisition[5] and recall after a delay[4] of information such as a list of words. This deficit is demonstrated most clearly on the more-detailed assessments such as the CERAD battery,[4] but is evident even on the brief screening instruments such as the MMSE[25] and the Short Blessed Test.[11] The reason for this deficit is probably that early AD is associated with neuropathologic change in the medial temporal regions of the brain necessary for forming permanent memory traces. Speeded performance on complex psychomotor tests such as Trailmaking is also impaired relatively early in AD.[26] The reason for this impairment is not obvious, although these tests do place heavy demands on attention and working memory, that part of the memory system used to hold information temporarily while it is in consciousness.

c. Distinguishing Among the Dementias

The two kinds of dementing conditions which are most often confused with uncomplicated AD are vascular dementia and dementia associated with Parkinsonian changes. While pure, uncomplicated cases of each type of dementia can be identified, there is often overlap between AD and vascular and between AD and Parkinsonian dementia. Autopsy studies often find that AD patients have some vascular or Parkinsonian changes in brain.[27] The extent to which these vascular and Parkinsonian changes affect the clinical and neuropsychological presentation of AD patients is not known precisely. Clinical descriptions indicate that patients with uncomplicated AD, vascular dementia, and mixed dementia usually present with the same types of cognitive and behavioral impairments.[28] Furthermore, Parkinsonian patients who develop a progressive dementia have problems with memory, language, praxis, orientation, and attention, just as patients with uncomplicated AD do.[29] Few studies have tried to compare the neuropsychological profiles of patients with AD, vascular, and Parkinsonian dementia. None of the widely used dementia assessment batteries has been shown to distinguish these patient groups.

Nevertheless, there are probably some neuropsychological differences on average between uncomplicated AD and the other common dementias. Both vascular and Parkinsonian dementia are thought to have more prominent subcortical components than does uncomplicated AD. Subcortical dementias are usually associated with deficits in attention, attention switching, planning, and categorization that are more prominent than they are in uncomplicated AD.[29] Deficits of this type have been shown in both vascular[30] and Parkinsonian[29] dementia. A noticeable slowing of cognitive performance is also present in most Parkinsonian dementias.[29] These differences from AD are, however, a matter of degree and the overlap of neuropsychologic test scores between conditions is substantial. Distinguishing among the common dementias can be difficult and neuropsychologic test scores probably contribute only a modest amount to the information provided by the other aspects of the clinical evaluation.

Occasionally, neuropsychologic testing will show a pattern of deficits that is markedly different from that typically seen in AD or in one of the other common dementias. In such cases it is prudent to scrutinize the clinical and laboratory data carefully to determine whether the patient has one of the rarer types of dementia such as Pick's disease, Creutzfeld-Jacob disease, or Progressive Supranuclear Palsy.

d. Measuring Change

Sometimes it is important to have an accurate assessment of the direction and magnitude of change in a patient's cognitive state. Knowing the rate of deterioration may help a family plan for future caregiving needs. If a patient is being treated it is helpful to have an objective assessment of change in mental status. All of the commonly used dementia assessment instruments have been shown in longitudinal studies to measure change in clinical state reliably. It is known, for example, that AD patients deteriorate approximately two to three points per year on the MMSE.[31] More detailed batteries such as the ADAS show larger annual changes.[32] Both the MMSE and the ADAS are scored so that a single score represents the severity of cognitive impairment. This enables change to be expressed as a simple point difference and it is not necessary to look at each cognitive domain separately. For both the MMSE[31] and the ADAS[32] the expected rate of deterioration in untreated patients is slower for mildly demented patients than it is for more severely demented patients. This suggests that symptoms can be expected to worsen quickly after patients move through an early disease phase when symptoms worsen at a slow rate. The rate of cognitive deterioration does not seem to depend upon the patient's gender, age, family history, or type of residence.[31-33]

III. CONCLUSIONS

The pattern of neuropsychological deficits associated with AD is well known, and neuropsychological tests are quite useful in helping to distinguish early AD from benign age-related memory loss. A baseline evaluation of memory, language, attention, and praxis will also provide information to assess objectively any change in the patient's clinical state. If a patient's pattern of neuropsychological deficits is markedly different from that found in the typical AD patient, then another cause for the dementia should be suspected.

REFERENCES

1. American Psychiatric Association, *Diagnostic and Statistical Manual of Mental Disorders*, 4th ed., American Psychiatric Association, Washington, DC, 1994.
2. McKhann, G., Drachman, D. A., Folstein, M., Katzman, R., Price, D., and Stadlan, E. M., Clinical diagnosis of Alzheimer's disease: Report of the NINCDS-ADRDA Work Group under the auspices of Department of Health and Human Services Task Force on Alzheimer's Disease, *Neurology*, 34, 939, 1984.
3. Folstein, M. F., Folstein, S. E., and McHugh, P. R., Mini-Mental State: a practical method for grading the cognitive state of patients for the clinician, *J. Psychiatr. Res.*, 12, 189, 1975.
4. Welsh, K. A., Butters, N., Hughes, J., Mohs, R. C., and Heyman, A., Detection of abnormal memory decline in mild cases of Alzheimer's disease using CERAD neuropsychological measures, *Arch. Neurol.*, 48, 278, 1991.
5. Petersen, R. C., Smith, G. E., Ivnik, R. J., Kokmen, E., and Tangalos, E. G., Memory function in very early Alzheimer's disease, *Neurology*, 44, 867, 1994.
6. Mohs, R. C., Neuropsychological assessment of patients with Alzheimer's disease in *Psychopharmacology: The Fourth Generation of Progress*, Bloom, F. E. and Kupfer, D. J., Eds., Raven Press, New York, 1995, chap. 117.
7. Galasko, D., Corey-Bloom, J., and Thal, L. J., Monitoring progression in Alzheimer's disease, *J. Am. Geriatr. Soc.*, 39, 932, 1991.
8. Masur, D. M., Sliwinski, M., Lipton, R. B., Blau, A. D., and Crystal, H. A., Neuropsychological prediction of dementia and the absence of dementia in healthy elderly persons, *Neurology*, 44, 1427, 1994.
9. Evans, D. A., Funkenstein, H., Albert, M. S., Scherr, P. A., Cook, N. R., Chown, M. J., Hebert, L. E., Hennekens, C. H., and Taylor, J. O., Prevalence of Alzheimer's disease in a community population of older persons, *JAMA*, 262, 2551, 1989.
10. Skoog, I., Nilsson, L., Palmertz, B., Andreasson, L.-A., and Svanborg, A. A population-based study of dementia in 85-year-olds, *N. Engl. J. Med.*, 328, 153, 1993.
11. Katzman, R., Aronson, M. K., Fuld, P., Kawas, C., Brown, T., Morgenstern, H., Frishman, W., Gidez, L., Eder, H., and Ooi, W. L., Development of dementing illness in an 80-year-old volunteer cohort, *Ann. Neurol.*, 25, 317, 1989.
12. Blessed, G., Tomllinson, B. E., and Roth, M., The association of quantitative measures of dementia and of senile change in the cerebral grey matter of elderly subjects, *Br. J. Psychiat.*, 114, 797, 1968.
13. Katzman, R., Brown, T., Fuld, P., et al. Validation of a short orientation-memory-concentration test of cognitive impairment, *Am. J. Psychiat.*, 140, 734, 1983.
14. Folstein, M., Anthony, J. C., Parhad, I., Duffy, B., and Gruenberg, E. M., The meaning of cognitive impairment in the elderly. *J. Am. Geriatar. Soc.*, 33, 228, 1985.
15. Sunderland, T., Hill, J. L., Mellow, A. M., Lawlor, B. A., Gundersheimer, J., Newhouse, P. A., and Grafman, J. H., Clock drawing in Alzheimer's disease: a novel measure of dementia severity, *J. Am. Geriatr. Soc.*, 37, 725, 1989.
16. Rosen, W. G., Mohs, R. C., and Davis, K. L., A new rating scale for Alzheimer's disease, *Am. J. Psychiatr.*, 141, 1356, 1984.

17. Reitan, R. M., Validity of the Trail Making Test as an indicator of organic brain damage, *Percep. Motor Skills*, 8, 271, 1958.

18. Kahn, R. L., Goldfarb, A. I., Pollack, M., et al., Brief objective measures for the determination of mental status in the aged, *Am. J. Psychiat.*, 117, 326, 1960.

19. Pfeiffer, E., A Short Portable Mental Status Questionnaire for the assessment of organic brain deficit in elderly patients, *J. Am. Geriatr. Soc.*, 23, 433, 1975.

20. Morris, J. C., Heyman, A., Mohs, R. C., Hughes, J., van Belle, G., Fillenbaum, G., Mellits, E. D., Clark, C., and the CERAD investigators, The Consortium to Establish a Registry for Alzheimer's Disease (CERAD). I. Clinical and neuropsychological assessment of patients with Alzheimer's disease, *Neurology*, 39, 1159, 1989.

21. Coblentz, J. M., Mattis, S., Zingesser, L. H., Kasoff, S. S., Wisniewski, H. M., and Katzman, R., Presenile dementia: clinical aspects and evaluation of cerebrospinal fluid dynamics, *Arch. Neurol.*, 29, 299, 1973.

22. Erzigkeit, H., The SKT — a short cognitive performance test as an instrument for the assessment of clinical efficacy of cognitive enhancers, in *Diagnosis and Treatment of Senile Dementia*, Bergener, W. and Riesberg, B., Eds., Springer-Verlag, Heidelberg, 1989, 164.

23. Welsh, K. A., Butters, N., Mohs, R. C., Beekly, D., Edland, S., Fillenbaum, G., and Heyman, A., The Consortium to Establish a Registry for Alzheimer's Disease (CERAD). V. A normative study of the neuropsychological battery, *Neurology*, 44, 609, 1994.

24. Welsh, K. A., Fillenbaum, G., Wilkinson, W., Heyman, A., Mohs, R. C., Stern, Y., Harrell, L., Edland, S., and Beekly, D. S. Neuropsychological performance of African-American and White patients with Alzheimer's disease, *Neurology*, 45, 2207, 1995.

25. Fillenbaum, G. G., Wilkinson, W. E., Welsh, K. A., and Mohs, R. C., Discrimination between stages of Alzheimer's disease with subsets of Mini-Mental-State items: an analysis of CERAD data, *Arch. Neurol.*, 51, 916, 1994.

26. Storandt, M. and Hill, R. D., Very mild senile dementia of the Alzheimer type: psychometric test performance, *Arch. Neurol.*, 46, 383, 1989.

27. Mirra, S. S., Heyman, A., McKeel, D., Sumi, S. M., Crain, B. J., Brownlee, L. M., Vogel, F. S., Hughes, J. P., van Belle, G., Berg, L., and participating CERAD neuropathologists. The Consortium to Establish a Registry for Alzheimer's Disease (CERAD). II. Standardization of the neuropathologic assessment of Alzheimer's disease, *Neurology*, 41, 479, 1991.

28. Thal, L. J., Grundman, M., and Klauber, M. R., Dementia: characteristics of a referral population and factors associated with progression, *Neurology*, 38, 1083, 1988.

29. Huber, S. J. and Shuttleworth, E. C., Neuropsychological assessment of subcortical dementia, in *Subcortical Dementia*, Cummings, J. L., Ed., Oxford, University Press, New York, 1990, 71.

30. Kertesz, A. and Clydesdalle, S., Neuropsychological deficits in vascular dementia vs Alzheimer's disease, *Arch. Neurol.*, 51, 1226, 1994.

31. Morris, J. C., Edland, S., Clark, C., Galasko, D., Koss, E., Mohs, R., van Belle, G., Fillenbaum, G., and Heyman, A., The Consortium to Establish a Registry for Alzheimer's Disease (CERAD). IV. Rates of cognitive change in the longitudinal assessment of probable Alzheimer's disease *Neurology*, 34, 2457, 1993.

32. Stern, R. G., Mohs, R. C., Davidson, M., Schmeidler, J., Silverman, J. M., Kramer-Ginzberg, E., Searcey, T., Bierer, L. M., and Davis, K. L., A longitudinal study of Alzheimer's disease: measurement, rate, and predictors of cognitive deterioration. *Am. J. Psychiat.*, 151, 390, 1994.

33. Katzman, R., Brown, T., Thal, L. J., Fuld, P. A., Aronson, M., Butters, N., Klauber, M. R., Wiederholt, W., Ray, M., Renbing, X., Ooi, W. L., Hofstetter, R., and Terry, R. D., Comparison of rate of annual change of mental status score in four independent studies of patients with Alzheimer's disease, *Ann. Neurol.*, 24, 384, 1988.

Chapter 10

HETEROGENEITY OF ALZHEIMER'S DISEASE

_____ Albert Heyman

CONTENTS

I. INTRODUCTION

In the past decade, a number of studies have suggested that Alzheimer's disease (AD) does not consist of a single disorder but may comprise several different subtypes.[1] In most of these studies, the basis for subtyping is the presence of specific clinical features that appear to be associated with either a more rapid rate of progression of the dementing process or differences in the neuropathologic findings. It has been suggested, for example, that patients with AD who show prominent signs of extrapyramidal dysfunction, those with overt psychotic behavior, or those with severe language disability have more rapid cognitive decline and a higher mortality rate than those without such manifestations.[2-4] Many investigators maintain that these associations between specific clinical manifestations and the rate of progression of the disorder identify subtypes of AD. Others believe that AD is indeed a variable disorder but that there is no convincing evidence for qualitative subtypes.[5] Although a biological basis for heterogeneity of AD is now well established, with more than one genetic locus linked to early or late onset of the illness, the various genetic mutations do not appear to be associated with different clinical manifestations. With one exception, the associations between the clinical symptomatology of AD and the outcome events described above are no longer considered to represent heterogeneity of the disorder but reflect instead different stages in the course of the illness. This one exception relates to the evidence for a specific subtype of AD among demented patients with extrapyramidal dysfunction.

II. EXTRAPYRAMIDAL MANIFESTATIONS OF ALZHEIMER'S DISEASE

Mayeux[6] suggested that the presence of extrapyramidal manifestations in patients with AD was associated with greater severity of dementia and impairment in daily activities of living. The presence of these manifestations was thought to predict an increased rate of progression of intellectual deterioration, functional decline, and death. Other studies, however, suggest that extrapyramidal manifestations do not necessarily indicate the presence of a clinical subtype of AD, but represent a later stage of the disease.

Patients with AD and extrapyramidal signs have stimulated much interest in recent years. In many of these cases, autopsy examinations revealed not only patho-anatomic lesions of AD but also evidence of an additional neurodegenerative disorder characterized by the presence of Lewy bodies in the brain stem and in the cerebral cortex. This condition, now known as Lewy body variant of AD, has been found in 20 to 30% of autopsy examinations of patients with a clinical diagnosis of AD.[7] The neuropathological findings of AD in patients with both AD and Parkinsonism often differ from those with AD alone. In the former cases, senile plaque formation is readily apparent, but neurofibrillary tangles are often sparse.[8] Moreover, patients with both AD and Lewy body lesions at autopsy had, during life, a higher frequency of bradykinesia, muscular rigidity, and postural and gait disturbances than did patients with autopsy evidence of AD alone.[9] These clinical and neuropathological findings have led many investigators to the conclusion that the presence of extrapyramidal dysfunction in AD may represent the Lewy body variant, i.e., a specific subtype of this disorder. In many instances, patients with this subtype show behavioral or psychotic features such as paranoia and auditory or visual hallucinations.[10] In some studies, these patients show a more rapid progression of the illness than do those with Alzheimer's disease alone. In other studies, the duration of the dementing disorder is the same in both groups.[9]

III. BEHAVIORAL SYMPTOMS AND PERSONALITY CHANGES IN ALZHEIMER'S DISEASE

It has been reported that approximately 25% of subjects with mild AD and about 50% of those with severe AD have behavioral changes, e.g., hallucinations, delusions, misidentifications, and agitation.[3] The presence of such psychotic symptoms is thought by some investigators to delineate a subgroup of patients who have a faster rate of cognitive decline than do non-psychotic patients with AD. The biological significance of this association between behavior and cognition is unknown, but it seems reasonable to assume that pathological and biochemical changes in the brain relating to psychosis may also affect the rate of cognitive decline. Although the frequency of hallucinatory phenomena or other psychotic symptoms seems to increase with the duration of AD, these manifestations are often observed in earlier stages of the illness. A recent study of a large sample of patients at various stages of AD[11] showed that these patients had an average of 15 behavioral changes (e.g., depression, agitation, aggression) in the month prior to examination. Agitation and hallucinations have also been reported to be predictive of a faster rate of cognitive decline.[2]

IV. APHASIA IN ALZHEIMER'S DISEASE

A number of studies have reported that severe language disability in patients with AD is often associated with early age of onset, rapid progression of the illness, or death. A 9-year longitudinal study, for example, evaluated the various clinical factors affecting the course and survival of patients with AD.[4] This study showed, among other things, that severe language disability was the factor most significantly related to mortality, but that age of onset did not influence the outcome. In another report, however, younger persons with AD who manifested severe dysphasia had a higher rate of institutionalization and death than did older persons with AD and a similar degree of language impairment.[12] The fact that patients with early onset of AD have been found to have a higher frequency of language disorders than those with late-onset dementia[13] is evidence that aphasic manifestations of AD may relate to survival. Whether indeed the presence of language disability represents a distinct subtype of AD or is an example of the wide variability of the illness remains uncertain.

REFERENCES

1. Khachaturian, Z. S., An overview of scientific issues associated with the heterogeneity of Alzheimer's disease, in *Heterogeneity of Alzheimer's Disease,* Boller, F., et al., Eds., Springer-Verlag, Berlin, 1992.
2. Chui, H. C., Lyness, S., Sobel, E., and Schneider, L.S., Extrapyramidal signs and psychiatric symptoms predict faster rate of progression in Alzheimer's disease, *Arch. Neurol.,* 51, 676, 1994.
3. Rubin, E. H., Drevets, W. C., and Burke, W. J., The nature of psychotic symptoms in senile dementia of the Alzheimer type, *J. Geriat. Psych. Neurol.,* 1, 16, 1988.
4. Bracco, L., Gallato, R., Grigoletto, F., Lippi, A., Lepore, V., Bino, G., Lazzaro, M. P., Carella, F., Piccolo, T., Pozzilli, C., Giometto, B., and Amaducci, L., Factors affecting course and survival in Alzheimer's disease: 9-year longitudinal study, *Arch. Neurol.,* 51, 1213, 1994.
5. Jorm, A. F., Subtypes of Alzheimer's dementia: a conceptual analysis and critical review, *Psychol. Med.,* 15, 543, 1985.
6. Mayeux, R., Stern. Y., and Spanton, S., Heterogeneity in dementia of the Alzheimer type: evidence of subgroups, *Neurology,* 35, 453, 1985.
7. Katzman, R. and Jackson, J. E., Alzheimer's disease: basic and clinical advances, *JAGS,* 39, 516, 1991.
8. Hansen, L., Salmon, D., Galasko, D., Masliah, E., Katzman, R., DeTeresa, R., Thal, L., Pay, M. M., Hofstetter, R., Klauber, M., Rice, V., Butters, N., and Alford, M., The Lewy body variant of Alzheimer's disease: a clinical and pathologic entity, *Neurology,* 40, 1, 1990.
9. Hulette, C., Mirra, S. S., Wilkinson, W. E., Heyman, A., Fillenbaum, G , and Clark, C. M., A prospective clinical-neuropathological study of parkinson's features in Alzheimer's disease, IX. *Neurology,* 45, 1991, 1995.
10. McKeith, I. G., Perry, R. H., Fairbairn, A. F., Jabeen, S., and Perry, E. K., Operational criteria for senile dementia of Lewy body type (SDLT), *Psychol. Med.,* 22, 911, 1992.
11. Tariot, P. N., Mack, J. L., Patterson, M. B., Edland, S. D., Weiner, M. F., Fillenbaum, G., Blazina, L., Teri, L., Rubin, E., Mortimer, J. A., and Stern, Y., The CERAD Behavior Rating Scale for Dementia (BRSD), *Am. J. Psychiat.,* submitted.
12. Heyman, A., Wilkinson, W. E., Hurwitz, B. J., Helms, M. J., Haynes, C. S., Utley, C. M., and Gwyther, L. P., Early-onset Alzheimer's disease: clinical predictors of institutionalization and death, *Neurology,* 37, 980, 1987.
13. Koss, E., Edland, S., Fillenbaum, G., Mohs, R., Clark, C., Galasko, D., and Morris, J. C., Clinical differences between patients with earlier and later onset of Alzheimer's disease: a CERAD analysis. XIII, *Neurology,* 46, 136, 1996.

BIOLOGICAL MARKERS

Chapter 11

THE NEUROPATHOLOGY OF ALZHEIMER'S DISEASE: DIAGNOSTIC FEATURES AND STANDARDIZATION

Suzanne S. Mirra
William R. Markesbery

CONTENTS

I. INTRODUCTION

In the absence of a clinical test for diagnosing Alzheimer's disease (AD) and distinguishing it from other dementias, the diagnosis of AD currently relies upon examination of brain tissue by a pathologist, usually at the time of autopsy. Brain biopsies, i.e., small portions of cerebral cortex removed surgically, also suffice for diagnosis. This procedure is rarely performed in patients with AD, however, except in individuals with atypical presentations in whom other remediable disorders must be ruled out or as part of special research studies in which tissue confirmation of diagnosis is required prior to institution of a therapeutic modality.

AD families are often interested in having a definite diagnosis established and in making a contribution to research. Because of their commitment, the autopsy rate, i.e., number of autopsies per total deaths, at many AD centers is over 50%, far exceeding the dismally low national average of <10%. When standard clinical approaches to the diagnosis are applied, neuropathologists are able confirm the diagnosis of AD in approximately 87% of the cases. Thus, pathologists at AD centers usually encounter dozens of AD autopsies each year. In most instances, making the diagnosis is a relatively straightforward process, and a quick glance at a silver stain of most regions of cerebral cortex will readily reveal the diagnosis. Yet the recognition and diagnosis of other disorders or coexistent pathology, the study of the clinical and pathophysiologic significance of the changes, and the application of new scientific findings and methodologies to the work at hand enlivens the neuropathologist's job.

II. EXTERNAL EXAMINATION

For many reasons, including expediency and economy, autopsies in dementia patients are often limited to removal of the brain. A complete autopsy, while of general interest, is often not performed. Families usually understand when they consent to an autopsy that the tissues will be used for diagnosis, teaching, and research. Thus, upon removal of the brain under the supervision of a physician, it may be partially dissected, frozen, or placed in fixatives for ongoing or anticipated research studies. The remainder of the brain is generally fixed in a formaldehyde solution for about a week prior to further examination. At this point, the pathologist assesses the appearance of the brain externally and on cut sections. While this process may take place in relative isolation in a research laboratory, the gross examination often occurs in the setting of a "brain cutting conference" attended by neuropathologists, nonspecialist pathologists, neurologists, other physicians, and students. On the wall of the autopsy suite in the Atlanta VA Medical Center, a plaque bears the Latin phrase, *Mortui Vivis Praecipiant* (Let the dead instruct the living). Indeed, something of value can be learned from each autopsy case.

Certain features seen grossly enable the neuropathologist to predict with reasonable certainty that the clinical diagnosis of AD was correct. Atrophy of the frontal, temporal, and parietal cortex manifested by narrowing of the gyri that form the convolutions of the brain, and widening of the spaces between them, or sulci, is common (Figure 1). Sections of the brain may additionally reveal narrowing of the entorhinal cortex, a part of the paleocortex, i.e., a portion of the cortex phylogenetically older than the external neocortex as well as atrophy (shrinkage) of the hippocampus and amygdala, other key sites involved in memory.

Another characteristic feature is enlargement of the ventricular system that contains the cerebrospinal fluid, with disproportionate enlargement of the ventricular extension of the temporal lobe, i.e., the temporal horn of the lateral ventricle (Figure 2). Finally, pallor of the locus ceruleus, in the upper brain stem, a nucleus with neuromelanin-containing brain cells, occurs with such consistency in AD patients with longstanding dementia that a normally pigmented locus ceruleus appropriately raises doubt as to the accuracy of the diagnosis (Figure 3). Still another neuromelanin-containing structure, the substantia nigra in the midbrain, may exhibit pallor in some cases with

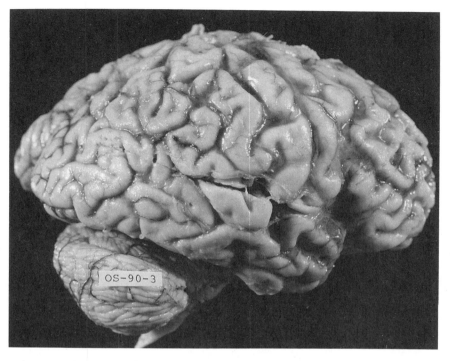

FIGURE 1 The external apearance (lateral view) of the brain of a patient with Alzheimer's disease. Note the widening of spaces between the convolutions involving the frontal and temporal lobes (on the right side of the photograph).

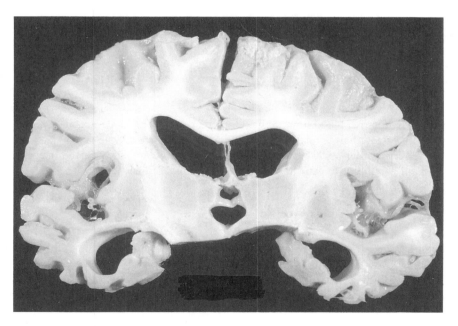

FIGURE 2 A coronal or cross section through the brain of a patient with Alzheimer's disease reveals enlargement of the lateral ventricles, particularly involving the temporal horn. The hippocampus is small and the parahippocampal cortex is narrowed.

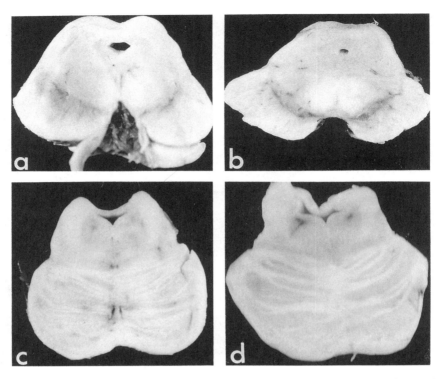

FIGURE 3   A pale or depigmented substantia nigra in the midbrain (a) and a pale locus ceruleus in the pons (c) in Alzheimer's disease are compared with their normal appearing counterparts (b and d).

loss of its normal black color. This pallor is commonly associated with microscopically detected loss of neurons and with inclusions within the pigmented nerve cells known as "Lewy bodies".

Other distinctive gross features of the brain may suggest different diagnoses. Pick's disease, a rare neurodegenerative disorder, is characterized by lobar rather than generalized atrophy with predominant involvement of the frontal and temporal lobes. In such cases, microscopic examination reveals the classic Pick bodies, cytoplasmic inclusions in nerve cells that stain dark brown-black on silver preparations.

The finding of multiple "strokes " or infarcts, i.e., vascular lesions caused by blood clots or abnormal vessels impairing blood flow, in the brain of a person with dementia, alerts the pathologist to the possibility of vascular dementia. Such brains may exhibit multiple small "lacunes" or lake-like lesions, reflecting their cystic nature, that are found predominantly in the deep gray matter such as the basal ganglia or thalamus, or within the cerebral white matter.

III. MICROSCOPIC EXAMINATION

Although careful assessment of the gross features of the brain is essential, the final neuropathological diagnosis of AD and many other dementias rests upon microscopic examination. Thus, at the time of brain cutting, pathologists take representative sections of multiple areas of the brain. The sections are dehydrated and embedded in wax, cut to a thickness of about 8 μm of a microtome, and stained using a variety of dyes and other chemicals highlighting various features under the microscope. While the diagnosis of AD can easily be made by examining one silver-stained section from neocortex, a more detailed assessment is important if other features or concomitant pathologies are to be appreciated. In addition, comprehensive characterization beyond diagnosis of the distribution and severity of the AD-related or other changes is valuable for clinical-pathological, molecular genetic, and other studies.

Although two major neuropathological features of AD, i.e., senile plaques and neurofibrillary tangles, have been recognized for decades, new information related to these structures continues to emerge. Two major subtypes of senile plaques are generally recognized — neuritic and diffuse (Figure 4). *Neuritic plaques* are spherical structures about 80 μm in diameter with thickened neurites, i.e., neuronal processes that may surround a central core of an abnormal protein known as "amyloid". Electron microscopic examination reveals that plaque neurites contain dense bodies thought to be lysosomes, mitochondria, and paired helical filaments. These neurites surround wisps or dense cores of fibrillar amyloid. In contrast, *diffuse plaques* lack the abnormal neurites and on silver stain have a softer, more amorphous appearance. Although both plaque subtypes label with antibodies to β-amyloid, little or no fibrillar amyloid is found in diffuse plaques by electron microscopy. Both neuritic and diffuse plaques occur in varying proportions in neocortex and other regions in AD and diffuse plaques predominate in some areas. Thought by some to represent an early stage in senile plaque evolution, diffuse plaques are not uncommon in brains derived from cognitively normal individuals or those with other neurodegenerative disorders.

The second major neuropathologic feature of AD is the *neurofibrillary tangle*, a silver-staining fibrillar structure within the cytoplasm of neurons (see Figure 4). While invariably occurring in AD, tangles are also found in the brains of cognitively normal or mildly impaired elderly individuals in regions prone to develop early neurofibrillary change, e.g., the entorhinal cortex. Under the electron microscope, AD tangles are composed primarily of *paired helical filaments*, spiral strands with characteristic periodicity composed predominantly of an abnormally phosphorylated form of tau, a protein associated with microtubules. Neurofibrillary tangles also staining with tau antibodies characterize other disorders as well, e.g., a form of parkinsonism often associated with mild dementia known as progressive supranuclear palsy (see below).

A third neuropathological feature of AD, also found in the brains of aged individuals, is that of amyloid angiopathy, i.e., amyloid deposition in blood vessels (Figure 4). Amyloid, an abnormal protein with characteristic physical, chemical, and morphologic properties, deposits within the walls of blood vessels in the meninges (brain coverings) and cortex. The severity of this deposition varies widely from case to case and may, when severe, be associated with intracerebral hemorrhages.

The hierarchical progression and anatomical distribution of AD changes have been of great interest. Work by the Braaks suggests that there is a predictable progression of neurofibrillary changes in AD. Although additional clinical-pathological studies are necessary to establish clearcut stages of progression, tangles and neuropil threads (another degenerative change in AD and other disorders) occur early in the region of the entorhinal cortex. The impact of neuropathological changes on neuronal circuitry must also be considered. For example, Hyman demonstrated that AD pathology affects both afferent and efferent pathways of the hippocampus, effectively isolating this important memory center.

Although senile plaques and neurofibrillary tangles dominate the microscopic landscape in AD, these readily visible changes do not tell the whole story. Loss of synapses, connections between nerve cells, correlates well with the degree of cognitive decline. Neuronal cell bodies, too, are lost from cortical and subcortical sites and potential mechanisms for this cell death are being investigated. Moreover, the role of nonneuronal cells, i.e., astrocytes and microglia, in the pathogenesis of AD is still being explored.

IV. STANDARDIZATION OF THE DIAGNOSIS OF ALZHEIMER'S DISEASE

Most neuropathologists looking at a section of neocortex laden with senile plaques and neurofibrillary tangles in a patient with dementia would agree on the diagnosis of AD. Neuropathological criteria

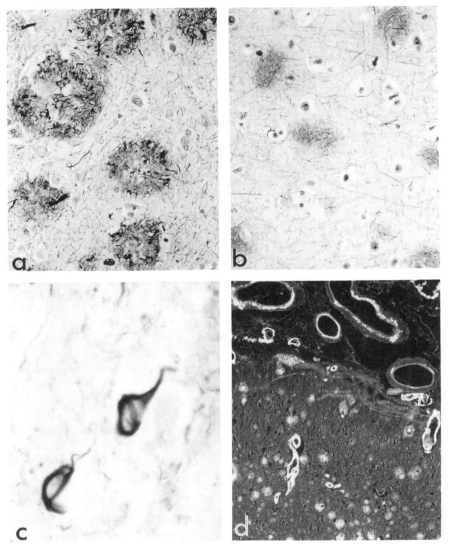

FIGURE 4 Microscopic features of Alzheimer's disease. (a) Several neuritic plaques within the cerebral cortex are seen on this silver stain. (b) Diffuse plaques predominate in this field of cerebral cortex. Silver stain. (c) Two neurofibrillary tangles are seen on silver stain. (d) A fluorescent stain (thioflavine S) reveals the ring-like profiles of amyloid within blood vessel walls in the meninges or coverings of the brain. The underlying cortical blood vessels also evidence amyloid angiopathy. Senile plaques in the cortex are also seen on this preparation.

for diagnosis, however, are not uniformly applied; technical and interpretive differences have militated against a standardized approach and pooling of data among centers. In a consensus report, neuropathologists convened by the National Institute on Aging in 1985, recommended minimal age-dependent senile plaque counts. These criteria, while applicable for the majority of cases of AD, did not allow for characterization of borderline cases, e.g., those with insufficient plaque frequency to merit a diagnosis, or those with many plaques but without a history of dementia. Nor were differences in technique that might affect plaque counts considered in establishing specific quantitative criteria.

In response to the need for a standardized neuropathology instrument for the evaluation of autopsy brains derived from patients clinically diagnosed as having AD and to facilitate pooling

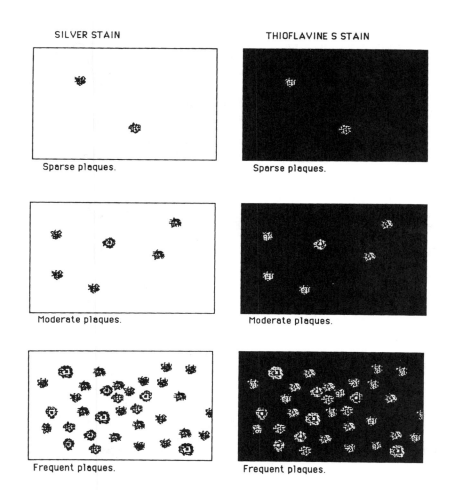

FIGURE 5 This cartoon depicts the scheme for semiquantitative rating of plaque frequency used by the Consortium to Establish a Registry for Alzheimer's Disease (CERAD). (From Mirra, S. S., Heyman, A., McKeel, D., et al., *Neurology,* 41, 479, 1991. With permission.)

of meaningful data among centers, a task force was formed by the Consortium to Establish a Registry for Alzheimer's Disease (CERAD), a longitudinal multicenter study sponsored by the National Institute on Aging. A neuropathology protocol consisting of an illustrated guide book and data entry forms was developed and tested. The protocol calls for participating neuropathologists to use their own routine fixation and staining methods to examine multiple regions of neocortex, entorhinal cortex, hippocampus, and subcortical structures. The evaluation includes (1) semiquantitative assessment of senile plaque and neurofibrillary tangle frequency in cortical and other structures (Figures 5 and 6); (2) determination of an age-related plaque score based on the age at death and the semiquantitative measure of neuritic plaques in neocortex; and (3) integration of the age-related plaque score with clinical information regarding the presence or absence of dementia to determine the level of certainty of the neuropathological diagnosis of AD. This assessment employs semiquantitative rather than strict quantitative measures of plaque and tangle frequency; the validity of this approach was affirmed by a CERAD study undertaken by 24 neuropathologists at 18 centers that demonstrated reasonable inter-rater reliability for semiquantitative measures of plaque and tangle frequency, but found significant inter-rater differences for quantitative plaque and tangle counts.

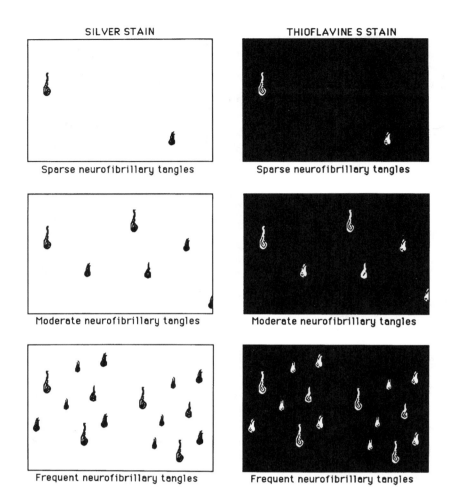

FIGURE 6 This cartoon depicts the scheme for semiquantitative rating of tangle frequency used by the Consortium to Establish a Registry for Alzheimer's Disease (CERAD) (From Mirra, S. S., Heyman, A., McKeel, D., et al., *Neurology,* 41, 479, 1991. With permission.)

V. THE HETEROGENEITY OF ALZHEIMER'S DISEASE AND OVERLAP WITH OTHER DISORDERS

A. OVERLAP WITH PARKINSON'S DISEASE — LEWY BODY DISEASES

Until recently, degeneration of the substantia nigra, a dopaminergic nucleus in the midbrain along with the microscopic finding of Lewy bodies, round concentric cytoplasmic inclusions in pigmented neurons in this region and other subcortical sites, was widely regarded as the morphologic correlate of idiopathic Parkinson's disease (Figure 7). Patients with this disorder classically present with extrapyramidal signs including bradykinesia (slow movement), rigidity, and tremor. Over the past few years, however, there has been increased recognition that patients with cognitive impairment resembling AD as well as certain additional clinical features including fluctuation in cognition and hallucinations may show similar neuropathology. The classification of this entity in which the presence of cortical Lewy bodies is emphasized (they have also been reported in idiopathic Parkinson's disease) is controversial as exemplified by the numerous appellations applied to it, e.g.,

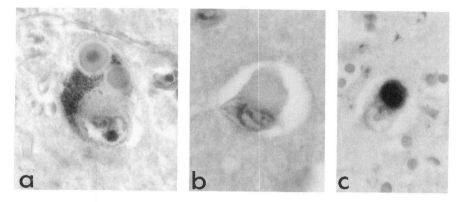

FIGURE 7   The microscopic appearance of Lewy bodies. (a) Two Lewy bodies are observed in a pigmented neuron of the substantia nigra. Note the typical concentric pattern with peripheral halo. (b) A cortical Lewy body is seen within a neuron. Hematoxylin-eosin. (c) A cortical Lewy body is noted on ubiquitin immunohistochemistry.

diffuse Lewy body disease, Lewy body variant of AD, AD plus Parkinson's disease, and senile dementia of the Lewy body type. The crux of the debate revolves around whether this form of Lewy body disease is indeed a variant of AD or whether it represents a distinctive clinical and neuropathological entity. It seems reasonable to consider the Lewy body diseases as a clinical-pathological spectrum, ranging from idiopathic Parkinson's disease, the movement disorder, at one end to a primary dementia with similar pathology, i.e., diffuse Lewy body disease (with or without coexistent AD) at the other end.

Regardless of classification, there is no question that nigral degeneration and Lewy bodies at multiple sites are observed in a substantive percentage of cases fulfilling conventional neuropathological criteria for AD, albeit with fewer neurofibrillary tangles than cases of "pure AD". In the multicenter CERAD autopsy series, concomitant Lewy body changes were observed in 21% of cases meeting criteria for definite AD. In our experience, only a small minority of patients diagnosed clinically as having probable AD turn out at autopsy to have exclusively PD features, i.e., brainstem and neocortical Lewy bodies and nigral degeneration without cortical plaques or tangles.

B.   OVERLAP WITH OTHER NEURODEGENERATIVE DISORDERS

Another neurologic disorder showing significant overlap with AD and other neurodegenerative disorders is progressive supranuclear palsy, characterized by supranuclear gaze palsy, postural instability, extrapyramidal signs, and cognitive dysfunction. Although the neuropathological features of progressive supranuclear palsy are relatively stereotypical, concomitant changes of AD, Parkinson's disease, corticobasal degeneration, and other disorders are not uncommon. It is unclear whether this neuropathological overlap represents the coincidental occurrence of disorders frequently encountered in the elderly or whether they implicate common pathogenetic pathways. These disorders all share cytoskeletal pathology and tau-positive inclusions in neurons.

C.   VASCULAR DEMENTIA

There are various cerebrovascular diseases and vascular-induced cerebral lesions that cause alterations in intellectual function and behavior. Patients with this compendium of problems may be diagnosed as having vascular dementia or occasionally, less precisely, multi-infarct dementia. Basically, vascular dementia is defined as acquired intellectual impairment resulting from brain injury caused by a cerebrovascular disorder. It is not a specific disease but a heterogeneous syndrome of multiple clinical and pathological manifestations and causes. Clinical studies have suggested that the frequency of vascular dementia ranges from 4.5 to 39%. Autopsy studies, however, have indicated that only between 1 to 22% of demented subjects in fact evidence cerebrovascular disease as the underlying cause. Overall, it is more likely that vascular dementia accounts for 10% or less of cases of dementia in the elderly.

The clinical diagnosis of vascular dementia is made by determining the presence of dementia and establishing its relationship to cerebrovascular lesions. This process entails the exclusion of many other potential causes of dementia as well as the demonstration of vascular lesions on brain imaging studies. Typically, the intellectual deficit is characterized by a loss of memory with deficits in two or more other cognitive functions severe enough to interfere with functioning in daily living. These include orientation, language, visuo-spatial abilities, calculations, motor control, praxis, abstraction and judgment. Most patients with vascular dementia have one or more focal neurologic deficits. These include motor signs (weakness, spasticity, hyperactive deep tendon reflexes, and Babinski responses), visual field defects, sensory changes, dysphagia, dysarthria, emotional instability, and gait disturbances. In this regard, patients with vascular dementia are quite different from patients with uncomplicated AD who most often do not have focal neurologic signs and symptoms. The Hachinski Ischemic Score utilizes a list of 13 characteristics that serve to separate vascular dementia from primary degenerative diseases such as AD.

The risk factors for vascular dementia include the risk factors for stroke — hypertension, congestive heart failure, atrial fibrillation, coronary artery disease, diabetes, cigarette smoking, and hypercholesterolemia. In addition, age, lower educational attainment, and non-white race are associated with vascular dementia.

One of the important gaps in our knowledge about vascular dementia is the lack of specific criteria for the pathological diagnosis. Two recent reports have proposed criteria for the pathological diagnosis of vascular dementia. A diagnosis of *definite* vascular dementia requires histopathologic examination of the brain to confirm the presence of vascular lesions. Also, the frequency of neuritic plaques and neurofibrillary tangles should be insufficient to warrant a diagnosis of AD and pathologic features of other dementing disorders should be absent.

The pathological characteristics of vascular dementia include small or large infarcts in the cerebral cortex, deep gray matter (basal ganglia and thalamus), and white matter as shown in Figures 8 and 9. In addition, there may be small or large hemorrhages in the cerebral hemispheres. The lesions in blood vessels are most commonly atherosclerotic occlusions of large or medium size intracranial or cervical arteries, or sclerotic occlusions of smaller arteries or arterioles. The latter is commonly seen in association with hypertension and diabetes. In addition, emboli from the heart or atherosclerotic lesions in the cervical arteries are encountered commonly. Several factors may be important in determining whether a patient develops vascular dementia. These include the *size* (volume) of the vascular lesions(s), the specific *location* of the lesion in brain regions critical to memory and other cognitive functions, and the *number* of vascular lesions. It is clear that dementia can result from destruction of a significant volume of brain in some subjects. Early studies suggested 100 ml or more of infarcted brain were associated with dementia. However, it is most likely that the location of the lesion is of greater importance.

Cerebrovascular disease and AD are common disorders in the elderly and it is not unexpected that there is considerable overlap between the two entities. Patients with both AD and vascular lesions are said to have a "mixed" dementia contributing to the heterogeneity of AD. The frequency of mixed dementia is not known because of a lack of crisp criteria for this diagnosis and many confounding factors such as inclusion criteria used in various clinical-pathological studies. Autopsy series reveal a range of 0 to 32% for mixed dementia, with a mean of 15%. Thus, many cases diagnosed clinically as having vascular dementia prove in fact to have mixed AD and vascular dementia. In our experience, this combined pathology is far more common than "pure" vascular dementia.

At autopsy the brains of patients with mixed dementia not only contain abundant senile plaques and neurofibrillary tangles, meeting the criteria described above for AD, but also display variable numbers of infarcts or hemorrhages. Whether these cerebrovascular lesions complicate long-standing AD without contributing to the intellectual decline or serve as additive factors in hastening the intellectual decline is not known. It is most likely that multiple vascular lesions or lesions located

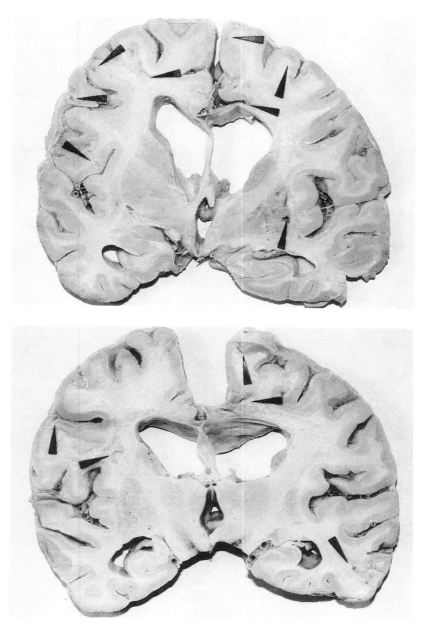

FIGURES 8 and 9   Sections from the brain of a patient with vascular dementia show multiple white matter, and basal ganglia stroke-like lesions or infarcts (arrowheads).

in regions critical to memory significantly increase the cognitive decline. Similarly, patients with multiple or critically located infarcts may show more impairment of cognitive functions if their brain contains moderate numbers of senile plaques and neurofibrillary tangles, but too few for a diagnosis of AD. Only through rigorous studies using standardized clinical and neuropathological approaches can the significance of vascular dementia be determined.

Leukoaraiosis is a term used to describe the diffuse periventricular white matter alterations found on computerized tomography scan and magnetic resonance imaging in patients with AD and in intellectually normal elderly individuals. It has been suggested that these changes are ischemic in nature, resulting from hypoperfusion in the distal zone of penetrating blood vessels. Microscopically these zones show pallor, mild myelin loss, gliosis, ependymal breakdown, and hyalinization, fibrosis, and luminal narrowing of arterioles. The importance of these lesions in cognitive function is not known, especially in regard to vascular dementia, AD, and mixed forms of dementia.

D. NEW DEVELOPMENTS RELATED TO THE NEUROPATHOLOGY OF ALZHEIMER'S DISEASE

The finding of Roses and co-workers that ε4 allele or gene variant of apolipoprotein E (apoE) is a risk factor for late-onset familial and sporadic AD and subsequent confirmation by many groups has stimulated additional studies examining the relationship of the apoE protein and its receptors to the neuropathology of AD. ApoE and β-amyloid colocalize in blood vessels and senile plaques in AD (Figure 10), and the severity of amyloid deposition in vessels (amyloid angiopathy) as well as the frequency of cortical plaques apparently increase with ε4 dosage. Despite the finding of Strittmatter and co-workers that there are isoform-specific differences in binding to nonphosphorylated tau *in vitro*, suggesting that ApoE genotype may influence neurofibrillary tangle formation, quantitative difference in tangles are not detected between those cases with or without the ε4 allele. The mechanism by which ApoE genotype conveys risk for the development of AD is still under investigation.

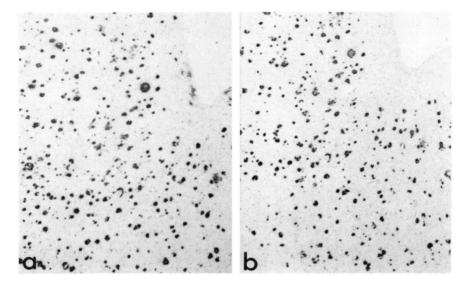

FIGURE 10   Immunohistochemical preparations using antibodies to βA4 amyloid (a) and apolipoprotein E (b) show similar label of senile plaques in the cerebral cortex.

ACKNOWLEDGMENTS

Supported by National Institutes of Health grants AG06790, AG10130, P01AG05119, and P50AGO5144 and a Veterans Affairs Merit Award.

SUGGESTED READING

Braak, H. and Braak, E., Neuropathological stageing of Alzheimer-related changes, *Acta Neuropathol.*, 82, 239, 1991.

Chui, H. C., Victoroff, J. I., Margolin, D., Jagust, W., Shankle, R., and Katzman, R., Criteria for the diagnosis of ischemic vascular dementia proposed by the State of California Alzheimer's Disease Diagnostic and Treatment Centers, *Neurology*, 42, 473, 1992.

Gearing, M., Mirra, S. S., Hansen, L. A., Hedreen, J. C., Sumi, S. M., and Heyman, A., Neuropathology confirmation of the clinical diagnosis of Alzheimer's disease: CERAD (Consortium to Establish a Registry for Alzheimer's Disease). X, *Neurology*, 45, 461, 1995.

Gearing, M., Rebeck, W., Hyman, B. T., Tigges, J., and Mirra, S. S., Neuropathology of aged chimpanzees and apolipoprotein E: implications for Alzheimer's disease, *Proc. Nat. Acad. Sci. U.S.A.,* 91, 9382, 1994.

Hachinski, V. C., Iliff, L. D., Zilhka, G. H., et al. Cerebral blood flow in dementia, *Arch. Neurol.,* 32, 632, 1975.

Hansen, L. A., Crain, B. J., Practical topics in neuropathology: making the diagnosis of mixed and non-Alzheimer's dementias, *Arch. Pathol. Lab. Med.,* 119, 1023, 1995.

Hyman, B. T., Van Hoesen, G. W., Damasio, A. R., and Barnes, C. L., Alzheimer's disease: cell specific pathology isolates the hippocampal formation, *Science,* 225, 1168, 1984.

Khachaturian, Z. S., Diagnosis of Alzheimer's disease, *Arch. Neurol.,* 42, 1097, 1985.

Mirra, S. S., Gearing, M., Hughes, J., et al., Inter-laboratory comparison of neuropathology assessments in Alzheimer's disease: a multicenter study of the Consortium to Establish a Registry for Alzheimer's Disease (CERAD). *J. Neuropathol. Exp. Neurol.,* 53, 303, 1994.

Mirra, S. S., Hart, M. N., and Terry, R. D., Making the diagnosis of Alzheimer's disease: a primer for practicing pathologists, *Arch. Pathol. Lab. Med.,* 117, 132, 1993.

Mirra, S. S., Heyman, A., McKeel, D., et al. CERAD. II. Standardization of the neuropathological assessment of AD, *Neurology,* 41, 479, 1991.

Roman, G. C., Tatemichi, T. K., Erkinjuntti, T., et al., Vascular dementia: diagnostic criteria for research studies, *Neurology,* 43, 250, 1993.

Tatemichi, T. K., Sacktor, N., and Mayeux, R., Dementia associated with cerebrovascular disease, other degenerative diseases, and metabolic disorders, in *Alzheimer Disease,* Terry, R. D., Katzman, R., and Bick, K. L., Eds., Raven Press, New York, 1994, chap. 9.

Chapter 12

PATHOLOGY, NEUROBIOLOGY, AND ANIMAL MODELS OF ALZHEIMER'S DISEASE

Juan C. Troncoso
Barbara J. Crain
Sangram S. Sisodia
Donald L. Price

CONTENTS

0-8493-8997-6/97/$0.00+$.50
© 1996 by CRC Press, Inc.

I. INTRODUCTION

This chapter deals with three principal issues in Alzheimer's disease (AD): neuropathological hallmarks and their importance for post-mortem diagnosis and pathogenesis of the dementia; biological processes that underlie these pathological features; and the current status of animal models.

II. THE HISTOPATHOLOGICAL FEATURES OF ALZHEIMER'S DISEASE

In reporting the index case of AD in 1907,[1] Alois Alzheimer established that presenile dementia and psychosis were associated with neocortical senile plaques (SP) and neurofibrillary tangles (NFT). In 1910, Kraepelin introduced the term "Alzheimer's Disease" to delineate the clinical-pathological entity.[2] Although Alzheimer was the first to identify NFT, SP had been recognized earlier by Blocq and Marinesco in 1892[3] and Emil Redlich in 1898[4] and were called SP by Simchowicz, who described SP as present in large numbers in the brains of patients with senile dementia.[2] Over the next few decades, the relationship between presenile and senile dementias was the subject of debate, because SP and NFT are present in both entities. Clinical and pathological evidence had begun to emerge to suggest that presenile and senile dementias shared a common pathogenesis. For example, clinicians observed senile dementia in a father and presenile dementia in his son, and pathologists viewed the differences between the two disorders as quantitative, not qualitative, in nature.[5] Nonetheless, investigators were reluctant for many years to attribute a pathogenic role to SP in dementia for two reasons: the frequent coexistence of cerebrovascular disease and degenerative changes in older demented individuals and the observation of SP in older nondemented subjects.[5] Although Oskar Fischer[6] proposed in 1907 that SP correlated with the severity of memory loss and dementia, it was not until the early 1960s that the relationship between SP and cognitive decline became widely accepted based on the observations and careful clinical-pathological correlations of Roth[7] and Tomlinson.[8]

Roth et al.[9] first described an approximately linear correlation between cognitive scores for dementia and counts of SP in the neocortex of elderly subjects. Moreover, these investigators suggested that further studies of the formation of SP, using techniques more precise than those used in their investigation, would provide insight into age-associated disorders.[9] Subsequently, Tomlinson et al.[10] confirmed the presence of SP, NFT, and granuolovacuolar degeneration as the histopathological hallmarks of senile dementia. However, at the same time, they recognized that all of these histological changes could also occur in nondemented old people, albeit to a lesser extent.[8,10] These observations eventually led to new clinical-pathological studies of dementia demonstrating that the major cause of dementia in the elderly was AD[11,12] — investigations that invigorated all aspects of research in this disorder.

Over the last 15 years, significant new information has become available on AD: neuronal circuits and populations vulnerable to the disease;[13-18] pharmacological abnormalities;[19-24] the biology of cerebral amyloid;[25] and, most importantly, the genetic underpinnings of the disease.[26-30] At the same time that new insights were being gained in the neurobiology and genetics of AD, investigators continued to report abundant SP in nondemented subjects.[31,32] Such observations raised fundamental questions concerning the importance of cerebral amyloid and SP in the pathogenesis of AD. All of these factors, combined with the development of the National Institute on Aging sponsored Alzheimer's Disease Research Centers throughout the country, contributed to the need to establish common criteria for the clinical[33] and neuropathological diagnoses of AD.[34]

III. DEVELOPMENT OF STANDARD CRITERIA FOR PATHOLOGICAL DIAGNOSIS OF ALZHEIMER'S DISEASE

In 1985, the National Institute on Aging (NIA) and other agencies sponsored a conference to foster investigation on AD and to advance the progress of research on the diagnosis of this disorder.[34] Neuropathologists at this conference developed the first autopsy criteria for the diagnosis of AD in patients with moderate or advanced dementia. These criteria were based primarily on the number of SPs in neocortex, adjusted by age, factoring in NFT and the clinical history of dementia. Panel members agreed that, in any microscopic field encompassing 1 mm^2 of tissue, a minimum number of SP are necessary for a diagnosis of AD (Table 1). The conferees also agreed that further clinical-pathological correlations would be necessary to establish a histological diagnosis in the early phases of AD.

TABLE 1   NIA (KHACHATURIAN) Criteria for a Diagnosis of AD

Age (years)	Number of SP/mm^2 (200× magnification)
<50	>2–5
50–65	>8
66–75	>10
>75	>15

Several years after the formulation of the NIA (Khachaturian) criteria, the Consortium to Establish a Registry for AD (CERAD) was established as a joint effort of many medical and research institutions across the U.S. and abroad to standardize the clinical and pathological diagnoses of AD. CERAD has formulated a diagnostic algorithm for the diagnosis of AD based on semiquantitative assessment of SP in neocortex, the age of the patient, and the clinical history of dementia (Table 2).[35,36] A unique feature of this system is that it directly confronts the issue of borderline cases. Diagnostic outcomes from this classification include definite, probable, and possible AD, as well as normal. In addition, CERAD has strived to assess the types and frequencies of other dementing disorders that may occur separately or in conjunction with AD (e.g., multiinfarct dementia, Parkinson's disease, Lewy body disease, and progressive supranuclear palsy).

TABLE 2   CERAD Criteria Age-Related SP Score for Individuals with History of Dementia

Age	Frequency of Neuritic SP			
	None	Sparse	Moderate	Frequent
<50	0	C	C	C
50–75	0	B	C	C
>75	0	A	B	C

Note: C, indicative of AD (in the presence of clinical history of dementia); B, suggestive of AD; A, uncertain evidence of AD; O, no evidence of AD.

IV. CURRENT ISSUES IN THE AUTOPSY DIAGNOSIS OF ALZHEIMER'S DISEASE

A. THE ROLE OF QUANTITATION

An ongoing source of controversy is whether the diagnosis of AD should depend on quantitative assessment of one or more histopathological changes. The single strongest argument in favor of quantitation is that each pathological marker of the disease (i.e., β-amyloid [Aβ] deposits, SP, and NFT) also occurs to some extent in apparently normal aging.[31,32] Thus, to be of practical use, any diagnostic criteria need to be at least semiquantitative. However, serious problems arise in deciding which pathological changes to measure. NFT are usually present in neocortex in AD and appear to correlate better with the severity of dementia than SP.[37] However, there are also cases lacking NFT in which the diagnosis of AD is based unquestionably on clinical grounds and the presence of neocortical SP.[38] Furthermore, there is growing evidence that the loss of neurons and synapses correlates better with cognitive decline than either SP or NFT.[39] Moreover, the former features are far from specific for AD and could not be used alone as diagnostic features. Finally, the technical and practical aspects of establishing scientifically valid and reproducible procedures for quantitation across laboratories should not be underestimated.

At this point, we believe that CERAD's simple semiquantitative assessment of SP in neocortex is practical and sufficient for routine diagnostic purposes. On the other hand, the establishment of reliable procedures for quantitating multiple histological markers of AD may prove to be extremely useful for grading the severity of the disease process in individual patients and for correlating the histological features of AD with other biological markers of disease in a research setting.

B. THE IMPORTANCE OF CLINICAL INFORMATION FOR AN AUTOPSY DIAGNOSIS OF ALZHEIMER'S DISEASE

Current diagnostic criteria for AD take into consideration the subject's history of cognitive decline.[34,35] Khachaturian[34] proposed that in the presence of a positive clinical history of AD, the severity of cortical lesions required for diagnosis (see Table 2) could be reduced 50%. CERAD criteria[35] use the clinical history to classify cases as definite, probable, or possible AD and explicitly preclude a diagnosis of definite AD in the absence of clinically documented dementia, although a diagnosis of "possible AD" is allowed. Thus, both sets of criteria imply that a diagnosis of AD could be made in the absence of a clinical history of dementia. However, there is no study to date to support the formulation of the diagnosis of AD in the absence of clinical evidence of dementia. Such a capability would be important for studies that utilize archival material and eventually for forensic purposes. Clinical-pathological correlations of subjects in longitudinal studies of aging (e.g., Baltimore Longitudinal Study of Aging [BLSA], Framingham study, Bronx study) may contribute to the development of such criteria.

C. BEYOND THE CURRENT CRITERIA FOR AN AUTOPSY DIAGNOSIS OF ALZHEIMER'S DISEASE

In practice, neuropathologists seldom have a problem with the diagnosis of AD in cases of moderate or advanced dementia. Most problems arise in the diagnosis of individuals who have a history of mild cognitive decline (i.e., deficit limited to memory) or mild dementia (loss in two cognitive domains, CDR = 0.5),[40,41] in putative "control" subjects, or in cases where detailed clinical information is lacking. The issues are particularly complex in very old subjects (i.e., >85 years).

From our experience with the BLSA,[42] it appears that the common denominator in elderly individuals (80 to 98 years of age) with early or mild dementia (Blessed Information-Memory-Concentration scores = 4 to 10) is the presence of widely distributed, rare-to-moderate SP (5 to 25 SP/mm^2) in all neocortical regions examined. In these same regions, NFTs are absent or rare. Either the CERAD or Khachaturian criteria could be modified to include these early cases by reducing the density of neocortical SP required for diagnosis and, at the same time, introducing a factor to account for the widespread distribution of lesions. However, such a change would miscategorize those well-demonstrated cases of cognitively intact individuals with abundant SP.[31,32] Thus, in the absence of clinical history, the inclusion of NFT, neuronal, or synaptic counts might be necessary adjuncts to assessment of SP for an accurate diagnosis.

V. THE BIOLOGY OF BRAIN ABNORMALITIES IN ALZHEIMER'S DISEASE

This section focuses on vulnerable neuronal systems and structural abnormalities in the brains of individuals with AD. First, neurons in multiple regions of the central nervous system become dysfunctional and die, leading to alterations in synaptic inputs, predominantly in the amygdala, hippocampus, and neocortex.[15,16,39] Second, cell bodies and proximal dendrites of these vulnerable neurons contain NFT, comprised of paired helical filaments (PHFs),[43] the principal component of which is hyperphosphorylated tau, a microtubule-binding protein.[43-45] Finally, the brains of cases of AD show extracellular deposits of Aβ, usually associated in SP with abnormal neuronal processes (i.e., neurites) as well as glia and microglia.[46,47] Aβ is also present in preamyloid parenchymal deposits and within the walls of leptomeningeal and cerebral vessels.[48]

A. VULNERABLE NEURONAL SYSTEMS

Neuronal loss is a well-recognized histological feature of AD. However, cell death is neither ubiquitous nor uniform in its extent. Rather, clinical symptoms and signs in AD are associated with abnormalities of specific neuronal systems in the neocortex, hippocampus, amygdala, basal forebrain cholinergic system, anterior thalamus, and monoaminergic brainstem systems (Figure 1).[15-17,23,49-54]

In the neocortex, degenerative changes in AD involve both the large glutamatergic pyramidal neurons of layers III and V[24,55-57] and various populations of interneurons, some of which use somastostatin or corticotropin-releasing factor as transmitters.[20,22,23,58,59]

In hippocampus and medial temporal lobe, abnormalities occur in pyramidal neurons, particularly those of entorhinal cortex and hippocampal areas CA1 and CA2,[14,17,18,49,57] as well as in neurons of the amygdala.[17,60,61] Recent stereological studies of hippocampus in AD have shown that the most distinctive abnormality is age-independent loss of neurons in CA1 region.[18] Lesions of entorhinal cortex and other limbic structures, potentially important in the genesis of memory impairments, may serve to disconnect hippocampus and neocortex.[16,62]

In the basal forebrain, degenerative changes are prominent in the medial septum, diagonal band, and nucleus basalis, which provide the principal cholinergic innervation of amygdala, hippocampus, and neocortex.[63,64]

Neurons of the locus coeruleus and raphe also exhibit perikaryal pathology (i.e., NFT). Axons and terminals of these cells may form dystrophic neurites, and noradrenergic and serotoninergic markers may be decreased in target fields.[14,50,65,66]

VI. CYTOSKELETAL PATHOLOGY

The pathology of AD is characterized by conspicuous perturbations of the cytoskeleton and its protein constituents. The most prominent abnormality of the neuronal cytoskeleton in AD are NFTs. Closely related to NFT are dystrophic neurites and neuropil threads. Other abnormal inclusions in affected neurons are Hirano bodies and granulovacuolar degeneration, which contain different cytoskeletal proteins (Figure 2).

Structural and immunocytochemical studies of human post-mortem tissues have identified the proteins that participate in these cytoskeletal abnormalities in AD. However, elucidation of the

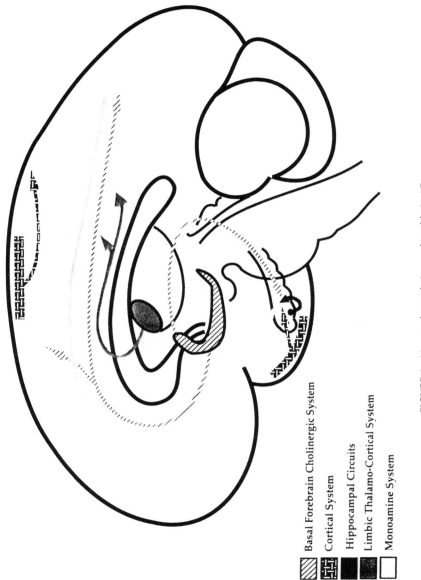

FIGURE 1 Neuronal populations vulnerable in AD.

Basal Forebrain Cholinergic System

Cortical System

Hippocampal Circuits

Limbic Thalamo-Cortical System

Monoamine System

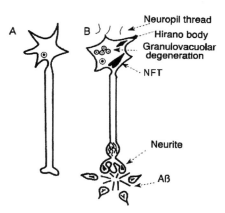

FIGURE 2 Schematic drawing of a normal nerve cell (A) and a neuron exhibiting abnormalities that occur in AD (B).

biochemical mechanisms that underlie formation is difficult in autopsy tissues and will eventually require complementary investigations in natural and transgenic animal models.

The principal ultrastructural components of NFT are the intracellular accumulations of insoluble PHF and 15-nm straight filaments. PHFs, which are also important constituents of neuropil threads and dystrophic neurites, are comprised principally of abnormally hyperphosphorylated isoforms of tau.[43,45,67-72]

Down-regulation of phosphatases (i.e., PP2A and PP2B) in AD brain may contribute to the hyperphosphorylated status of tau and its decreased binding to microtubules, thus, leading to the aggregation and transformation of tau into PHF/NFT.[73] Aberrant phosphorylation of tau may also promote the formation of the straight filaments that become increasingly modified and cross linked to form insoluble PHF.[74] Other NFT-associated epitopes include ubiquitin, microtubule-associated protein (MAP-2), neurofilament proteins (particularly phosphorylated epitopes of the 200-kDa protein), and, possibly, Aβ.[43,75-80] Although still controversial,[81] NFT may also contain aluminum and iron;[82] these metals may promote the aggregation of some cytoskeletal proteins. Recent studies suggest that aluminum binds to phosphorylated or PHF tau, induces these proteins to aggregate, and retards their proteolysis.[83]

Dystrophic neurites are enlarged neuronal processes that contain PHF, 15-nm straight filaments, and various organelles, including mitochondria, membranous inclusions, lysosomes, and, in some cases, synaptic vesicles.[43,45,69,71,75,77-79,84-88] Neuropil threads, another altered neuronal process, are predominantly dendrites;[89-91] although some may represent aberrant axonal sprouts.[92]

Because NFT, neurites, and neuropil threads contain similar cytoskeletal constituents, it is likely that these fibrillar inclusions result from common mechanisms. Moreover, NFT and neuropil threads exhibit similar characteristic distributions over time;[57] involvement proceeds from the transentorhinal region to entorhinal cortex and then to Ammon's horn and isocortex.[57] The severity of these lesions in cerebral cortical regions appears to correlate with hierarchies of cortical-cortical connections, and nerve cells of associated cortices exhibit the greatest vulnerability.[93]

VII. AMYLOIDOGENESIS

Molecular mechanisms that lead to the formation and deposition of cerebral amyloid are the focus of intense investigation in AD. Although these mechanisms remain unclear, substantial progress has been made over the last 10 years in this area of research.

Amyloid is a generic term that describes fibrillar aggregates which have a common β-pleated sheet structure; these aggregates exhibit birefringent properties in the presence of Congo Red and polarized light.[25] Aβ, an ~4-kDa peptide derived from larger amyloid precursor proteins (APP), is

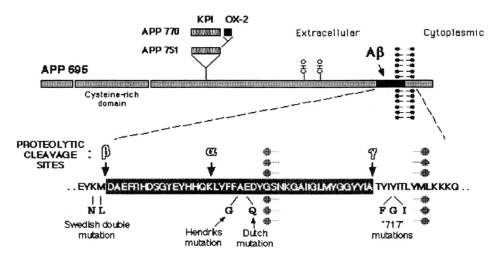

FIGURE 3 Schematic representation of APP. Phosphorylation sites and NPXY internalization signal are located in the C-terminal portion of molecules. Note location of the Aβ peptide, sites of α, β, and γ secretase, and several mutations linked to Aβ amyloidogenesis.

the principal constituent of amyloid in SP in AD[94] and in congophilic angiopathy.[25] The 39 to 43 amino acid span of Aβ is comprised of 11 to 15 amino acids from the transmembrane domain and 28 amino acids from the extracellular domain of APP (Figure 3).

The *APP* gene, encompassing ~400 kilobases of DNA,[95] is on human chromosome 21.[96] APP pre-mRNA is spliced alternatively to generate several transcripts that encode a family of Aβ-containing proteins of between 695 and 770 amino acids.[96-100] APP is expressed ubiquitously and is highly conserved in vertebrates; proteins homologous to APP have also been identified in such evolutionarily divergent organisms as *Drosophila*[101] and *Caenorhabditis elegans*.[102] Recent studies have documented the expression of novel APP-like proteins (APLP) in human and mouse tissues,[103-106] indicating that vertebrate APP is a member of a larger family of related molecules. Notably, APLP differ from APP by the conspicuous absence of the Aβ region.

The function(s) of APP in the nervous system is not well defined. Indirect evidence has supported a role for APP in cell adhesion,[107] in the growth of neuronal and nonneuronal cells,[108,109] and in signal transduction pathways.[110] A truncated and soluble derivative of APP-751 is identical to "protease nexin II" or "factor XIa inhibitor", a molecule involved in wound healing and hemostasis.[111-113]

APPs are type-I integral membrane glycoproteins that mature through the constitutive secretory pathway.[111,114-116] Depending on cell type and level of expression, a fraction (~10 to 30%) of newly synthesized APP may appear on the cell surface;[114,117,118] some of these molecules are cleaved[117,118] between positions 16 and 17 of Aβ,[119-122] resulting in the release of soluble APP (APP[s]) into the conditioned medium. The presence of APP[s] in human cerebrospinal fluid that contains Aβ epitopes suggests that similar processing events occur *in vivo*.[123] This important processing pathway precludes Aβ amyloidogenesis by directing cleavage within the Aβ peptide region. The protease responsible for the endoproteolytic cleavage of APP at the cell surface has not been identified and, for convenience, has been termed "α-secretase".[119]

Given the general observation that a large fraction of newly synthesized APP fails to be released into the extracellular medium, alternative routes of APP trafficking and metabolism have been investigated. Cell-surface APP is internalized by endocytosis.[117] APP is also processed in endosomal/lysosomal compartments and degraded to a complex set of membrane-bound fragments, some of which contain the entire Aβ sequence.[117,124] Current ideas about the role of these fragments in the pathogenesis of Aβ formation are discussed below.

Until recently, many investigators believed that Aβ was generated by aberrant metabolism of the precursor. This concept had to be reevaluated when it was discovered that Aβ was detectable in the conditioned medium of a wide variety of cultured cells and in human cerebrospinal fluid.[125-128] The vast majority of Aβ peptides secreted in these settings is Aβ1-40.[125,126] Significantly, Aβ1-42/43, admixed with smaller amounts of Aβ1-40, appears to be the predominant Aβ species in SP amyloid.[94,129,130] Most importantly, Aβ1-42/43 nucleates rapidly into amyloid fibrils and may serve as a seed for the aggregation and subsequent deposition of Aβ.[131] The notion that the production of long Aβ (i.e., 1-42/43) causes or contributes to amyloidogenesis is supported by studies of cells transfected with APP cDNA encoding the "717" substitutions characteristic of some families with early-onset autosomal dominant AD.[27,132,133] These cells secrete a higher percentage of long Aβ peptides (i.e., Aβ1-42) relative to cells expressing wild-type APP,[134] suggesting that Aβ1-42 or Aβ1-43, rather than Aβ1-40, may be the pathogenic peptide in AD. Further support for this hypothesis comes from immunocytochemical studies of the brains of individuals with AD that demonstrate convincingly that the bulk (>95%) of SP consists of Aβ1-42.[130]

Molecular mechanisms involved in the production of Aβ remain unclear. However, accumulated evidence currently favors the hypothesis that Aβ may be generated intracellularly in acidic compartments (i.e., endosome or late Golgi)[125,127] rather than in the endosomal/lysosomal pathways[125,128,135] and that the reinternalization of APP from the cell surface may favor the generation of Aβ.[135,136] Supporting this model are recent studies that demonstrate the secretion of iodinated Aβ from APP labeled on the cell surface.[137] Surprisingly, with only one notable exception,[138] Aβ has not been detected intracellularly.[125,127,139] Thus, despite the demonstration of Aβ production by cultured cells, the intracellular sites in which Aβ is actually generated have not yet been identified.

Moreover, Aβ may interact with other moieties (e.g., apolipoprotein E [apoE], apoliprotein J [apoJ])[30,140,141] to enhance the formation of Aβ fibrils.

A. ApoE
1. Evidence for a Role of ApoE in Alzheimer's Disease

There is an increased prevalence of the apoE4 allele (or a reduced prevalence of apoE3) in late-onset familial AD as well as sporadic AD.[30,142,143] The mechanisms by which the characteristics of the apoE4 alleles are linked to the structural alterations that occur in AD are not known,[144] but several lines of evidence (outlined below) implicate apoE in the amyloidogenesis and pathogenesis of AD.

ApoE is a 34-kDa glycoprotein and a component of very low-, intermediate-, and high-density lipoproteins and chylomicrons, which transport cholesterol and other lipids.[145,146] ApoE, which serves as a ligand for receptor-mediated removal of lipoproteins from plasma, may play roles in immunoregulation and cell proliferation and differentiation.[146] ApoE is expressed at high levels in the liver and nervous system and is also the major apolipoprotein in human cerebrospinal fluid.[147,148] In the central nervous system, apoE is synthesized and secreted by astrocytes[149] and is up-regulated in response to neuronal damage and deafferentation.[150,151] Thus, ApoE is implicated in the growth and repair of the nervous system.

The three major structural alleles of apoE (i.e., E2, E3, and E4)[152-154] are products of a single gene. The E3 allele is the most common allele in the human population with an allelic frequency of 0.78, whereas the allelic frequency for E4 is 0.14. This allelic variation may be associated with significant differences in plasma low-density lipoprotein levels.[155] E2, with an allelic frequency 0.08, is the least common allele and is associated with increased risk of hyperlipoproteinemia.[156]

The mechanisms by which apoE4 is linked to the structural alterations that occur in AD are not known. *In vitro* binding studies[30] using synthetic amyloid Aβ peptide carried out in the presence of either apoE3 or apoE4 showed that the binding of Aβ was saturable at 0.1 mM peptide. However, the binding of apoE4 was much more rapid than that of apoE3 (minutes vs. hours). In addition, apoE3 bound Aβ from pH 7.6 to 4.6, whereas apoE4 failed to bind Aβ at pH <6.6. These results indicate differences in the two isoforms in binding to Aβ and suggest that isoform-specific effects may be involved in the pathogenesis of AD.

Immunocytochemical analysis also suggests a role for apoE in AD. Like antiserum to Aβ, antiserum to apoE labels amyloid plaques and vascular amyloid deposits in brain sections from aged lemurs and patients with AD.[157,158] Moreover, the presence of apoE immunoreactivity within some neurons has been interpreted to mean that apoE may be associated with NFT. Interestingly, the intensity of apoE staining of amyloid correlates with allele type. Brains from homozygous apoE4 patients with AD[143] showed more SP, apoE, and Aβ staining of congophilic angiopathy than did the brains from apoE3 homozygotes. Moreover, individuals with apoE4 AD showed greater numbers of SP than AD patients with one or no apoE4 allele.

VIII. ANIMAL MODELS

A. TRANSGENIC MICE

Transgenic strategies provide a unique opportunity to determine the mechanisms of Aβ deposition *in vivo*. Over the past few years, various laboratories have attempted to generate mouse models of AD using standard pronuclei injection-based transgenic technologies (Table 3).

TABLE 3   Published Reports of APP or Aβ Transgenic Mice

APP	Promotor	Levels of Transgenic mRNA	Levels of Transgenic Protein	Pathology	Ref.
APP-751	Neuron-specific enolase	+	?	Increased APP in neurons; ? extracellular deposits; ? A68 in neuronal processes	159
Aβ	~1.8 kb of human APP	1/50 of endogenous APP	Not examined	Clusters of intracytoplasmic inclusions visualized with a variety of polyclonal antibodies, including anti-Aβ, but immunoreactivity also seen in controls	160
C-100	Thy-1	+	Not detectable	NFT, neurites, and Aβ deposits reported but not reproducible (paper retracted)	161
C-100	Dystrophin	+	Not detectable	? Aβ deposits in cells and neuropil; thioflavin staining of some vessels	162
C-100	JC virus early region	+	?	Not detailed	163
C-99 with APP signal sequence	β-Actin (MSV enhancer)	+++	Twofold increase (14 kDa)	No pathology in brain at 13 months	Fukuchi and Martin (personal communication)
400 kb of APP	APP	Similar to endogenous	Similar to endogenous	Distribution of transgene products similar to endogenous; no pathology in one 3-month-old animal	95
Murine Aβ	Neuro filament NF-L	++	Not examined	Neuronal degeneration, apoptosis, gliosis, apparent Aβ deposits in neuropil	164
APP 717V→F	(PDGF)-β	++	++	Aβ deposits, Aβ plaques, dystrophic neurites, gliosis	165

These attempts to develop a model of Aβ deposition have utilized various transgenes, including the wild-type and mutated human APP gene or the sequence encoding the 4-kDa Aβ peptide, under the control of various promoters. Although several investigators have been able to establish a number of transgenic lines,[166,167] few of these animals manifest neuropathological changes relevant to AD.[159,164,165]

1. Mice Carrying APP Transgenes

Because the level of APP-751 mRNA was increased in subsets of affected neurons in AD,[168] Quon and colleagues[159] set out to test whether the overexpression of APP-751 could facilitate the formation of Aβ. They established mice that expressed a human APP-751 cDNA under the control of a neuron-specific enolase promoter. Although some extracellular Aβ deposits in hippocampus and cortex were documented in these mice, absolute levels of the transgene product were not determined.

Because it has been difficult to overexpress APP using conventional transgenic technologies, Lamb and co-workers[95] recently used yeast artificial chromosome-embryonic stem (YAC-ES) technologies to express human APP in mice. A 650-kb YAC containing the entire unrearranged 400-kb APP gene was transferred by lipid-mediated transfection into ES cells. Cells that expressed human APP were then introduced into mouse blastocytes to generate chimeric mice. Subsequent breeding efforts resulted in mice that harbor human sequences in the germline. Levels of transgene expression in the brain and peripheral tissues of these animals are approximately equivalent to the mouse endogenous APP level. These mice are still too young to be expected to develop Aβ deposits. However, these animals will be valuable for breeding to the apoE transgenic mice to test the hypothesis that multiple factors are necessary to produce neuropathological abnormalities.

Recently, Games et al.[165] reported that transgenic mice expressing high levels of human mutant APP (717V→F) develop extracellular thioflavin S-positive Aβ deposits as well as dystrophic neurites. The construct used to generate these mice utilized the platelet-derived growth factor (PDGF-β) promoter driving a human APP minigene encoding the APP (717V→F) mutation associated with familial AD. The construct contained APP introns 6 to 8, which allow alternative splicing of exons 7 and 8. Southern blots disclosed ~40 copies of the transgene inserted at a single site and transmitted in a stable fashion. Levels of human APP mRNA and proteins were significantly greater than endogenous; the three major splicing variants of APP were demonstrable. Significantly, levels of the transgene product were tenfold higher than endogenous mouse APP. Moreover, a 4-kDa Aβ-immunoreactive peptide was identified in the brains of these animals. By 8 months of age, Aβ deposits were seen in the hippocampus, corpus callosum, and cerebral cortex; these deposits increased in number over time. Deposits ranged from diffuse irregular types to compacted plaques with cores. Amyloid deposition was confirmed by thioflavin, Congo red, and Bielschowsky methods. Many SP showed glial fibrillary acid protein-positive astrocytes as well as microglial cells. NFT and tau-positive neurites were absent, although distorted neurites were often present in proximity to the SP. The densities of synapses and dendrites were reduced. To date, there have been no behavioral abnormalities documented nor have there been quantitative estimates of cell loss.

2. Mice Carrying a Transgene Encoding for Aβ

Several laboratories have generated mice harboring a transgene encoding the 4-kDa Aβ peptide with variable success as models of AD.[160-164] Mice reported by Wirak and colleagues[160] expressed the transgene at <0.02 the level of endogenous APP mRNA and showed small foci of Aβ immunoreactivity in hippocampus. However, wild-type C57BL/6J mice (the same strain used to generate these transgenic lines) also developed age-related clusters of intracytoplasmic inclusions in astrocytic processes that immunostain nonspecifically with a number of polyclonal antibodies, including Aβ antibodies. Recently, LaFerla and colleagues[164] have generated a line of mice carrying a transgene encoding for the murine homologue of Aβ1-42 under the control of the 68-kDa polypeptide neurofilament promoter (NF-L). Expression of the transgene was confirmed by Northern analysis and positive *in situ* hybridization in hippocampus and cerebral cortex. Neuropathological examination of these animals, which suffered seizures and died at higher rates than controls, showed extensive cell death, apoptosis, and intense gliosis in cerebral cortex and hippocampus. No SPs were identified by silver staining, but apparent extracellular Aβ immunostaining was detected in the neuropil.

B. AGED NONHUMAN PRIMATES
1. Behavioral and Cognitive Changes

At present, *Macaca mulatta*, with an estimated life span of >35 years, is the best available model for the age-associated behavioral and brain abnormalities that occur in aged humans and individuals with AD. This model is the most useful for examining the role of age in the pathogenesis of AD-type abnormalities. Behavioral investigations indicate that cognitive and memory deficits in rhesus monkeys appear late in the 2nd decade and become more evident in the mid to late twenties.[169-173] Interestingly, different aspects of cognition may decline at different rates. Impairments in performance of certain spatial abilities occur in some animals in their late teens; however, in other test categories (i.e., visual recognition memory task), behavior is not altered until the 3rd decade of life. Variations in performance among aged animals and among tasks are similar to those observed in aged humans.

2. Brain Abnormalities: Alterations in Specific Populations of Neurons and in Neurotransmitter Markers

In older rhesus monkeys, cholinergic and monoaminergic markers are reduced in some regions of cortex.[170,174-177] Cholinergic neurons are reduced in number in the medial septal nucleus.[178] Moreover, abnormal neurites in cortex are derived, in part, from cholinergic, monoaminergic, serotoninergic, GABAergic, and peptidergic neurons.[179-185] The brains of some older monkeys show decreased concentrations of dopamine and norepinephrine in certain regions of cortex.[174,175,177]

3. Dystrophic Neurites and Senile Plaques

These older monkeys also show more specific AD-type lesions.[48,170,186-190] The earliest structural changes in the parenchyma of cortex are slightly enlarged neurites (i.e., distal axons, nerve terminals, and dendrites) and preamyloid deposits.[48,86,88,184,186,191] Abnormal neurites often contain membranous elements, mitochondria (some degenerating), lysosomes, APP, phosphorylated neurofilaments, synaptophysin, and transmitter markers.[88] In individual SP, APP- and synaptophysin-immunoreactive neurites are often surrounded by a halo of distorted neuropil and Aβ immunoreactivity.[88] The presence of APP-like immunoreactivity in neuronal perikarya, axons, and neurites within Aβ-containing SP suggests that neurons can serve as one source for some Aβ deposits. Recent observations in the cerebral cortices of older macaques indicate that morphological abnormalities at synapses precede the accumulation of APP within neurites and extracellular Aβ deposits. Furthermore, these Aβ deposits are preceded by the appearance of nonfibrillar Aβ within neurons and glia.[190] In addition, the proximity of Aβ to reactive astrocytes and microglia and to vascular cells suggests that these populations of nonneuronal cells may participate in the formation of Aβ.[30,46,47,192-199] Consistent with this idea is the finding that α1-antichymotrypsin, the serine protease inhibitor that colocalizes with deposits of Aβ, is derived, in part, from astrocytes.[86,187,194,200]

IX. CONCLUSIONS

In the coming years, we envision that the efforts of scientists from diverse disciplines will contribute to unravel the genetic, cellular, and molecular mechanisms that underlie AD. The availability of transgenic animal models will allow faster testing of hypotheses for the pathogenesis of AD and the development of strategies to prevent or retard specific pathological processes (i.e., neuronal degeneration, Aβ deposits/senile plaques). Eventually, some of these strategies will reach the clinical arena for testing and use in patients with AD or, ideally, in nondemented subjects at high risk of developing the disease.

ACKNOWLEDGMENTS

This work was supported by grants from the U.S. Public Health Service (NS 20471, NS 07179, AG 05146), The Robert L. & Clara G. Patterson Trust, The Metropolitan Life Foundation, the American Health Assistance Foundation, the Charles A. Dana Foundation, the Alzheimer's Association, and funds from the Claster family. Dr. Price is the recipient of a Leadership and Excellence in Alzheimer's Disease (LEAD) award (NIA AG 07914) and a Javits Neuroscience Investigator Award (NIH NS 10580).

REFERENCES

1. Alzheimer, A., Über eine eigenartige Erkrankung der Hirnrinde, *Allg. Z. Psychiat. Psych.-Gerich. Med.* 64, 146, 1907.
2. Finger, S., *Origins of Neuroscience. A History of Explorations into Brain Function*, Oxford University Press, New York, 1994,
3. Blocq, P. and Marinesco, G., Sur les lésions et la pathogénie de l'épilepsie dite essentielle, *Sem. Med.,* 12, 445, 1892.
4. Randolph, M. and Semmes, J., Behavioral consequences of selective subtotal ablations in the postcentral gyrus of *Macaca mulatta*, *Brain Res.,* 70, 55, 1974.
5. Rothschild, D., Pathologic changes in senile psychoses and their psychobiologic significance, *Am. J. Psychiat.,* 93, 757, 1937.
6. Fischer, O., Miliare Nekrosen mit drusigen Wucherungen der Neurofibrillen, eine regelmässige Veränderung der Hirnrinde bei seniler Demenz, *Monatsschr. Psychiatr. Neurol.,* 22, 361, 1907.
7. Roth, M., Correlation between scores for dementia and counts of "senile plaques" in cerebral gray matter of elderly subjects, *Nature,* 209, 109, 1966.
8. Tomlinson, B. E., Blessed, G., and Roth, M., Observations on the brains of non-demented old people, *J. Neurol. Sci.,* 7, 331, 1968.
9. Roth, M., Tomlinson, B. E., and Blessed, G., Correlation between scores for dementia and counts of 'senile plaques' in cerebral grey matter of elderly subjects, *Nature,* 209, 109, 1966.
10. Tomlinson, B. E., Blessed, G., and Roth, M., Observations on the brains of demented old people, *J. Neurol. Sci.,* 11, 205, 1970.
11. Amaducci, L. and Lippi, A., Descriptive and analytic epidemiology of Alzheimer's disease, in *Alzheimer's Disease*, Maurer, K., Riederer, P., and Beckmann, H., Eds., Springer-Verlag, Vienna, 1990, 41.
12. Häfner, H., Epidemiology of Alzheimer's disease, in *Alzheimer's Disease. Epidemiology, Neuropathology, Neurochemistry, and Clinics*, Maurer, K., Riederer, P., and Beckmann, H., Eds., Springer-Verlag, Vienna, 1990, 23.
13. Ball, M. J., Neuronal loss, neurofibrillary tangles and granulovacuolar degeneration in the hippocampus with ageing and dementia. A qualitative study, *Acta Neuropathol.,* 37, 111, 1977.
14. Tomlinson, B. E., Irving, D., and Blessed, G., Cell loss in locus coeruleus in senile dementia of Alzheimer type, *J. Neurol. Sci.,* 49, 419, 1981.
15. Whitehouse, P. J., Price, D. L., Struble, R. G., Clark, A. W., Coyle, J. T., and DeLong, M. R., Alzheimer's disease and senile dementia: loss of neurons in the basal forebrain, *Science,* 215, 1237, 1982.
16. Hyman, B. T., Van Hoesen, G. W., Damasio, A. R., and Barnes, C. L., Alzheimer's disease: cell-specific pathology isolates the hippocampal formation, *Science,* 225, 1168, 1984.
17. Kemper, T., Neuroanatomical and neuropathological changes in normal aging and in dementia, in *Clinical Neurology of Aging*, Albert M. L., Ed., Oxford University Press, New York, 1984, 9.
18. West, M. J., Coleman, P. D., Flood, D. G., and Troncoso, J. C., Differences in the pattern of hippocampal neuronal loss in normal ageing and Alzheimer's disease, *Lancet,* 344, 769, 1994.
19. Davies, P. and Maloney, A. J. F., Selective loss of central cholinergic neurons in Alzheimer's disease, *Lancet,* 2, 1403, 1976.
20. Davies, P., Katzman, R., and Terry, R. D., Reduced somatostatin-like immunoreactivity in cerebral cortex from cases of Alzheimer's disease and Alzheimer senile dementia, *Nature,* 288, 279, 1980.
21. McGeer, P. L., McGeer, E. G., Suzuki, J., Dolman, C. E., and Nagai T., Aging, Alzheimer's disease, and the cholinergic system of the basal forebrain, *Neurology,* 34, 741, 1984.
22. Beal, M. F., Mazurek, M. F., Tran, V. T., Chattha, G., Bird, E. D., and Martin J. B., Reduced numbers of somatostatin receptors in the cerebral cortex in Alzheimer's disease, *Science,* 229, 289, 1985.

23. De Souza, E. B., Whitehouse, P. J., Kuhar, M. J., Price, D. L., and Vale, W. W., Reciprocal changes in corticotrophin-releasing factor (CRF)-like immunoreactivity and CRF receptors in cerebral cortex of Alzheimer's disease, *Nature,* 319, 593, 1986.

24. Kowall, N. W. and Beal M. F., Glutamate-, glutaminase-, and taurine-immunoreactive neurons develop neurofibrillary tangles in Alzheimer's disease, *Ann. Neurol.,* 29, 162, 1991.

25. Glenner, G. G. and Wong, C. W., Alzheimer's disease: initial report of the purification and characterization of a novel cerebrovascular amyloid protein. *Biochem. Biophys. Res. Commun.,* 120, 885, 1984.

26. St George-Hyslop, P. H., Tanzi, R. E., Polinsky, R. J., Haines, J. L., Nee, L., Watkins, P. C., Myers, R. H., Feldman, R. G., Pollen, D., Drachman, D., Growdon, J., Bruni, A., Foncin, J.-F., Salmon, D., Frommelt, P., Amaducci, L., Sorbi, S., Piacentini, S., Stewart, G. D., Hobbs, W. J., Conneally, P. M., and Gusella J. F., The genetic defect causing familial Alzheimer's disease maps on chromosome 21, *Science,* 235, 885, 1987.

27. Goate, A., Chartier-Harlin, M.-C., Mullan, M., Brown, J., Crawford, F., Fidani, L., Giuffra, L., Haynes, A., Irving, N., James, L., Mant, R., Newton, P., Rooke, K., Roques, P., Talbot, C., Pericak-Vance, M., Roses, A., Williamson, R., Rossor, M., Owen, M., and Hardy, J., Segregation of a missense mutation in the amyloid precursor protein gene with familial Alzheimer's disease, *Nature,* 349, 704, 1991.

28. Tanzi, R. E. and Hyman. B. T., Alzheimer's mutation, *Nature,* 350, 564, 1991.

29. Schellenberg, G. D., Payami, H., Wijsman, E. M., Orr, H. T., Goddard, K. A. B., Anderson, L, and Nemens E., Chromosome 14 and late-onset familial Alzheimer's disease (FAD), *Am. J. Hum. Genet.,* 53, 619, 1993.

30. Strittmatter, W. J., Saunders, A. M., Schmechel, D., Pericak-Vance, M., Enghild, J., Salvesen, G. S., and Roses, A. D. Apolipoprotein E: high-avidity binding to β-amyloid and increased frequency of type 4 allele in late-onset familial Alzheimer's disease, *Proc. Natl. Acad. Sci. U.S.A.,* 90, 1977, 1993.

31. Katzman, R., Terry, R., DeTeresa, R., Brown, T., Davies, P., Fuld, P., Renbing, X., and Peck, A., Clinical, pathological, and neurochemical changes in dementia: a subgroup with preserved mental status and numerous neocortical plaques, *Ann. Neurol.,* 23, 138, 1988.

32. Dickson, D. W., Crystal, H. A., Mattiace, L. A., Masur, D. M., Blau, A. D., Davies, P., Yen, S.-H., and Aronson M. K., Identification of normal and pathological aging in prospectively studied nondemented elderly humans, *Neurobiol. Aging,* 13, 179, 1991.

33. McKhann, G., Drachman, D., Folstein, M., Katzman, R., Price, D., and Stadlan, E. M., Clinical diagnosis of Alzheimer's disease: report of the NINCDS-ADRDA Work Group under the auspices of the Department of Health and Human Services Task Force on Alzheimer's Disease, *Neurology,* 34, 939, 1984.

34. Khachaturian, Z., Diagnosis of Alzheimer's disease, *Arch. Neurol.,* 42, 1097, 1985.

35. Mirra, S. S., Heyman, A., McKeel, D., Sumi, S. M., Crain, B. J., Brownlee, L. M., Vogel, F. S., Hughes, J. P., van Belle, G., Berg, L., and et al. The consortium to establish a registry for Alzheimer's disease (CERAD). II. Standardization of the neuropathologic assessment of Alzheimer's disease, *Neurology,* 41, 479, 1991.

36. Mirra, S. S., Hart, M. H., and Terry, R. D., Making the diagnosis of Alzheimer's disease. A primer for practicing pathologists, *Arch. Pathol. Lab. Med.,* 117, 132, 1993.

37. Arriagada, P. V., Growdon, J. H., Hedley-Whyte, E. T., and Hyman B. T., Neurofibrillary tangles but not senile plaques parallel duration and severity of Alzheimer's disease, *Neurology,* 42, 631, 1992.

38. Terry, R. D., Hansen, L. A., DeTeresa, R., Davies, P., Tobias, H., and Katzman, R., Senile dementia of the Alzheimer type without neocortical neurofibrillary tangles, *J. Neuropathol. Exp. Neurol.,* 46, 262, 1987.

39. Terry, R. D., Masliah, E., Salmon, D. P., Butters, N., DeTeresa, R., Hill, R., Hansen, L. A., and Katzman. R., Physical basis of cognitive alterations in Alzheimer's disease: synapse loss is the major correlate of cognitive impairment, *Ann. Neurol.,* 30, 572, 1991.

40. Berg, L. Clinical dementia rating (CDR), *Psychopharmacol. Bull.,* 24, 637, 1988.

41. Morris, J. C. and Fulling, K., Early Alzheimer's disease. Diagnostic considerations, *Arch. Neurol.,* 45, 345, 1988.

42. Troncoso, J. C., Martin, L. J., Dal Forno, G., and Kawas, C. H., Cognitive states and neuropathology in controls and demented subjects from the Baltimore Longitudinal study of aging, *Neurobiol. Aging,* 1995.

43. Grundke-Iqbal, I., Iqbal, K., Quinlan, M., Tung, Y.-C., Zaidi, M. S., and Wisniewski, H. M., Microtubule-associated protein tau. A component of Alzheimer paired helical filaments, *J. Biol. Chem.,* 261, 6084, 1986.

44. Goedert, M., Spillantini, M. G., Cairns, N. J., and Crowther, R. A., Tau proteins of Alzheimer paired helical filaments: abnormal phosphorylation of all six brain isoforms, *Neuron,* 8, 159, 1992.

45. Lee, V. M.-Y., Balin, B. J., Otvos, L., Jr., and Trojanowski. J. Q., A68: a major subunit of paired helical filaments and derivatized forms of normal tau, *Science,* 251, 675, 1991.

46. Wisniewski, H. M., Wegiel, J., Wang, K. C., Kujawa, M., and Lach, B., Ultrastructural studies of the cells forming amyloid fibers in classical plaques, *Can. J. Neurol. Sci.,* 16, 535, 1989.

47. Frackowiak, J., Wisniewski, H. M., Wegiel, J., Merz, G. S., Iqbal, K., and Wang. K. C., Ultrastructure of the microglia that phagocytose amyloid and the microglia that produce β-amyloid fibrils, *Acta Neuropathol.,* 84, 225, 1992.

48. Selkoe, D. J., Bell, D. S., Podlisny, M. B., Price, D. L., and Cork, L. C., Conservation of brain amyloid proteins in aged mammals and humans with Alzheimer's disease, *Science,* 235, 873, 1987.

49. Hyman, B. T., Van Hoesen, G. W., Kromer, L. J., and Damasio, A. R., Perforant pathway changes and the memory impairment of Alzheimer's disease, *Ann. Neurol.,* 20, 472, 1986.

50. D'Amato, R. J., Zweig, R. M., Whitehouse, P. J., Wenk, G. L., Singer, H. S., Mayeux, R., Price, D. L., and Snyder, S. H., Aminergic systems in Alzheimer's disease and Parkinson's disease, *Ann. Neurol.,* 22, 229, 1987.

51. Zweig, R. M., Ross, C. A., Hedreen, J. C., Steele, C., Cardillo, J. E., Whitehouse, P. J., Folstein, M. F., and Price, D. L., The neuropathology of aminergic nuclei in Alzheimer's disease, *Ann. Neurol.,* 24, 233, 1988.

52. Hyman, B. T., Van Hoesen, G. W., and Damasio, A. R., Memory-related neural systems in Alzheimer's disease: an anatomic study, *Neurology,* 40, 1721, 1990.

53. Vogels, O. J. M., Broere, C. A. J., Ter Laak, H. J., Ten Donkelaar, H. J. Nieuwenhuys, R., and Schultz, B. P. M., Cell loss and shrinkage in the nucleus basalis Meynert complex in Alzheimer's disease, *Neurobiol. Aging,* 11, 3, 1990.

54. Braak, H. and Braak, E., Alzheimer's disease affects limbic nuclei of the thalamus, *Acta Neuropathol.,* 81: 261, 1991.

55. Hardy, J., Cowburn, R., Barton, A., Reynolds, G., Lofdahl, E., O'Carroll, A.-M., Webster, P., and Winblad, B., Region-specific loss of glutamate innervation in Alzheimer's disease, *Neurosci. Lett.,* 73, 77, 1987.

56. Mann, D. M. A., Marcyniuk, B., Yates, P. O., Neary, D., and Snowden, J. S., The progression of the pathological changes of Alzheimer's disease in frontal and temporal neocortex examined both at biopsy and at autopsy, *Neuropathol. Appl. Neurobiol.,* 14, 177, 1988.

57. Braak, H. and Braak, E., Neuropathological stageing of Alzheimer-related changes, *Acta Neuropathol.,* 82, 239, 1991.

58. Rossor, M. N., Emson, P. C., Mountjoy, C. Q., Roth, M., and Iversen, L. L., Reduced amounts of immunoreactive somatostatin in the temporal cortex in senile dementia of Alzheimer type, *Neurosci. Lett.,* 20, 373, 1980.

59. Ferrier, I. N., Cross, A. J., Johnson, J. A., Roberts, G. W., Crow, T. J., Corsellis, J. A. N., Lee, Y. C., O'Shaughnessy, D., Adrian, T. E., McGregor, G. P., Baracese-Hamilton, A. J., and Bloom, S. R., Neuropeptides in Alzheimer type dementia, *J. Neurol. Sci.,* 62, 159, 1983.

60. Herzog, A. G. and Kemper, T. L., Amygdaloid changes in aging and dementia, *Arch. Neurol.,* 37, 625, 1980.

61. Scott, S. A., DeKosky, S. T., Sparks, D. L., Knox, C. A., and Scheff, S. W., Amygdala cell loss and atrophy in Alzheimer's disease, *Ann. Neurol.,* 32, 555, 1992.

62. De LaCoste, M.-C. and White, C. L., III., The role of cortical connectvity in Alzheimer's disease pathogenesis: a review and model system. *Neurobiol. Aging* 14, 1, 1993.

63. Lehmann, J., Struble, R. G., Antuono, P. G., Coyle, J. T., Cork, L. C., and Price, D. L., Regional heterogeneity of choline acetyltransferase activity in primate neocortex. *Brain Res.,* 322, 361, 1984.

64. Struble, R. G., Lehmann, J., Mitchell, S. J., McKinney, M., Price, D. L., Coyle, J. T., and DeLong, M. R., Basal forebrain neurons provide major cholinergic innervation of primate neocortex, *Neurosci. Lett.,* 66, 215, 1986.

65. Bondareff, W., Mountjoy, C. Q., and Roth, M., Loss of neurons of origin of the adrenergic projection to cerebral cortex (nucleus locus ceruleus) in senile dementia, *Neurology,* 32, 164, 1982.

66. Curcio, C. A. and Kemper, T., Nucleus raphe dorsalis in dementia of the Alzheimer type: neurofibrillary changes and neuronal packing density, *J. Neuropathol. Exp. Neurol.,* 43, 359, 1984.

67. Wolozin, B. L., Pruchnicki, A., Dickson, D. W., and Davies, P., A neuronal antigen in the brains of Alzheimer patients, *Science,* 232, 648, 1986.

68. Kosik, K. S., Orecchio, L. D., Binder, L., Trojanowski, J. Q., Lee, V. M.-Y., and Lee, G., Epitopes that span the tau molecule are shared with paired helical filaments, *Neuron,* 1, 817, 1988.

69. Brion, J.-P. Molecular pathology of Alzheimer amyloid and neurofibrillary tangles, *Semin. Neurosci.,* 2, 89, 1990.

70. Greenberg, S. G. and Davies, P., A preparation of Alzheimer paired helical filaments that displays distinct τ proteins by polyacrylamide gel electrophoresis, *Proc. Natl. Acad. Sci. U.S.A.,* 87, 5827, 1990.

71. Goedert, M., Sisodia, S. S., and Price, D. L., Neurofibrillary tangles and β-amyloid deposits in Alzheimer's disease, *Curr. Opin. Neurobiol.,* 1, 441, 1991.

72. Lee, V. M.-Y. and Trojanowski, J. Q., The disordered neuronal cytoskeleton in Alzheimer's disease, *Curr. Opin. Neurobiol.,* 2, 653, 1992.

73. Matsuo, E. S., Shin, R.-W., Billingsley, M. L., Van de Voorde, A., O'Connor, M., Trojanowski, J. Q., and Lee, V. M.-Y., Biopsy-derived adult human brain tau is phosphorylated at many of the same sites as Alzheimer's disease paired helical filament tau, *Neuron,* 13, 989, 1994.

74. Grunke-Iqbal, I., Iqbal, K., Tung, Y.-C., Quinlin, M., Wisniewski, H. M., Binder, L. I., Abnormal phosphorylation of the microtubule-associated protein τ (tau) in Alzheimer cytoskeletal pathology, *Proc. Natl. Acad. Sci., U.S.A,.* 83, 4913, 1986.

75. Anderton, B. H., Breinburg, D., Downes, M. J., Green, P. J., Tomlinson, B. E., Ulrich, J., Wood, J. N., and Kahn, J., Monoclonal antibodies show that neurofibrillary tangles and neurofilaments share antigenic determinants, *Nature,* 298, 84, 1982.

76. Masters, C. L., Multhaup, G., Simms, G., Pottgiesser, J., Martins, R. N., and Beyreuther, K., Neuronal origin of a cerebral amyloid: neurofibrillary tangles of Alzheimer's disease contain the same protein as the amyloid of plaque cores and blood vessels, *EMBO J.,* 4, 2757, 1985.

77. Cork, L. C., Sternberger, N. H., Sternberger, L. A., Casanova, M. F., Struble, R. G., and Price, D. L., Phosphorylated neurofilament antigens in neurofibrillary tangles in Alzheimer's disease, *J. Neuropathol. Exp. Neurol.,* 45, 56, 1986.

78. Kosik, K. S., Joachim, C. L., and Selkoe, D. J., Microtubule-associated protein (tau) is a major antigenic component of paired helical filaments in Alzheimer's disease, *Proc. Natl. Acad. Sci. U.S.A.* 83, 4044, 1986.

79. Perry, G., Friedman, R., Shaw, G., and Chau, V., Ubiquitin is detected in neurofibrillary tangles and senile plaque neurites of Alzheimer's disease brains, *Proc. Natl. Acad. Sci. U.S.A.,* 84, 3033, 1987.

80. Wischik, C. M., Novak, M., Thogersen, H. C., Edwards, P. C., Runswick, M. J., Jakes, R., Walker, J. E., Milstein, C., Roth, M., and Klug, A., Isolation of a fragment of tau derived from the core of the paired helical filament of Alzheimer's disease, *Proc. Natl. Acad. Sci. U.S.A.*, 85, 4506, 1988.

81. Lovell, M. A., Ehmann, W. D., and Markesbery, W. R., Laser microprobe analysis of brain aluminum in Alzheimer's disease, *Ann. Neurol.*, 33, 36, 1993.

82. Good, P. F., Perl, D. P., Bierer, L. M., and Schmeidler, J., Selective accumulation of aluminum and iron in the neurofibrillary tangles of Alzheimer's disease: a laser microprobe (LAMMA) study, *Ann. Neurol.*, 31, 286, 1992.

83. Shin, R.-W., Lee, V. M.-Y., and Trojanowski, J. Q., Aluminum modifies the properties of Alzheimer's disease PHFτ proteins *in vivo* and *in vitro*, *J. Neurosci.*, 14, 7221, 1994.

84. Wisniewski, H. M. and Terry, R. D., Reexamination of the pathogenesis of the senile plaque, in *Progress in Neuropathology*, Zimmerman, H. M., Ed., Grune & Stratton, New York, 1973, 1.

85. Armstrong, D. M., Bruce, G., Hersh, L. B., and Terry, R. D., Choline acetyltransferase immunoreactivity in neuritic plaques of Alzheimer brain, *Neurosci. Lett.*, 71, 229, 1986.

86. Cork, L. C., Masters, C., Beyreuther, K., and Price, D. L., Development of senile plaques. Relationships of neuronal abnormalities and amyloid deposits. *Am. J. Pathol.*, 137, 1383, 1990.

87. Cras, P., Kawai, M., Lowery, D., Gonzalez-DeWhitt, P., Greenberg, B., and Perry, G., Senile plaque neurites in Alzheimer's disease accumulate amyloid precursor protein, *Proc. Natl. Acad. Sci. U.S.A.*, 88, 7552, 1991.

88. Martin, L. J., Sisodia, S. S., Koo, E. H., Cork, L. C., Dellovade, T. L., Weidemann, A., Beyreuther, K., Masters, C., and Price, D. L., Amyloid precursor protein in aged nonhuman primates, *Proc. Natl. Acad. Sci. U.S.A.*, 88, 1461, 1991.

89. McKee, A. C., Kosik, K. S., and Kowall, N. W., Neuritic pathology and dementia in Alzheimer's disease, *Ann. Neurol.*, 30, 156, 1991.

90. Perry, G., Kawai, M., Tabaton, M., Onorato, M., Mulvihill, P., Richey, P., Morandi, A., Connolly, J. A., and Gambetti. P., Neuropil threads of Alzheimer's disease show a marked alteration of the normal cytoskeleton, *J. Neurosci.*, 11, 1748, 1991.

91. Masliah, E., Ellisman, M., Carragher, B., Mallory, M., Young, S., Hansen, L., DeTeresa, R., and Terry, R. D., Three-dimensional analysis of the relationship between synaptic pathology and neuropil threads in Alzheimer's disease, *J. Neuropathol. Exp. Neurol.*, 51, 404, 1992.

92. Masliah, E., Mallory, M., Hansen, L., Alford, M., Albright, T., DeTeresa, R., Terry, R., Baudier, J., and Saitoh, T., Patterns of aberrant sprouting in Alzheimer's disease, *Neuron*, 6, 729, 1991.

93. Arnold, S. E., Hyman, B. T., Flory, J., Damasio, A. R., and Van Hoesen, G. W., The topographical and neuroanatomical distribution of neurofibrillary tangles and neuritic plaques in the cerebral cortex of patients with Alzheimer's disease, *Cereb. Cortex*, 1, 103, 1991.

94. Roher, A., Wolfe, D., Palutke, M., and KuKurga, D., Purification, ultrastructure, and chemical analysis of Alzheimer's disease amyloid plaque core protein, *Proc. Natl. Acad. Sci. U.S.A.*, 83, 2662, 1986.

95. Lamb, B. T., Sisodia, S. S., Lawler, A. M., Slunt, H. H., Kitt, C. A., Kearns, W. G., Pearson, P. L., Price, D. L., and Gearhart, J. D., Introduction and expression of the 400 kilobase *precursor amyloid protein* gene in transgenic mice, *Nat. Genet.*, 5, 22, 1993.

96. Kang, J., Lemaire, H.-G., Unterbeck, A., Salbaum, J. M., Masters, C. L., Grzeschik, K.-H., Multhaup, G., Beyreuther, K., and Müller-B., Hill, The precursor of Alzheimer's disease amyloid A4 protein resembles a cell-surface receptor, *Nature*, 325, 733, 1987.

97. Kitaguchi, N., Takahashi, Y., Tokushima, Y., Shiojiri, S., and Ito, H., Novel precursor of Alzheimer's disease amyloid protein shows protease inhibitory activity, *Nature*, 331, 530, 1988.

98. Ponte, P., Gonzalez-DeWhitt, P., Schilling, J., Miller, J., Hsu, D., Greenberg, B., Davis, K., Wallace, W., Lieberburg, I., Fuller, F., and Cordell, B., A new A4 amyloid mRNA contains a domain homologous to serine proteinase inhibitors, *Nature*, 331, 525, 1988.

99. Tanzi, R. E., McClatchey, A. I., Lampert, E. D., Villa-Komaroff, L., Gusella, J. F., and Neve, R. L., Protease inhibitor domain encoded by an amyloid protein precursor mRNA associated with Alzheimer's disease, *Nature*, 331, 528, 1988.

100. König, G., Mönning, U., Czech, C., Prior, R., Banati, R., Schreiter-Gasser, U., Bauer, J., Masters, C. L., and Beyreuther, K., Identification and differential expression of a novel alternative splice isoform of the βA4 amyloid precursor protein (APP) mRNA in leukocytes and brain microglial cells, *J. Biol. Chem.*, 267, 10804, 1992.

101. Rosen, D. R., Martin-Morris, L., Luo, L., and White, K., A *Drosophila* gene encoding a protein resembling the human-amyloid protein precursor, *Proc. Natl. Acad. Sci. U.S.A.*, 86, 2478, 1989.

102. Daigle, I. and Li, C., *Apl-1* a *Caenorhabditis elegans* gene encoding a protein related to the human β-amyloid protein precursor, *Proc. Natl. Acad. Sci. U.S.A.*, 90, 12045, 1993.

103. Wasco, W., Bupp, K., Magendantz, M., Gusella, J. F., Tanzi, R. E., and Solomon, F., Identification of a mouse brain cDNA that encodes a protein related to the Alzheimer's disease-associated amyloid-beta-protein precursor, *Proc. Natl. Acad. Sci. U.S.A.*, 89, 10758, 1992.

104. Wasco, W., Gurubhagavatula, S., Paradis, M. D., Romano, D. M., Sisodia, S. S., Hyman, B. T., Neve, R. L., and Tanzi, R. E., Isolation and characterization of *APLP2* encoding a homologue of the Alzheimer's associated amyloid β protein precursor, *Nature Genet.*, 5, 95, 1993.

105. Sprecher, C. A., Grant, F. J., Grimm, G., O'Hara, P. J., Norris, F., Norris, K., and Foster, D. C., Molecular cloning of the cDNA for a human amyloid precursor protein homolog: evidence for a multigene family, *Biochemistry*, 32, 4481, 1993.

106. Slunt, H. H., Thinakaran, G., von Koch, C., Lo, A. C. Y., Tanzi, R. E., and Sisodia. S. S., Expression of a ubiquitous, cross-reactive homologue of the mouse β-amyloid precursor protein (APP), *J. Biol. Chem.*, 269, 2637, 1994.

107. Schubert, D., Jin, L.-W., Saitoh, T., and Cole, G., The regulation of amyloid β protein precursor secretion and its modulatory role in cell adhesion, *Neuron*, 3, 689, 1989.

108. Saitoh, T., Sundsmo, M., Roch, J.-M., Kimura, T., Cole, G., Schubert, D., Oltersdorf, T., and Schenk, D. B., Secreted form of amyloid β protein precursor is involved in the growth regulation of fibroblasts, *Cell*, 58, 615, 1989.

109. Klier, F. G., Cole, G., Stalleup, W., and Schubert, D., Amyloid β-protein precursor is associated with extracellular matrix, *Brain Res.*, 515, 336, 1990.

110. Nishimoto, I., Okamoto, T., Matsuura, Y., Takahashi, S., Murayama, S., and Ogata, E., Alzheimer amyloid protein precursor complexes with brain GTP-binding protein G_o, *Nature*, 362, 75, 1993.

111. Oltersdorf, T., Fritz, L. C., Schenk, D. B., Lieburg, I., Johnson-Wood, K. L., Beattie, E. C., Ward, P. J., Blacher, R. W., Dovey, H. F., and Sinha, S., The secreted form of the Alzheimer's amyloid precursor protein with the Kunitz domain is protease nexin-II, *Nature*, 341, 144, 1989.

112. Smith, R. P., Higuchi, D. A., and Broze, G. J., Jr., Platelet coagulation factor XI_a-inhibitor, a form of Alzheimer amyloid precursor protein, *Science*, 248, 1126, 1990.

113. Van Nostrand, W. E., Schmaier, A. H., Farrow, J. S., and Cunningham, D. D., Protease nexin-II (amyloid-protein precursor): a platelet-granule protein, *Science*, 248, 745, 1990.

114. Weidemann, A., König, G., Bunke, D., Fischer, P., Salbaum, J. M., Masters, C. L., and Beyreuther, K., Identification, biogenesis, and localization of precursors of Alzheimer's disease A4 amyloid protein, *Cell*, 57, 115, 1989.

115. Hung, A. Y. and Selkoe, D. J., Selective ectodomain phosphorylation and regulated cleavage of β-amyloid precursor protein, *EMBO J.*, 13, 534, 1994.

116. Caporaso, G. L., Takei, K., Gandy, S. E., Matteoli, M., Mundigl, O., Greengard, P., and De Camilli, P., Morphologic and biochemical analysis of the intracellular trafficking of the Alzheimer β/A4 amyloid precursor protein, *J. Neurosci.*, 14, 3122, 1994.

117. Haass, C., Koo, E. H., Mellon, A., Hung, A. Y., and Selkoe, D. J., Targeting of cell-surface β-amyloid precursor protein to lysosomes: alternative processing into amyloid-bearing fragments, *Nature*, 357, 500, 1992.

118. Sisodia, S. S., β-Amyloid precursor protein cleavage by a membrane-bound protease, *Proc. Natl. Acad. Sci. U.S.A.*, 89, 6075, 1992.

119. Esch, F. S., Keim, P. S., Beattie, E. C., Blacher, R. W., Culwell, A. R., Oltersdorf, T., McClure, D., and Ward, P. J., Cleavage of amyloid β peptide during constitutive processing of its precursor, *Science*, 248, 1122, 1990.

120. Sisodia, S. S., Koo, E. H., Beyreuther, K., Unterbeck, A., and Price, D. L., Evidence that β-amyloid protein in Alzheimer's disease is not derived by normal processing, *Science*, 248, 492, 1990.

121. Anderson, J. P., Esch, F. S., Keim, P. S., Sambamurti, K., Lieburg, I., and Robakis, N. K., Exact cleavage site of Alzheimer amyloid precursor in neuronal PC-12 cells, *Neurosci. Lett.*, 128, 126, 1991.

122. Wang, R., Meschia, J. F., Cotter, R. J., and Sisodia, S. S., Secretion of the β/A4 amyloid precursor protein. Identification of a cleavage site in cultured mammalian cells, *J. Biol. Chem.*, 266, 16960, 1991.

123. Pasternack, J. M., Palmert, M. R., Usiak, M., Wang, R., Zurcher-Neely, H., Gonzalez-DeWhitt, P. A., Fairbanks, M. B., Cheung, T., Blades, D., Heinrikson, R. L., Greenberg, B. D., Cotter, R. J., and Younkin, S. G., Alzheimer's disease and control brain contain soluble derivatives of the amyloid protein precursor that end within the β amyloid protein region, *Biochemistry*, 31, 10936, 1992.

124. Golde, T. E., Estus, S., Younkin, L. H., Selkoe, D. J., and Younkin, S. G., Processing of the amyloid protein precursor to potentially amyloidogenic derivatives, *Science*, 255, 728, 1992.

125. Haass, C., Schlossmacher, M. G., Hung, A. Y., Vigo-Pelfrey, C., Mellon, A., Ostaszewski, B. L., Lieburg, I., Koo, E. H., Schenk, D., Teplow, D. B., and Selkoe, D. J., Amyloid β-peptide is produced by cultured cells during normal metabolism, *Nature*, 359, 322, 1992.

126. Seubert, P., Vigo-Pelfrey, C., Esch, F., Lee, M., Dovey, H., Davis, D., Sinha, S., Schlossmacher, M., Whaley, J., Swindlehurst, C., McCormack, R., Wolfert, R., Selkoe, D., Lieburg, I., and Schenk D., Isolation and quantification of soluble Alzheimer's β-peptide from biological fluids, *Nature*, 359, 325, 1992.

127. Shoji, M., Golde, T. E., Ghiso, J., Cheung, T. T., Estus, S., Shaffer, L. M., Cai, X.-D., McKay, D. M., Tintner, R., Frangione, B., and Younkin, S. G., Production of the Alzheimer amyloid β protein by normal proteolytic processing, *Science*, 258, 126, 1992.

128. Busciglio, J., Gabuzda, D. H., Matsudaira, P., and Yankner, B. A., Generation of β-amyloid in the secretory pathway in neuronal and nonneuronal cells, *Proc. Natl. Acad. Sci. U.S.A.*, 90, 2092, 1993.

129. Masters, C. L., Simms, G., Weinman, N. A., Multhaup, G., McDonald, B. L., and Beyreuther, K., Amyloid plaque core protein in Alzheimer's disease and Down syndrome, *Proc. Natl. Acad. Sci. U.S.A.*, 82, 4245, 1985.

130. Iwatsubo, T., Odaka, A., Suzuki, N., Mizusawa, H., Nukina, N., and Ihara, Y., Visualization of Aβ42(43)-positive and Aβ40-positive senile plaques with end-specific Aβ-monoclonal antibodies: evidence that an initially deposited Aβ species is Aβ1-42(43), *Neuron*, in press.

131. Jarrett, J. T. and Lansbury, P. T., Jr., Seeding "one-dimensional crystallization" of amyloid: a pathogenic mechanism in Alzheimer's disease and scrapie?, *Cell*, 73, 1055, 1993.

132. Chartier-Harlin, M.-C., Crawford, F., Houlden, H., Warren, A., Hughes, D., Fidani, L., Goate, A., Rossor, M., Roques, P., Hardy, J., and Mullan, M., Early-onset Alzheimer's disease caused by mutations at codon 717 of the β-amyloid precursor protein gene, *Nature*, 353, 844, 1991.

133. Naruse, S., Igarashi, S., Kobayashi, H., Aoki, K., Inuzuka, T., Kaneko, K., Shimizu, T., Iihara, K., Kojima, T., Miyatake, T., and Tsuji, S., Mis-sense mutation Val→Ile in exon 17 of amyloid precursor protein gene in Japanese familial Alzheimer's disease, *Lancet*, 337, 978, 1991.

134. Suzuki, N., Cheung, T. T., Cai, X.-D., Odaka, A., Otvos, L., Jr., Eckman, C., Golde, T. E., and Younkin, S. G., An increased percentage of long amyloid β protein secreted by familial amyloid β protein precursor (βAPP_{717}) mutants, *Science*, 264, 1336, 1994.

135. Haass, C., Hung, A. Y., Schlossmacher, M. G., Teplow, D. B., and Selkoe, D. J., β-Amyloid peptide and a 3-kDa fragment are derived by distinct cellular mechanisms, *J. Biol. Chem.*, 268, 3021, 1993.

136. Citron, M., Oltersdorf, T., Haass, C., McConlogue, L., Hung, A. Y., Seubert, P., Vigo-Pelfrey, C., Lieberburg, I., and Selkoe, D. J., Mutation of the β-amyloid precursor protein in familial Alzheimer's disease increases β-protein production, *Nature*, 360, 672, 1992.

137. Koo, E. H. and Squazzo, S. L., Evidence that production and release of amyloid β-protein involves the endocytic pathway, *J. Biol. Chem.*, 269, 17386, 1994.

138. Wertkin, A. M., Turner, R. S., Pleasure, S. J., Golde, T. E., Younkin, S. G., Trojanowski, J. Q., and Lee, V. M.-Y., Human neurons derived from a teratocarcinoma cell line express solely the 695-amino acid amyloid precursor protein and produce intracellular β-amyloid or A4 peptides, *Proc. Natl. Acad. Sci. U.S.A.*, 90, 9513, 1993.

139. Haass, C. and Selkoe, D. J., Cellular processing of β-amyloid precursor and the genesis of amyloid β-peptide, *Cell*, 75, 1039, 1993.

140. Wisniewski, T. and Frangione, B., Apolipoprotein E: a pathological chaperone protein in patients with cerebral and systemic amyloid, *Neurosci. Lett.*, 135, 235, 1992.

141. Ghiso, J., Matsubara, E., Koudinov, A., Choi-Miura, N. H., Tomita, M., Wisniewski, T., and Frangione, B., The cerebrospinal-fluid soluble form of Alzheimer's amyloid beta is complexed to SP-40,40 (apolipoprotein J), and inhibitor of the complement membrane-attack complex, *Biochem. J.*, 293, 27, 1993.

142. Corder, E. H., Saunders, A. M., Strittmatter, W. J., Schmechel, D. E., Gaskell, P. C., Small, G. W., Roses, A. D., Haines, J. L., and Pericak-Vance, M. A., Gene dose of apolipoprotein-E type 4 allele and the risk of Alzheimer's disease in late onset families, *Science*, 261, 921, 1993.

143. Rebeck, G. W., Reiter, J. S., Strickland, D. K., and Hyman, B. T., Apolipoprotein E in sporadic Alzheimer's disease: allelic variation and receptor interactions, *Neuron*, 11, 575, 1993.

144. Maestre, G., Ottman, R., Stern, Y., Gurland, B., Chun, M., Tang, M.-X., Shelanski, M., Tycko, B., and Mayeux, R., Apolipoprotein E and Alzheimer's disease: ethnic variation in genotypic risks, *Neurol.*, 37, 254, 1995.

145. Breslow, J. L., Human apolipoprotein molecular biology and genetic variation, *Annu. Rev. Biochem.*, 54, 699, 1985.

146. Mahley, R. W., Apolipoprotein E: cholesterol transport protein with expanding role in cell biology, *Science*, 240, 622, 1988.

147. Roheim, P. S., Carey, M., Forte, T., and Vega, G. L., Apolipoproteins in human cerebrospinal fluid, *Proc. Natl. Acad. Sci. U.S.A.*, 76, 4646, 1979.

148. Pitas, R. E., Boyles, J. K., Lee, S. H., Hui, D., and Weisgraber, K. H., Lipoproteins and their receptors in the central nervous system, *J. Biol. Chem.*, 262, 14352, 1987.

149. Pitas, R. E., Boyles, J. K., Lee, S. H., Foss, D., and Mahley, R. W., Astrocytes synthesize apolipoprotein E and metabolize apolipoprotein E-containing lipoproteins, *Biochim. Biophys. Acta*, 917, 148, 1987.

150. Ignatius, M. J., Gebicke-Härter, P. J., Pate Skene, J. H., Schilling, J. W., Weisgraber, K. H., Mahley, R. W., and Shooter, E. M., Expression of apolipoprotein E during nerve degeneration and regeneration, *Proc. Natl. Acad. Sci. U.S.A.*, 83, 1125, 1986.

151. Snipes, G. J., McGuire, C. B., Norden, J. J., and Freeman, J. A., Nerve injury stimulates the secretion of apolipoprotein E by nonneuronal cells, *Proc. Natl. Acad. Sci. U.S.A.*, 83, 1130, 1986.

152. Utermann, G., Langenbeck, U., Beisiegel, U., and Weber, W., Genetics of the apolipoprotein E system in man, *Am. J. Hum. Genet.*, 32, 339, 1980.

153. Utermann, G., Steinmetz, A., and Weber, W., Genetic control of human apolipoprotein E polymorphism: comparison of one- and two-dimensional techniques of isoprotein analysis, *Hum. Genet.*, 60, 344, 1982.

154. Zannis, V. I., Breslow, J. L., Utermann, G., Mahley, R. W., Weisgraber, K. H., Havel, R. J., Goldstein, J. L., Brown, M. S., Schonfeld, G., Hazzard, W. R., and Blum, C., Proposed nomenclature of apoE isoproteins, apoE genotypes, and phenotypes, *J. Lipid Res.*, 23, 911, 1982.

155. Davignon, J., Gregg, R. E., and Sing, C. F., Apolipoprotein E polymorphism and atherosclerosis, *Arteriosclerosis*, 8, 1, 1988.

156. Weintraub, M. S., Eisenberg, S., and Breslow, J. L., Different patterns of postprandial lipoprotein metabolism in normal, type IIa, type III, and type IV hyperlipoproteinemic individuals, *J. Clin. Invest.*, 79, 1110, 1987.

157. Namba, Y., Tomonaga, M., Kawasaki, H., Otomo, E., and Ikeda, K., Apolipoprotein E immunoreactivity in cerebral amyloid deposits and neurofibrillary tangles in Alzheimer's disease and kuru plaque amyloid in Creutzfeldt-Jakob disease, *Brain Res.,* 541, 163, 1991.
158. Strittmatter, W. J., Weisgraber, K. H., Huang, D. Y., Dong, L.-M., Salvesen, G. S., Pericak-Vance, M., Schmechel, D., Saunders, A. M., Goldgaber, D., and Roses, A. D., Binding of human apolipoprotein E to synthetic amyloid β peptide: isoform-specific effects and implications for late-onset Alzheimer's disease, *Proc. Natl. Acad. Sci. U.S.A.,* 90, 8098, 1993.
159. Quon, D., Wang, Y., Catalano, R., Scardina, J. M., Murakami, K., and Cordell, B., Formation of β-amyloid protein deposits in brains of transgenic mice, *Nature,* 352, 239, 1991.
160. Wirak, D. O., Bayney, R., Ramabhadran, T. V., Fracasso, R. P., Hart, J. T., Hauer, P. E., Hsiau, P., Pekar, S. K., Scangos, G. A., Trapp, B. D., and Unterbeck, A. J., Deposits of amyloid β protein in the central nervous system of transgenic mice, *Science,* 253, 323, 1991.
161. Kawabata, S., Higgins, G. A., and Gordon, J. W., Amyloid plaques, neurofibrillary tangles and neuronal loss in brains of transgenic mice overexpressing a C-terminal fragment of human amyloid precursor protein, *Nature,* 354, 476, 1991.
162. Kammesheidt, A., Boyce, F. M., Spanoyannis, A. F., Cummings, B. J., Ortegón, M., Cotman, C., Vaught, J. L., and Neve, R. L., Deposition of β/A4 immunoreactivity and neuronal pathology in transgenic mice expressing the carboxyterminal fragment of the Alzheimer amyloid precursor in the brain, *Proc. Natl. Acad. Sci. U.S.A.,* 10857, 1992.
163. Sandhu, F. A., Salim, M., and Zain, S. B., Expression of the human β-amyloid protein of Alzheimer's disease specifically in the brains of transgenic mice, *J. Biol. Chem.,* 266, 21331, 1991.
164. LaFerla, F. M., Tinkle, B. T., Bieberich, C. J., Haudenschild, C. C., and Jay, G., The Alzheimer's Aβ peptide induces neurodegeneration and apoptotic cell death in transgenic mice, *Nat. Genet.,* 9, 21, 1995.
165. Games, D., Adams, D., Alessandrini, R., Barbour, R., Berthelette, P., Blackwell, C., Carr, T., Clemens, J., Donaldson, T., Gillespie, F., Guido, T., Hagopian, S., Johnson-Wood, K., Khan, K., Lee, M., Leibowitz, P., Lieberburg, I., Little, S., Masliah, E., McConlogue, L., Montoya-Zavala, M., Mucke, L., Paganini, L., Penniman, E., Power, M., Schenk, D., Seubert, P., Snyder, B., Soriano, F., Tan, H., Vitale, J., Wadsworth, S., Wolozin, B., and Zhao, J., Alzheimer-type neuropathology in transgenic mice overexpressing V717F β-amyloid precursor protein, *Nature,* 373, 523, 1995.
166. Sisodia, S. S. and Price, D. L., Amyloidogenesis in Alzheimer's disease: basic biology and animal models, *Curr. Opin. Neurobiol.,* 2, 648, 1992.
167. Price, D. L. and Sisodia, S. S., Cellular and molecular biology of Alzheimer's disease and animal models, *Annu. Rev. Med.,* 45, 435, 1994.
168. Johnson, S. A., McNeill, T., Cordell, B., and Finch, C. E., Relation of neuronal APP-751/APP-695 mRNA ratio and neuritic plaque density in Alzheimer's disease, *Science,* 248, 854, 1990.
169. Presty, S. K., Bachevalier, J., Walker, L. C., Struble, R. G., Price, D. L., Mishkin, M., and Cork, L. C., Age differences in recognition memory of the rhesus monkey (Macaca mulatta), *Neurobiol. Aging,* 8, 435, 1987.
170. Walker, L. C., Kitt, C. A., Struble, R. G., Wagster, M. V., Price, D. L., and Cork, L. C., The neural basis of memory decline in aged monkeys, *Neurobiol. Aging,* 9, 657, 1988.
171. Rapp, P. R. and Amaral, D. G., Evidence for task-dependent memory dysfunction in the aged monkey, *J. Neurosci.,* 9, 3568, 1989.
172. Bachevalier, J., Landis, L. S., Walker, L. C., Brickson, M., Mishkin, M., Price, D. L., and Cork, L. C., Aged monkeys exhibit behavioral deficits indicative of widespread cerebral dysfunction, *Neurobiol. Aging,* 12, 99, 1991.
173. Rapp, P. R. and Amaral, D. G., Recognition memory deficits in a subpopulation of aged monkeys resemble the effects of medial temporal lobe damage, *Neurobiol. Aging,* 12, 481, 1991.
174. Goldman-Rakic, P. S. and Brown, R. M., Regional changes of monoamines in cerebral cortex and subcortical structures of aging rhesus monkeys, *Neuroscience,* 6, 177, 1981.
175. Wenk, G. L., Pierce, D. J., Struble, R. G., Price, D. L., and Cork, L. C., Age-related changes in multiple neurotransmitter systems in the monkey brain, *Neurobiol. Aging,* 10, 11, 1989.
176. Wagster, M. V., Whitehouse, P. J., Walker, L. C., Kellar, K. J., and Price, D. L., Laminar organization and age-related loss of cholinergic receptors in temporal neocortex of rhesus monkey, *J. Neurosci.,* 10, 2879, 1990.
177. Beal, M. F., Walker, L. C., Storey, E., Segar, L., Price, D. L., and Cork, L. C., Neurotransmitters in neocortex of aged rhesus monkeys, *Neurobiol. Aging,* 12, 407, 1991.
178. Stroessner-Johnson, H. M., Rapp, P. R., and Amaral, D. G., Cholinergic cell loss and hypertrophy in the medial septal nucleus of the behaviorally characterized aged rhesus monkey, *J. Neurosci.,* 12, 1936, 1992.
179. Kitt, C. A., Price, D. L., Struble, R. G., Cork, L. C., Wainer, B. H., Becher, M. W., and Mobley, W. C., Evidence for cholinergic neurites in senile plaques, *Science,* 226, 1443, 1984.
180. Struble, R. G., Hedreen, J. C., Cork, L. C., and Price, D. L., Acetylcholinesterase activity in senile plaques of aged macaques, *Neurobiol. Aging,* 5, 191, 1984.
181. Kitt, C. A., Struble, R. G., Cork, L. C., Mobley, W. C., Walker, L. C., Joh, T. H., and Price, D. L., Catecholaminergic neurites in senile plaques in prefrontal cortex of aged nonhuman primates, *Neuroscience,* 16, 691, 1985.
182. Walker, L. C., Kitt, C. A., Struble, R. G., Schmechel, D. E., Oertel, W. H., Cork, L. C., and Price, D. L., Glutamic acid decarboxylase-like immunoreactive neurites in senile plaques, *Neurosci. Lett.,* 59, 165, 1985.

183. Walker, L. C., Kitt, C. A., Schwam, E., Buckwald, B., Garcia, F., Sepinwall, J., and Price, D. L., Senile plaques in aged squirrel monkeys, *Neurobiol. Aging*, 8, 291, 1987.

184. Walker, L. C., Kitt, C. A., Cork, L. C., Struble, R. G., Dellovade, T. L., and Price, D. L., Multiple transmitter systems contribute neurites to individual senile plaques, *J. Neuropathol. Exp. Neurol.*, 47, 138, 1988.

185. Kitt, C. A., Walker, L. C., Molliver, M. E., and Price, D. L., Serotoninergic neurites in senile plaques in cingulate cortex of aged nonhuman primate, *Synapse*, 3, 12, 1989.

186. Struble, R. G., Price, Jr., Cork, L. C., and Price, D. L., Senile plaques in cortex of aged normal monkeys, *Brain Res.*, 361, 267, 1985.

187. Abraham, C. R., Selkoe, D. J., Potter, H., Price, D. L., and Cork, L. C., α_1-antichymotrypsin is present together with the β-proten in monkey brain amyloid deposits, *Neuroscience*, 32, 715, 1989.

188. Price, D. L., Martin, L. J., Sisodia, S. S., Wagster, M. V., Walker, L. C., Koliatsos, V. E., and Cork, L. C., Aged nonhuman primates: an animal model of age-associated neurodegenerative disease, *Brain Pathol.*, 1, 287, 1991.

189. Price, D. L., Martin, L. J., Clatterbuck, R. E., Koliatsos, V. E., Sisodia, S. S., Walker, L. C., and Cork, L. C., Neuronal degeneration in human diseases and animal models, *J. Neurobiol.*, 23 1277, 1992.

190. Martin, L. J., Pardo, C. A., Cork, L. C., and Price, D. L., Synaptic pathology and glial responses to neuronal injury precede the formation of senile plaques and amyloid deposits in the aging cerebral cortex, *Am. J. Pathol.*, 145, 1358, 1994.

191. Struble, R. G., Cork, L. C., Whitehouse, P. J., and Price, D. L., Cholinergic innervation in neuritic plaques, *Science*, 216, 413, 1982.

192. Pasternack, J. M., Abraham, C. R., Van Dyke, B. J., Potter, H., and Younkin, S. G., Astrocytes in Alzheimer's disease gray matter express α_1-antichymotrypsin mRNA, *Am. J. Pathol.*, 135, 827, 1989.

193. Wegiel, J. and Wisniewski, H. M., The complex of microglial cells and amyloid star in three-dimensional reconstruction, *Acta Neuropathol.*, 81, 116, 1990.

194. Koo, E. H., Abraham, C. R., Potter, H., Cork, L. C., and Price, D. L., Developmental expression of α_1-antichymotrypsin in brain may be related to astrogliosis, *Neurobiol. Aging*, 12, 495, 1991.

195. Wisniewski, H. M. and Wegiel, J., Spatial relationships between astrocytes and classical plaque components, *Neurobiol. Aging*, 12, 593, 1991.

196. Wisniewski, H. M., Barcikowska, M., and Kida, E., Phagocytosis of β/A_4 amyloid fibrils of the neuritic neocortical plaques, *Acta Neuropathol.*, 81, 588, 1991.

197. Johnson, S. A., Lampert-Etchells, M., Pasinetti, G. M., Rozovsky, I., and Finch, C. E., Complement mRNA in the mammalian brain: responses to Alzheimer's disease and experimental brain lesioning, *Neurobiol. Aging*, 13, 641, 1992.

198. Miyakawa, T., Katsuragi, S., Yamashita, K., and Ohuchi. K., Morphological study of amyloid fibrils and preamyloid deposits in the brain with Alzheimer's disease, *Acta Neuropathol.*, 83, 340, 1992.

199. Wisniewski, H. M., Wegiel, J., Wang, K. C., and Lach, B., Ultrastructural studies of the cells forming amyloid in the cortical vessel wall in Alzheimer's disease, *Acta Neuropathol.*, 84, 117, 1992.

200. Abraham, C. R., Selkoe, D. J., and Potter, H., Immunocytochemical identification of the serine protease inhibitor α_1-antichymotrypsin, in the brain amyloid deposits of Alzheimer's disease, *Cell*, 52, 487, 1988.

Chapter 13

NEUROIMAGING APPLICATIONS FOR THE STUDY OF ALZHEIMER'S DISEASE

_____Thomas F. Budinger

CONTENTS

I. INTRODUCTION

Noninvasive studies of brain anatomy changes in Alzheimer's disease (AD) started in the mid 1970s after the introduction of X-ray computed tomography (CT). These anatomical studies showing generalized atrophy were followed by positron emission tomography (PET) glucose studies in the early 1980s and by magnetic resonance imaging (MRI) in the mid 1980s. The PET and MRI modalities have dominated the research activities over the last 15 years. Other noninvasive modalities such as functional magnetic resonance imaging, magnetic resonance spectroscopy of selected volumes, computerized electroencephalography frequency maps, and magnetic source imaging (magnetic encephalography) have been added to the exploration of the characteristics of the central nervous system in dementia. Figure 1 illustrates schematically the different imaging modalities which have been employed in studying AD.

The plan of this chapter is to first present the physics and engineering of each technique and then to describe applications to anatomy, perfusion, metabolism, chemical content, and neuroreceptors in *in vivo* studies of the AD brain. This chapter presents the physical principles underlying six noninvasive imaging modalities and summarizes how these modalities are being used to study the AD patient's brain. The intent is to give the readers an explanation of what the different methods can measure and how they have contributed to characterization of AD. As will be seen, contemporary methods are useful now but can be expected to improve in resolution by a factor of three in the next few years.

II. DESCRIPTION OF IMAGING METHODS USED TO STUDY BRAIN ANATOMY AND FUNCTION

A. X-RAY CT

X-ray transmission CT gives anatomical information on the positions of air, soft tissues, and bone based mainly on the scattering of X-ray photons by electrons. The denser the electrons, the more the X-ray beams are scattered or attenuated. In addition, the absorption of X-rays due to the photoelectric effect differences in elemental composition has important effects for imaging bone or calcium deposits because this absorption process is dependent on the atomic number as well as the density. Indeed, the reason there are small differences between gray and white matter in the brain in CT images is that the H, C, N, O, and P contents for gray and white matter differ slightly, resulting in about 3% changes between gray and white matter. Thus, X-ray CT gives information on the density of tissue and shows average elemental composition differences. Very little contrast is observable between blood and muscle as the density (about 1.05 gm/cm^3) and the elemental compositions are very similar. To provide image contrast between the blood vasculature and surrounding tissue, a dense fluid with elements of high atomic number (e.g., iodine, barium) can be injected or swallowed during the X-ray exposures. The movement through the body vasculature of a "contrast agent" such as an iodinated compound can be visualized by acquiring a sequence of images. The iodine agent absorbs photons more than blood and tissue because the density is higher and the element iodine has a high atomic number giving rise to more photoelectric absorption than

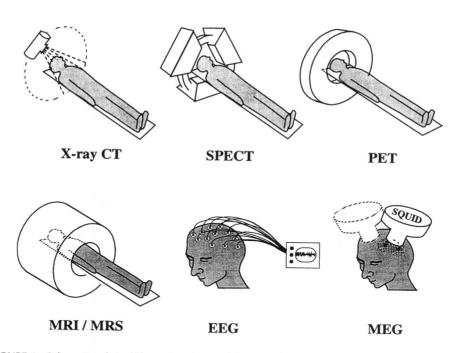

X-ray CT **SPECT** **PET**

MRI / MRS **EEG** **MEG**

FIGURE 1 Schematic of six different imaging modalities used in medical research to study the brain.

is the case for H, C, N, O, or P. The contemporary trend for X-ray CT is to acquire finer resolution at high speed. These innovations have application to moving organs and are not expected to have an impact on AD evaluation or therapy.

B. SPECT

Emission computed tomography (ECT) involves detection of photons from radionuclide distributions in the body after injection of a radionuclide. There are two general classes of emission tomography (SPECT and PET). Single photon emission computed tomography (SPECT) dates from the early 1960s, when the idea of emission transverse section tomography was presented by Kuhl and Edwards.[1] As in X-ray CT, SPECT involves rotation of a photon detector array around the body to acquire data from multiple angles (see Figure 1).

In emission tomography, we seek the position and concentration of radionuclide distribution. This task is far more difficult than that of X-ray tomography, wherein the source position and strength are known at all times and only the attenuation coefficients need to be determined. The reconstruction algorithms are similar to those for X-ray CT with the exception of the need to compensate for this attenuation. Attenuation effects have until recently been ignored in commercial SPECT. To some extent clinical results were acceptable because the resulting reconstruction, although not quantitative, shows relative concentrations if the activity distribution is concentrated in the central portion of the section. Now SPECT methods incorporate some mathematical methods to compensate for attenuation.[2] The usual strategy is to acquire volumetric data using one or more gamma cameras mounted on a rotating gantry. The data are organized into a series of slice projections, each corresponding to a section of 10- to 20-mm thickness. Each section is computed separately. A comprehensive discussion of the mathematics is found in Reference 3.

The quantitative accuracy in emission tomography with attenuation compensation depends on the size of the object relative to the resolution. In fact, the accuracy or bias related to correct sampling of data is quite different from the precision of a measurement that is dependent on statistics. This important concept can be seen from the simulations shown in Figure 2. As the sampling resolution decreases from 10 to 2 mm, the reconstruction data have more statistical

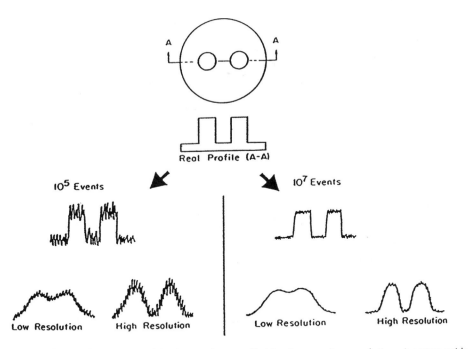

FIGURE 2   The quantitative accuracy of the images is controlled by the sampling resolution. A system with good resolution will channel the events into the regions of interest from which they originate; however, a system with poor resolution will spread the data outside the anatomic region of interest, owing to blurring in the poor-resolution system. Statistical uncertainty is a separate consideration.

fluctuation (less precision), but in a region of interest corresponding to the region of the source the mean value becomes closer to the actual value (more accuracy). Commercially available instruments have resolutions of 7 to 10 mm. Thus, objects less than 15 mm in size will not be quantitatively imaged. This problem is particularly important for tracers which localize in the cerebral gray matter wherein activity within the 3.5 mm wide cerebral cortical ribbon cannot be quantitatively compared to activity in the much larger central gray regions (e.g., caudate nucleus, putamen).

SPECT has been thought to be substantially inferior to PET because of attainable resolution and sensitivity. However, these differences have usually been exaggerated. Sensitivity is the number of events detected from a specified source of radiation and depends mainly on the solid angle of detection. For SPECT, collimation is necessary to increase the in-plane resolution, and this results in a decrease in the solid angle and a loss in sensitivity by a larger factor than is the case for PET. The solid angle factor is the ratio of the area of detector available to a source anywhere in the imaging volume to the area of a sphere with radius R from the center of the volume to the imaging detectors. For example, if 1 cm × 1 cm is the area of detection for a single gamma camera for an object with a radius of 15 cm from the detector, the single photon solid angle factor is

$$\frac{1\,\text{cm}^2}{4\pi R^2\,\text{cm}^2} = \frac{1}{2835}$$

Because the positron device can have a ring of detector area, for example, 1 cm thick around the entire circumference, the solid angle factor is

$$\frac{1 \times 2\pi R}{4\pi R^2} = \frac{1}{30}$$

or almost 100 times better than that of the single photon system for 1-cm resolution. It was on the basis of this incomplete argument that many concluded that SPECT would never compete with PET. However, there are many other factors that must be taken into account. If 4 arrays of detectors are placed around the object this advantage is reduced to 25. Secondly, for PET, the probability of positron detection is the product of the probability of detection by each opposing crystal; thus a crystal efficiency of 80% leads to a PET efficiency of 0.8^2 which is only 64%. The attenuation losses are associated with the total path length through the object in PET and thus are greater in PET than in SPECT. In addition to the efficiency and attenuation differences, the positron tomograph requires a larger diameter (e.g., 60 cm for PET and 30 cm for SPECT for the head). Thus, instead of a sensitivity ratio of 100, the expected sensitivity ratio for 1-cm resolution in an instrument for head imaging is:

$$\frac{S(\text{PET})}{S(\text{SPECT})} = \frac{15}{a}$$

where S is sensitivity and a (cm) is the in-plane resolution. Having 15 times less sensitivity is not a serious deterrent to SPECT of the brain, but the relative sensitivity for a resolution of 5 mm is 30 and this difference makes SPECT less practical at high resolution. Whereas the SPECT sensitivity in terms of detected events for a given amount of radionuclide is less than PET, the availability of new SPECT radiopharmaceuticals, particularly for the brain and head, and the practical and economic aspects of SPECT instrumentation make this mode of emission tomography attractive for clinical studies of the brain.

C. PET

Positron emission tomography (PET) utilizes the fact that the annihilation photons of 511 keV arising from the positron-electron interaction are emitted 180° one from the other; thus, the electronic detection of photons in two detectors of an array gives the line through the object along which the radionuclide must be (Figure 3). By observing the coincident pairs for thousands of events we can locate the points of radionuclide concentration. The general approach is similar to that of X-ray CT and SPECT, but as in the case of SPECT, the information being sought is the position and intensity of the gamma radiation emitted by the isotope. The radiated photons are attenuated by the soft tissues between the sources and the detectors. Incorporation of attenuation compensation is much simpler in PET than SPECT and this along with the 10- to 20-fold increase in sensitivity and the availability of C, N, and O radioisotopes has lead to the claim that PET is much more informative than SPECT.

At present, the resolution of 2.6 mm has been achieved in a PET system which images only one layer at a time.[4] New technology gives promise that volume imaging at 2-mm resolution is possible. This technology requires the development of new detector systems to overcome the inherent resolution penalties of less-expensive commercial systems and the need to achieve improved resolution (2 mm × 2 mm × 2 mm).[5]

1. Emission Tomography (PET, SPECT) vs. Magnetic Resonance (MRI, MRS)

A major difference between PET or SPECT and magnetic resonance techniques is that PET gives information on nanomolar concentrations of substances in the brain, whereas magnetic resonance methods require millimolar concentrations for reliable detection. PET information is based on where a specific tracer tag accumulates, even in nanomolar concentrations; magnetic resonance spectroscopy identifies specific molecules, but with a sensitivity which requires millimolar concentrations. This difference in sensitivity gives PET and SPECT an advantage in imaging those neurochemicals that are submillimolar in the brain. However, PET measures where the tracer is located and not the chemical composition. The unique capability of magnetic resonance spectroscopy is the capability of measuring the local concentration of many compounds in the brain.

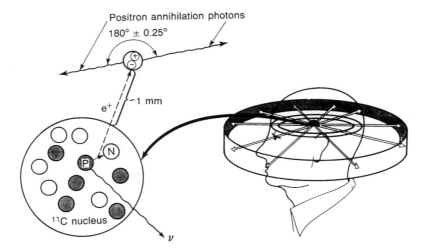

FIGURE 3   The concept of positron emission tomography (PET).

D. MAGNETIC RESONANCE
1. Magnetic Resonance Imaging

The physical principle that forms the basis of magnetic resonance imaging (MRI) is the interaction of nuclei which have a magnetic moment with a magnetic field.[6] The nucleus of an atom such as the hydrogen atom of water has a positive charge and is considered as a charge spinning about an axis. This motion of the nucleus is equivalent to an electric current flowing in a loop of wire and this generates a small magnetic field. The small fields line up with an externally applied magnetic field like a bar magnet would line up; however, as the nuclear field is generated by rotation the interaction of the nuclear field with the magnetic field results in a precession in the same way a rotating top precesses about the Earth's gravitational field. The frequency of this precession is specific for each nuclear species and proportional to the external magnetic field. Thus, for a field of 1.5 T (15000 gauss) the frequency is 63 MHz. The basic relation is $v = \gamma'B$, where v is the resonant frequency of the precession oscillation, γ' is the usual gyromagnetic rate divided by 2π and B is the field.

The quantum theory requires that for hydrogen two magnetic moment values occur resulting in an alignment of the nuclear spins with and against the external field. The hydrogen nuclei are said to populate corresponding lower and upper energy states with a very small population difference (about one in a million). If energy in the form of an externally applied rotating magnetic field, the RF pulse, whose frequency exactly matches the precession frequency is applied, then resonant absorption of energy takes place and this boosts nuclei from the lower state to the higher state. After this applied field is turned off, the excited "spins" return to their equilibrium position after losing energy by a relaxation process (the T1 relaxation). The signal received from the relaxation is the magnetic resonance signal. The more nuclei or the higher the water content (^{1}H nuclei), the greater the signal. The signal strength in MRI depends on the number of nuclei residing in the tissue volume and as the difference in the excited and lower states is only 1 in 1 million a strong signal requires a high concentration of nuclei. This is the case for hydrogen nuclei in tissue because the concentration of about 90 molar or about 10^{18} per cubic millimeter will give a substantial signal, yet the concentrations of phosphorous and sodium are 10,000 times less.

The time required for the nuclei to regain equilibrium after receiving a resonant RF pulse is dependent on the interaction of the resonant nuclei with the magnetic fields of the surrounding nuclei in the molecular matrix of the tissue. This is the T1 effect, and T1 is about 600 to 800 ms in the brain at 1.5T and 2000 ms in CSF. A second relaxation time known as T2 is caused by the interactions of the nuclear spin with adjacent nuclear spins which results in a loss of coherence or "in step" rotation of each nuclear spin in the ensemble. This effect is noted in the rate of decay of the emitted signal after the RF pulse. Because these two relaxation times vary with the type of tissue and even the state of tissue oxygenation, it is possible to glean image contrast from analysis of the received signals after sending in RF pulses of various durations and at various intervals.

The spatial information from MRI comes from the fact that the frequency of the signal varies with the local field. If the field through the patient is modified in a known direction and a known magnitude, then the received frequency will be proportional to the spatial position of the proton concentration in the magnetic field. The method of varying the external field is through field gradients applied successively and rapidly in different directions. It is also convenient to vary the phase of the resonant frequency in a known manner by pulses of gradient change to speed up the oscillations momentarily; thus, when the initial frequency returns to that of the static field, the phase will be advanced. Manipulations of this type of varying pulsed gradient fields in time and direction allow the acquisition of three-dimensional data.

Thus, the anatomical position of different tissues, mainly gray matter, white matter, and CSF, are determined at resolutions of less than 1 mm using routine MRI. In addition, it is possible to differentiate flow or motion in blood vessels and microscopic diffusion though observation of how the MRI signal changes after prescribed RF and gradient pulses. *In vivo* microscopy using MRI with sufficient resolution to evaluate the dynamic changes in amyloid plaque clusters in the cerebral cortex would require a coordinated national effort to build an 8- to 10-Tesla MRI/MRS system for human brain studies. The expected resolution for an 8-T system is 50 μm × 50 μm × 100 μm.

2. Magnetic Resonance Spectroscopy

Magnetic resonance spectroscopy (MRS) gives information on the chemical composition of a sample or a specific region in the body. Magnetic resonance spectroscopy provides a method for evaluation of neurochemical composition in localized regions (e.g., choline, choline-containing compounds, creatine, *N*-acetylaspartate, *N*-acetyl-containing compounds, glutamate, glutamine, gamma aminobutyric acid, lactate, etc.). With future increases in resolution and the resulting improvement in signal to noise, the prospects for quantitative evaluation of metabolites in AD are great at higher fields such as 4 T.

The principles of magnetic resonance discussed above state that the frequency of a particular element will be dependent on the magnetic field. However, the field at a specific nuclear site in a molecule is usually slightly different from the applied external field due to the local magnetic field from the orbiting electrons (Figure 4). The net effect is to shield the nucleus somewhat from the external field and this shielding will depend on the position in the molecule of the nucleus. For example, the resonant frequency for phosphorous at 1.5 T is 25.9 MHz, but the actual frequency for the three phosphorous nuclei in ATP and the one phosphorous of creatine phosphate will be slightly different from inorganic phosphorous due to the different electronic or magnetic field environments associated with the molecular positions. These differences in frequency are measured as parts per million differences from the resonance frequency of the unshielded nucleus as shown for the typical phosphorus spectrum in Figure 5. As discussed above the population difference between the nuclear spins in the upper and lower energy states is only about 1 in 10^6. Since the concentration of most metabolites in tissue is in the millimolar range as opposed to hydrogen which is in the 100 molar range, the signal from the different nuclei is about 10^4 times less than the proton signal used in imaging. To compensate for this low sensitivity it is necessary to use large volumes of tissue, particularly in *in vivo* studies at the conventional fields of 1.5 T. At higher fields such as 4 T there is an improvement in the signal in proportion to the increase in field, but even at these high fields the phosphorous and carbon spectral data acquisition requires volumes of tens of cubic centimeters and imaging resolution is too coarse for meaningful studies particularly of cerebral neocortex regions. However, meaningful studies of the brain composition of choline-containing compounds, creatinine, and *N*-acetyl-aspartate can be studied in 0.2-cc volumes (in 6 mm × 6 mm × 6 mm regions) because the proton (hydrogen nucleus) signal is 10,000 times greater than that from carbon and phosphorous compounds at the same magnetic field.

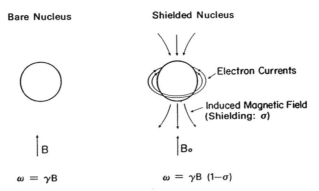

FIGURE 4   Electron shielding results in a small change in the magnetic field with a corresponding change in frequency.

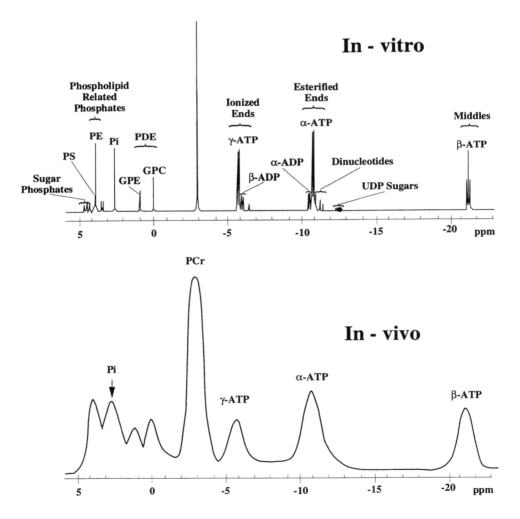

FIGURE 5   Schematic of an *in vitro* ^{31}P MRS spectrum of brain at 11.7 T (upper). Typical *in vivo* ^{31}P MRS spectrum of brain at 1.5 T (lower). Modified from Reference 6.

E. ELECTRICAL ACTIVITY MAPS AND ANALYSIS

Electrical recordings from the surface of the brain (electroencephalogram) or from the outer surface of the head demonstrate continuous electrical activity in the brain with a wide band of frequencies. The intensities of the brain waves on the surface of the scalp range from 0 to 300 μV and frequencies range from once every few seconds to 50 or more per second. The four frequency bands are delta: 0.4 to 3.6 Hz; theta: 4 to 7.6 Hz; alpha: 8 to 13.6 Hz; and beta: 14 to 24 Hz. Typically 16 to 20 electrodes are used. From the voltage oscillations during the awake state a Fourier transformation is made and the resulting spectrum squared to give the power spectrum. Quantitative EEG analysis involves determination of the power in four frequency bands for a multiple lead system and topographic brain maps can be constructed using the numerical data.[7] (Figure 6). The reconstruction of electric current sources from surface recordings is a very ill-posed mathematical problem and new approaches which high performance computers and prior MRI data might facilitate.[151]

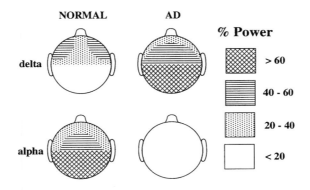

FIGURE 6 A simple topographic image schematic representing a ratio of power in frequency bands might be an important and inexpensive adjunct to quantifying the severity and response to therapy in AD.

F. MAGNETOENCEPHALOGRAPHY (MEG)

Ion currents arising in the neurons of the heart and the brain produce magnetic fields outside the body which can be measured by arrays of SQUID (Superconducting QUantum Interference Device) detectors placed near the head (see Figure 1). The recording of these magnetic fields over the head is known as magnetoencephalography (MEG). These fields result from the synchronous activity of tens or hundreds of thousands of neurons. The reconstruction of the most likely position in the brain for the current source or sources giving rise to the MEG is known as magnetic source imaging (MSI). Both magnetic source imaging and electrical source imaging seek to determine the location, orientation, and magnitude of current sources within the body. The magnetic field at the surface is most strongly determined by current sources directed parallel to the surface, but the electrical potentials are determined by current sources directed perpendicular to the surface. Other than the signal distortion from the heterogeneity of tissue conductivity, there is no clear physical reason why the clinical information produced by biomagnetic measurements could not as well be obtained from electric potential mapping.

An advantage of MSI is that all body tissues are magnetically transparent and the magnetic fields propagate to the surface without distortion. The electrical potentials at the surface, on the other hand, are distorted by conductivity variations within the body; this is especially true in the head, where the low conductivity of the skull both distorts and hides the electrical activity of the brain. A disadvantage of MSI is that the need for cryogenic cooling and a magnetically shielded room makes the procedure cumbersome with present technology.

A major strength of MSI is that it can resolve events separated by milliseconds, whereas other methods (e.g., MRI, MRS, PET, SPECT) have time resolutions of seconds to many minutes, depending on the information sought. A weakness of magnetic source imaging is that any magnetic field distribution on the surface of the head can be explained by an infinite number of current distributions inside the head. A successful source analysis is dependent on the availability of additional information suitable to constrain the inverse problem to be solved.[151]

The limited number of detectors and the low signal-to-noise ratio means that MSI has poorer spatial resolution (1 to 2 cm) than many other medical imaging modalities; furthermore, depending on the source strength, sources in the brain must be within several centimeters of the surface to be reliably detected; sources in the heart are stronger, and deeper sources can be detected there. The temporal resolution, however, is milliseconds or tens of milliseconds, which makes MSI attractive for neuroscience studies.

A current line of research is to improve the apparent spatial resolution of MSI by using prior knowledge of the anatomy obtained from MRI or CT to constrain to magnetic source reconstruction. One simple approach is simply to superimpose reconstructed dipole solutions on an MR image registered to the same coordinate system; dipole locations not consistent with the anatomy may then be rejected as artifacts. This has been done with dipole point sources and is useful in interpreting the reconstruction. As with electroencephalography and electrocardiology, clinical and scientific applications await less-expensive instrumentation as well as practical computational strategies for determining the spatial distribution of the current generators in the brain and heart.

The maps of magnetic field are usually made in response to a stimulus, and no reported work has been found on the application of this technique to AD. However, applications to other mental disorders in addition to seizure disorders give some basis for suspecting this method will reveal important biological attributes of dementia in the cooperative patient. This method gives good results for seizure foci, for mapping visual response activity in the occipital cortex, auditory activity in the temporal cortex, etc., and has the inherent property of good temporal resolution as is also the case for EEG mapping. However, the MSI method does not work well at present with distributed sources. This is an area of active research and the potential for combination of MSI with functional imaging using MRI has the potential for studies of the biology of dementia but these methods are unlikely candidates for AD evaluation due to the need for cooperation as the methods are very sensitive to motion artifacts.

III. NEUROIMAGING ANATOMICAL STUDIES

The two major modes of *in vivo* anatomical studies employed by the neuroradiologist and researchers are X-ray CT and MRI. For the majority of clinically indicated and research based anatomical studies, MRI is preferred over X-ray CT. However, the early findings from X-ray CT are worthy of note.

A. X-RAY COMPUTED TOMOGRAPHY ANATOMICAL STUDIES

Since the advent of X-ray CT investigations, the size of sulci and ventricles have been explored as possibly a sensitive tool for separation of AD from age-matched controls.[8-11] A careful study of measurable features of the X-ray CT such as the suprasellar cistern and the anterior temporal horn separation showed a classification accuracy of about 80%. As MRI systems become widely available, X-ray CT has been less a part of AD evaluation except in the case of long term follow-up of a large patient population.[12] Incidentally, it should be noted that intracerebral calcifications and anatomic abnormalities of the calvarium are not associated with AD.

B. MAGNETIC RESONANCE IMAGING ANATOMICAL STUDIES

MRI using protons has become an effective tool for imaging anatomy with very high resolution. These anatomical data serve as a neuroarchitectural study of longitudinal changes and also are useful for correcting the partial volume effects of the PET data. Studies of hippocampal anatomy by MRI show a correlation of hippocampal atrophy and Mini-Mental status as well as an age-related decrease of the hippocampus normalized to total brain volume.[13-18] With a Mini-Mental State Examination score greater than 21, the principal finding is a decrease in normalized volume of 36% for the hippocampal/intracranial volume and 25% for the hippocampal formation/intracranial volume. With scores less than 21, this atrophy increased to 40% for the amydala/intracranial volume and 45% for the hippocampal formation/intracranial volume. The caudate nucleus showed atrophy along with ventricular enlargement in the more demented patients. Though the sensitivity of differentiating AD from controls using temporal lobe measurements seems to be in the 90% range, there is not a consensus that MRI can be relied upon to separate AD from cognitively normal elderly subjects; as atrophy of temporal structures makes the diagnosis of AD likely, the absence does not rule out the possibility of early AD.[17]

Even at 1.5 T the cortical anatomy can be explored to some extent showing neocortical anatomy at 1.5 T using surface coils (see photo in Figure 10). Cortical changes such as gray matter thickness, or volume can be quantitated in longitudinal studies. Indeed, a demonstration of columnar modules and myelin septa perpendicular to the pia in the cerebral cortex has been made at 1.5 T using a spin echo sequence.[19] In another study, the stria of Gennari has been claimed to be visualized in the living striate cortex at 1.5T using a 5-in surface coil and a proton density, inversion recovery pulse sequence.[20]

In general, the findings of regional and generalized cerebral atrophy were as would be expected from post-mortem studies. The decline of hippocampal volumes by MRI has been correlated with aging and cognitive activity deterioration.[12] However, correlations between the degree of hippocampal atrophy and neocortex decrease in glucose metabolism by PET were not found.[13] The hippocampal signs were expected to precede neocortex pathology but even this is not consistent in Alzheimer's populations.[21] Studies testing the hypothesis that atrophy of the hippocampal formation in nondemented elderly individuals could predict subsequent Alzheimer's disease suggested strongly that dilatation of the perihippocampal fissures were a useful radiographic marker for identifying the early features of AD.[12] The existence of Alzheimer's subtypes is supported by cases of preserved hippocampal metabolism but neocortex decreases as well as cases of decreased hippocampal yet preserved neocortex metabolism.[21]

Whereas the past technologies MRI allowed successive 2D slices of the brain to be imaged it was not until recently that 3D MRI has been available at high resolution for accurate studies of the anatomy of AD. The availability and demonstrated capability of MRI techniques to acquire whole brain images with good gray-white matter and CSF separation with nearly 1mm isotropic resolution in less than 20 minutes has encouraged research using these anatomical studies on the correlation of atrophy with the progression of disease.[12, 22] For example, the progression of brain atrophy with age can be quantitated over the entire brain (Figure 7) or on a regional basis as shown for the hippocampus atrophy on Figure 8.

A resolution of approximately 400×400 μm can be achieved using different MRI methods which give different types of contrast between gray and white matter and cerebral spinal fluid (CSF). However, the section thickness or third dimension is usually over 1000 μm even for local imaging as in Figure 10. The resolution limitations of magnetic resonance are based on the sampling density, signal to noise including contrast mechanisms, and inherent physiological properties of the tissue (e.g.,. motion, flow diffusion, and susceptibility anisotropy). The signal to noise can be improved significantly using surface coils, thus at 1.5 T allowing 300 μm resolution studies of the cerebral cortex but not of the deeper tissues of the mesial temporal cortex are possible. To achieve higher resolution in three dimensions, higher magnetic fields and multiple coil arrangements are needed. The neocortex can be imaged more readily than the deepest lying hippocampus because the surface coils used are not sensitive to structures deep in the brain.

The proposal to image the concentration and change in concentration of amyloid plaques *in vivo* in the human cortex is motivated by the success of MRI in monitoring multiple sclerosis (MS) lesions as objective measures of the progression and regression of this disease.[23] However, amyloid plaques are 100 times smaller than the 2-mm lesions seen in MS. Therefore, amyloid plaque imaging

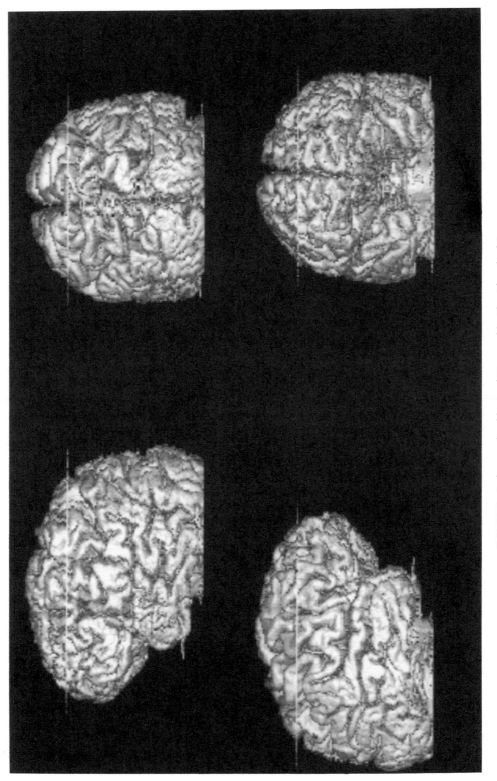

FIGURE 7 Surface-rendered brain of 86-year-old with widened sulci.

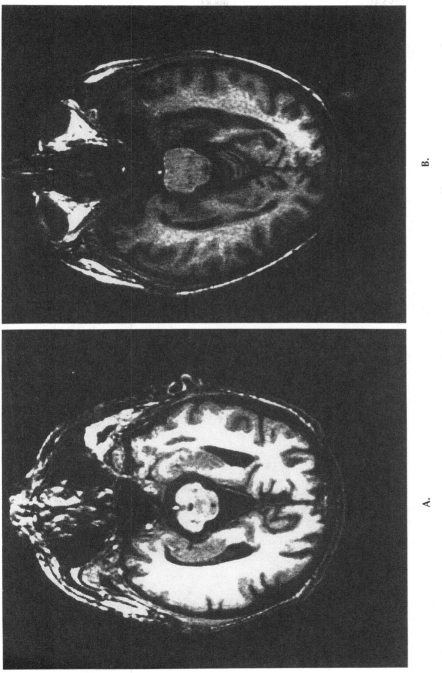

B.

A.

FIGURE 8 MRI of a normal aged 76 year old (A) and of a 77 year old with AD (B). MRI: Degeneration of hippocampus is seen in AD (B) but not in normal aged (A).

is beyond current technologies but not beyond the technology of magnetic resonance *in vivo* microscopy at 8 to 10 T. Most magnets are at 1.5 T with a few at 4 T. The argument of plausibility is as follows. Most amyloid plaques average about 30 μm in diameter (B. Hyman, personal communication) with some larger plaques at 42 μm.[24] The present capabilities of *in vivo* imaging at 1.5 T are such that the linea alba in the human cerebral cortex is easily discerned and less than 300 μm resolution can be obtained at least in two of three directions. For objects with magnetic susceptibility differences such as trabecular bone, the resolution can be 80 μm in a 15-minute imaging period with contrast developed through bone–tissue susceptibility differences. Assuming the susceptibility differences between amyloid plaques and surrounding tissues are large, and knowing the susceptibility effect increases with magnetic field increases, it will be possible to visualize the presence of plaques through the susceptibility contrast mechanism at fields of 8 T. The feasibility of building a magnet to operate at 8 to 10 T for safe studies of the human brain has been established through careful studies over the last 15 years.[25] The motivation to proceed with this project depends on a demonstration of the organized plaque MRI contrast attributes.

IV. NEUROIMAGING OF PERFUSION

Perfusion imaging is readily performed using both PET with ^{15}O-H_2O and SPECT labeled agents with the tracers ^{123}I or ^{99m}Tc. More recently, MRI has been used to infer perfusion from blood volume images after injection of susceptibility contrast material or T1 changes after tagging incoming blood with an MRI saturation pulse. In the normal brain as well as in AD, regional cerebral blood flow is coupled to metabolic demand. Thus, changes in cerebral flow reflect variation in neuronal metabolism.[26] As the SPECT studies can be easily performed in clinical practice, they have been widely applied to AD and have assisted in the differential diagnosis.[27] The degree and extent of decreased cerebral blood flow on SPECT has been correlated with AD severity.[28, 29] Some of the earliest imaging studies in AD used ^{15}O-H_2O with disappointing results due to the poor resolution of the instruments 10 years ago. Since that time, both FDG metabolism and flow have been shown to be decreased about 30% from normal in the parietal temporal regions of the cerebrum.

SPECT agents in common use for cerebral blood flow are *N*-isopropyl-*p*-[^{123}I]iodoamphetamine (IMP),[30,31] [^{123}I]hydroxyiodobenzylpropanediamine (HIPDM),[28] and the ^{99m}Tc-labeled hexamethyl-propyleneamine oxime (HMPAO).[32,33] The diffusible gas ^{133}Xe is also being used.[34-36] The possibility for revival in brain imaging using SPECT appears to be great because the new compounds concentrate in the brain in proportion to flow[37,38] and can be imaged over short periods of time (5 minutes) with a resolution of 7 mm full width at half-maximum with appropriate instrumentation.

Comparisons between SPECT flow imaging and PET FDG metabolism studies have shown similar characteristic temporoparietal abnormalities[29,39,40] but the presence of abnormalities in glucose metabolism are shown in other associative areas. These differences could be explained by an evaluation of the differences in resolution of the particular instruments involved in the comparative study. PET was found to be superior to SPECT for the differentiation of vascular dementia from AD.[40]

V. NEUROIMAGING OF BIOCHEMISTRY

A. GLUCOSE METABOLISM

A major advance in 1980 in the study of AD was the finding of parietal-temporal decreases in glucose metabolism using PET fluorodeoxyglucose (FDG) studies (Figure 9). Though these *in vivo* studies were considered a breakthrough in the early 1980s, they were not different from what would be expected from known pathology.[41] The interest in and possibility of early diagnosis[42] has been offset by the appreciation of the nonspecificity of reductions in parietal and temporal cerebral metabolic rates with other dementias.[43] What can be concluded now is that PET glucose metabolism

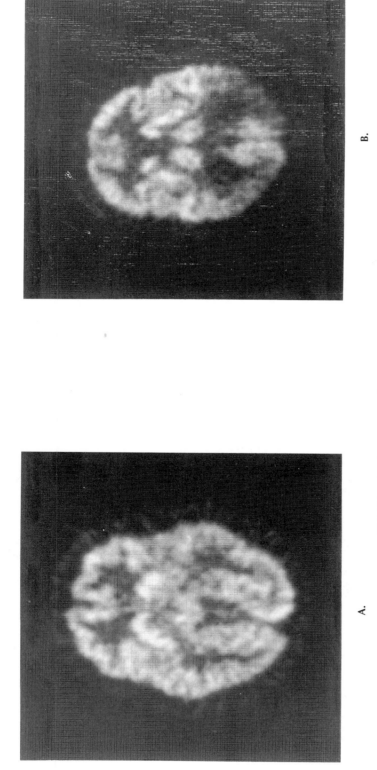

FIGURE 9 PET/FDG in normal (i.e., control) (A) and AD brains (B).

**TABLE 1   Potential Applications of Magnetic Resonance
in the Studies of Alzheimer's Disease**

Magnetic Resonance	Brain System
MRS	ATP
	Creatine phosphate
	Phosphodiesters
	Choline (containing compounds)
	N-Acetylaspartate
	GABA
	Glutamate
	Glutamine
	Taurine
	Lactate
	^{13}C-compounds
	pH
Ultrafast MRI	Patterns of brain activity stimulated by sensory, cognitive, and provoked responses
High field MRI	Subcortical *in vivo* microscopy at less than 100-μm resolution
	Intracellular K^+ and Na^+

decreases allow quantitation of the progression of the disease.[44,45] Of additional interest is the previous finding of Alzheimer's-like glucose metabolism reductions in a large portion of late Parkinson's disease patients[46, 47] which argues for subtypes of AD and challenges the specificity of FDG PET.

The future studies of brain metabolism need to go beyond our 16 years of FDG-PET observations to examine hypotheses regarding oxidative processes, mitochondrial mutations, transport pathologies, phosphorylation abnormalities, etc. The rationale for some of these directions is given below.

The chemical components of millimolar concentrations in the brain which can be studied by MRS are given in Table 1.

B. OXIDATIVE STATE MEASUREMENTS

A specific mitochondrial marker, 18F-rotenone, has recently been developed and characterized in animal studies.[48] This ligand has potential as a tracer of mitochondrial mass. The rationale for further development of mitochondrial probes for PET or SPECT imaging is given below.

The possibility of oxidative damage through mitochondrial dysfunction has been proposed with the expectation of a progressive impairment of oxidative phosphorylation.[49-51] Patients with defects in oxidative phosphorylation generate increased amounts of oxygen free radicals and these damage the mitochondrial DNA.[52] These observations are consistent with the large body of evidence regarding impairment of glucose metabolism using PET.

Studies of 8-hydroxy-2-deoxyguanosine, a biomarker of oxidative DNA damage, support this connection between mtDNA damage and oxidation in that the amount of 8-hydroxy-2-deoxyguanosine increases with normal aging in nuclear and mitochondrial DNA; however, the rate of increase is greater in mtDNA.[53] Recently, through the use of polymerase chain reaction (PCR),[54] deletion of mitochondrial DNA (mtDNA) has been discovered to increase in aging human brain neurons. One particular deletion (mtDNA4977) accumulates with age primarily in nondividing cells such as muscle and brain of normal individuals. The level of the deletion rises with age by more than 100-fold in the heart and brain and to a lesser extent in other tissues. Different regions of the brain have substantially different levels of deletion. The highest levels of the deletion mtDNA4977 are seen in the caudate, putamen, and substantia nigra in which there is high dopamine metabolism and corresponding monoamine oxidase activity that produces H_2O_2. This activity can lead to free radical formation. It has been proposed that oxidative damage to mtDNA may be "catastrophic"; mutations affecting mitochondrially encoded polypeptides involved in ion electron transport could increase free radical generation leading to more mtDNA damage.[54]

These observations have encouraged development of a marker of mitochondrial mass which could be used with PET and will cross the blood-brain barrier.[48] The new ligand is an inhibitor of complex I which is appropriate as the age-dependent decreases in mitochondrial respiration in the rodent are known to be associated with decline in complex I capacity.[55]

C. NEURORECEPTORS

Multiple neuroreceptor changes are present in AD based upon analyses from autopsy brain tissue; however, these receptor changes represent the final stage of the disease and might for the most part be epiphenomena. Because PET and SPECT have the capacity of evaluate neuroreceptors *in vivo*, these imaging modalities play an important role in the development of methods for early detection of AD and for longitudinal studies of the efficacy of proposed therapies.

The specificity and sensitivity of PET (detects nanomolar concentrations) for neuroreceptor studies gives this technique tremendous potential for studying the human brain; the spatial resolution of contemporary devices is inferior to the goal of quantitation in the regions of our greatest interests which are sublayers of the cerebral cortex, the hippocampal structures, and periaqueductal gray matter nuclei. In the near future we can expect PET will give us 2-mm resolution and allow quantitative imaging in regions such as the locus ceruleus. Now that we can expect the required resolution, what might be the strategy for exploring the neuroreceptors in AD?

Many neurochemical systems are abnormal in AD, including the well-described cholinergic and somatostatinergic systems as well as the biogenic amine systems (norepinephrine, serotonin, and dopamine). In each neurotransmitter system, considerable evidence suggests that the abnormality involves the presynaptic neuron. For example, the presynaptic nature of the cholinergic deficit is strongly supported by the frequently reported degeneration of basal forebrain projections. Each biogenic amine system studied in AD patients shows degeneration of the subcortical projection system, e.g., the locus ceruleus, raphe nucleus, and ventral tegmental area associated with evidence of loss of the corresponding projections to cerebral cortex, noradrenaline, serotonin, and dopamine. These presynaptic losses generally stand in distinct contrast to the more conflicting data regarding changes in postsynaptic receptors in the cholinergic, serotonergic, and adrenergic systems, where variable increases, decreases, or lack of change in the receptors have been noted.

In view of the morphological and chemical evidence of presynaptic loss in AD, it is reasonable to pursue *in vivo* measures of presynaptic function in order to map the degeneration in AD. The development of such markers would have important consequences for understanding the pathophysiology of AD, improving its diagnosis, and monitoring the effects of treatment. Selective markers offer the ability to relate changes in specific neurochemical systems to the biological heterogeneity of the disease. Specific ligands which are in development for the presynaptic systems of interest are L-dopa and *m*-tyrosine for the dopaminergic system, nitroquipazine for the serotonergic system,[56] and derivatives of vesamicol for the cholinergic system.[57] The latter two have been labeled for SPECT studies but have the potential for high-resolution PET studies. Even at poorer resolution, these two ligands have promise in investigations of the regional changes in serotonergic and cholinergic system. The α-adrenergic system represented in thin cortical layers and small nuclei of the periaqueductal gray is also a target for PET studies. In this case the available ligand is atipamezole an α_2 postsynaptic antagonist.[58]

A list of recently available ligands important for neurodegeneration studies is given in the Table 2.

TABLE 2   Radiolabeled Probes of the Brain Neurochemical Systems

Radioligand	Neurochemistry
^{18}F-benzamides	Dopaminergic D_2 receptors (high affinity)
^{11}C-PK 11195	Macrophage benzodiazepine receptors
^{11}C-carfentanil	Mu-opiate receptors
^{11}C-choline	Choline transport
^{11}C-diprenorphine	Mu, delta, and kappa-opiate receptors
^{11}C-deprenyl	Monamine oxidase tracer
^{11}C-leucine, ^{11}C-methionine	Amina acid and transport Protein synthesis
^{11}C-nicotine	Nicotinic/muscarinic receptors
^{11}C-N-methyl-spiperone	Serotonergic/dopaminergic D_2 receptors (high affinity)
^{11}C-raclopride	Dopaminergic D_1, D_2 receptors (low affinity)
^{18}F-17-β-estradiol	Estrogen receptors
^{18}F-yohimbine analogs	$α_2$-Adrenergic receptors
^{18}F-fluoro-atipamezole	$α_2$-Adrenergic receptors
^{18}F-dihydro-rhodamine/rotenone	Mitochondrial concentration or activity
^{18}F-fluoro-L-dopa	Presynaptic dopaminergic receptors
^{18}F-fluoro-misonidazole	Hypoxic tissues
^{18}F-fluorothienylcyclohexylpiperidine (FTCP)	N-methyl-D-aspartate (NMDA)-sensitive glutamate receptors
Labeled arginine analog	Nitric oxide synthase
^{124}I-labeled T-lymphocytes	Immunologically based pathologies
^{68}Ga-EDTA, ^{82}Rb	Blood-brain barrier permeability
^{123}I-iodobenzylvesamicol	Acetylcholine (presynaptic) receptors

1.   Muscarinic

The first target for noninvasive imaging studies of receptors is that of the cholinergic muscarinic system since decreases in the acylcholinesterase enzyme and in acetylcholine have been measured at autopsy. However, the debate concerning receptor abnormalities is unresolved. Dewey and co-workers showed a decline of muscarinic receptors with age.[61] PET receptor ligands used for the study of the muscarinic system are ^{11}C-benztropine,[61] ^{11}C-tropanyl benzilate,[62] and ^{11}C-scopolamine.[62] The studies with SPECT have centered around use of I-QNB.[63] These and other studies have shown preserved muscarinic receptors in AD subjects.[64, 65] The muscarinic antagonist quinuclidinyl benzilate labeled with ^{123}I [^{123}I(R,R)QNB] for SPECT imaging has shown a consistent regional pattern that correlated with the expected normal distribution from autopsy studies in normals but in AD some focal deficits were noted in frontal or posterior temporal cortex.[66] These and earlier studies suggested that decreases in local binding *in vivo* may characterize some patients with AD; however, there is no strong evidence of a cerebral gray matter distribution other than that related to perfusion in AD.[67] Thus, without normalization for the flow delivery of the receptor ligand by perfusion imaging, a reliable estimate of the muscarinic receptors cannot be made. In addition there is evidence that AD involves selective loss of muscarinic M2 but not M1 receptors in the posterior parietal cortex, but there is not yet available a specific M2-selective radioligand which will penetrate the blood-brain barrier, though the pharmacokinetics of ^{123}I(R,R)QNB for M1 and M2 are sufficiently different that some differential evaluation might be possible.[68] A new radioligand which binds to the acetylcholine transporter on presynaptic vesicles was evaluated in normal subjects. The radioligand (–) 5-iodobenzovesamicol (IBVM) distributes in the brain in proportion, to the vesicular acetylchlorine transporter (VACHT). The most recent studies of the acetylchorine system using "C-tropanyl benzilate" gives evidence that cerebral muscarinic receptor avaiability does not undergo a major decline with the normal aging of the adult brain.

2.   Serotonergic

Significant reduction in 5-HT2 receptor binding in the cerebral cortex has been observed using PET with the radioligand 18F setoperone.[69] These observations correspond to known decreases in receptors from autopsy patients. The development of radioligands for evaluation of presynaptic serotonin for both PET and SPECT is currently underway.[70-72] The reason we cannot visualize the neurorecptors in the cortex is that the receptor regions (e.g., 1 mm bands in the cortex) are blurred by the relatively poor resolution .

3. Dopaminergic

Much of the focus of neurochemistry studies of the past has been on the dopamine system of the central gray and the dopamine receptors of other areas has not been studied because of inferior resolution (Figure 10). The postsynaptic dopamine D_2 system has received extensive evaluation in other disorders using labeled spiperone, raclopride, and new highly specific ligand benzamides.[73] Even the most recent commercial PET systems cannot be expected to give quantitative results for receptor concentration in cortical gray, periaqueductal gray, and the neocortex because the resolution capabilities (e.g., 4.5 to 6 mm) are less by a factor of 2 than that necessary to visualize many of the layers and nuclei of interest to the neuroscientist.

True activity blurred into noise

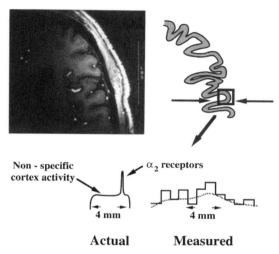

FIGURE 10   Spatial resolution of PET not adequate to see the fine details of the brain.

4. Nicotinic

Reduced numbers of nicotinic receptors have been reported from AD using PET studies wherein a lower uptake of (R)(+) ^{11}C-nicotine compared to (S)(–) [11]Ca-nicotine in patients with AD confirms lower nicotinic receptor activity from autopsy studies.[74] When ^{11}C-nicotine is injected into normal volunteers the subsequent brain distribution of activity corresponds to that expected from *in vitro* binding studies[75] with high uptake in the thalamus, putamen, and caudate nucleus and lower uptake in the frontal cortex, temporal cortex, and cerebellum. PET studies of the known nicotinic receptor losses[75] have been performed in AD patients at different stages of disease[76] and a significant correlation was found between the decrease of ^{11}C-nicotine uptake and the MMSE scores.[74]

5. Adrenergic

As with other neuroreceptor systems there is abnormal adrenergic activity in AD brains. Adrenergic receptors specific to noradrenaline and adrenaline are classified into four subtypes, i.e., α_1, α_2, β_1, and β_2.[77] The α_2 adrenergic system is found mainly in the presynaptic terminals in the locus ceruleus, nucleus tractis lateralis, hippocampus and frontal cortex. This system is implicated in hypertension, diabetes, drug abuse, depression, anxiety states and dementia, and, in addition to its presence in the brain, the α_2 system is found in arteries (e.g., basilar artery, pulmonary artery, aorta, and pancreas islet cells). The knowledge of the adrenal system in normal aging and AD is derived from chemical analyses of bioamines in the brain homogenates and neuroanatomical autoradiography.[58,78-86] In addition to the findings of a deficiency in the content of noradrenaline[87,88] and in the synthesizing enzymes, there is a degeneration of locus ceruleus which is also independently known to occur in dementia.[88,89] A reduction of the α_2 adrenergic receptor in the nucleus basalis of Meynert has also been observed.[80]

The decrease in frontal cortex α_2 density using *p*-aminoclonidine[90] was corroborated by an autoradiographic study using the agonist tritiated bromoxidine; a significant reduction in the density of α_2 adrenoreceptors was found in frontal cortex (layers I and III) and hippocampus (CA$_1$ and stratum granularis at the dentate gyrus) in AD compared to age-matched controls.[86]

There is evidence and a current contention that the loss of noradrenaline and α_2-adrenoceptors is secondary to the degeneration of cortical adrenergic terminals arising from the locus ceruleus.[86,91,92]

Most α_2-adrenoceptors are thought to correspond to the inhibitory presynaptic autoreceptors, thus stimulation would lead to a decrease in synaptic noradrenaline content.[93] An interesting observation of the effect of an α_2 agonist is the profound effect of dexmedetomidine on enhancing gas anesthesia and the antidotal effect of the antagonist atipamezole in reversing this effect. The high affinity of atipamezole, 0.2 nM, lead us to evaluate the ability of this ligand to quantitate the distribution of the α_2 system.[58] The observation that the antagonists label both high- and low-affinity states of the α_2 system has been forwarded as a rationale for favoring agonists rather than antagonists if the labeling chemistry and biodistribution kinetics are acceptable.

Exploitation of imaging techniques for the *in vivo* study of normal aging and dementia is in its infancy principally because of two limitations. First, until recently, the resolution of emission imaging systems is too poor to detect much less quantitate the concentration of a radiolabeled ligand for the α_2 system as the receptors in the cortical layers I and III, locus ceruleus, hippocampus dentate gyrus, and hippocampus CA$_1$ layers reside in regions less than 2 mm in width (Figure 10). Indeed, a major motivation for the construction of a 2-mm PET imaging system is the importance of imaging the α_2 system. Second, there has not yet been developed an appropriate labeled ligand for definitive *in vivo* studies. With respect to the PET labeled ligands candidates which have been evaluated are the antagonists yohimbine, atipamezole, idazoxan, rauwolscine, and the agonists clonidine, dexmedetomidine, bromoxidine, and *p*-aminoclonodine. Difficulties in labeling antagonists may be overcome by the recent discovery of yohimbine analogs, the "isoquinoaphthyridines", which have α_1/α_2 selectivities in the range of 2,000 to 15,000. The near-term expectations for study of the α_2 system in aging and dementia depends on the development of high-resolution PET and this development can now be realized as discussed under the PET technology section.

D. NEUROPEPTIDES

The neuropeptides found in high concentrations in cerebral cortex include somatostatin (SS), neuropeptide Y (NPY), cholecystokinin (CCK), vasoactive-intestinal polypeptide (VIP), and galanin. Important neuropeptides in lower concentration include corticotropin-releasing factor (CRF), substance P (SP), and neurotensin (VT). Neuropeptide-containing neurons are primarily found on the cerebral cortex (layers I, III, and VI).[94] Many of these local circuit neurons contain gamma-aminobutyric acid (GABA) as a transmitter. Neuropeptide changes have been reproducibly demonstrated in AD hippocampal areas and reductions are noted in neocortical SS and CRF concentrations.[95] The dysfunction of affected neurons containing SS and CRF could produce widespread failure of cerebral cortical functions, resulting in the various behavioral deficits seen in AD. Radioligands for somatostatin and substance P are available but little research has been done on brain uptake due to the limited blood-brain barrier transport. Banks and co-workers discovered that administration of some octapeptide analogs of somatostatin in a serum-free perfusate caused a 200× increase in the amount of material that crossed the blood-brain barrier.[96] This suggests that some serum-related factor, probably the previously described protein binding or an aggregation-promoting factor, is the main determinant in limiting the blood-to-brain passage of somatostatin analogs.

E. CHOLINE AND PHOSPHOLIPIDS

The importance of choline in AD is based on the known decreases in acetylcholine which along with phosphatidylcholine is formed from choline. It is known that choline is the rate-limiting step in the synthesis of acetylcholine and over 10 years ago it was hypothesized that when neurons which synthesize acetylcholine are deprived of choline, they will catabolize phosphatidylcholine or membrane choline compounds and use the choline for acetylcholine synthesis.[59] The study of choline content and transport in the human brain has been hampered by the fact that until recently there have been no methods to study these compounds *in vivo*, changes in acetylcholine and choline content are rapid after death, and the transport across the blood-brain barrier is slow. Imaging methods of MRS offer a noninvasive and potentially quantitative approach to the *in vivo* study of choline-containing compounds. Of the major choline-containing compounds — choline, acetylcholine, phosphorylcholine, glycerophosocholine, phosphatidylcholine, and sphingomyelin — only the latter two have concentrations sufficient to be revealed by proton magnetic resonance.[60]

There appears to be a major decrease in the transport of choline across the blood-brain barrier with aging. Males received 4 g of choline chloride (as free base) orally and brain levels of choline and its water-soluble metabolites were assessed using MRS. In young males brain levels of choline and its water-soluble metabolites doubled after 3 hours. In aged (mean age = 72 ± 7) men, comparable elevations occurred in plasma choline levels; however, brain water-soluble choline compounds increased by only 19%.[97] Comparable findings have also been reported in rats.[98] This age-related impairment of choline transport could underlie the age dependence of AD on choline transport. It is believed that compounds that interact with choline and with its precursors and metabolites may provide effective treatments for AD.[97] Of significance is the possible relationship of decreased transport of choline, decreased availability of choline as a substrate, and possible related findings of increased glycerophosphocholine (GPC) and glycerophosphoethanolamine (GPE).

MRS studies from cortical areas of post-mortem brains have shown a decrease in phosphatidylcholine and phosphatidylethanolamine, choline, and ethanolamine, and increases in the phospholipid deacylation product, glycerophosphocholine.[99] Enzyme studies of increased glycerol-3-phosphorylcholine and phosphodiesterase and decreased choline kinase activities in AD brain samples[100] also lend support for the importance of membrane composition studies in the evaluation of AD including evaluation of proposed treatments.

The study of ^{11}C-choline by PET for evaluation of uptake or conversion to ^{11}C-acetylcholine is hampered by the low brain penetration (approximately 0.2% of injected dose) and the rapid incorporation of ^{11}C into metabolic products.[101,102] The half life of ^{11}C of only 20 minutes severely limits the use of this tracer for transport studies.

F. GABA-ACETYLCHOLINE SYSTEM

The relation of GABA to AD is through the effect of increased activity of GABA on the acetylcholine neurotransmitter release.[103]

PET studies have investigated the effects of two noncholinergic drugs on the release of acetylcholine. By examining the effects of gamma-vinyl GABA (a GABA transaminase inhibitor) or altanserin (a serotonergic antagonist) on the regional binding of ^{11}C-benztropine in the primate brain (Papio anubis), it was demonstrated that drugs acting upon either GABAergic or serotonergic neurons produce profound regional changes in acetylcholine release.[105] After administration of the gamma-vinyl GABA the accumulation of the PET ligand "C-benztropine" was less, indicating an endogenous increase of acetylcholine due to GABA increases. The acetylcholine is thought to be competitive to the PET tracer, thus the lower uptake. Striatal binding was decreased 47% and cortical binding decreased by 26% with no changes in thalamic and cerebellar binding. This type of study shows the power of PET to trace the effect of one neurotransmitter system on another system, in this case gives warning that agents which decrease GABA activity may enhance cholinergic hypofunction in Alzheimer's patients. It is also found in the studies with agonists and antagonists of 5HT that agents which increase serotonergic activity might also decrease cholinergic activity.[103,104]

These findings indicate that the mechanisms of action and the subsequent therapeutic efficacy of these centrally acting drugs may be linked to their multitransmitter effects. This application of PET represents a very promising experimental approach that can be directed toward elucidating abnormalities in neurotransmitter modulation relevant to disease progression and pharmacologic treatment.[105]

G. N-ACETYLASPARATE

Among its interesting features is the fact that *N*-acetylaspartate (NAA) is found only within the nervous system, with only trace amounts seen in the periphery.[106] NAA has been found by MRI in glia and neurons but not in astrocytes. For this reason the level of NAA has been proposed as an index of neuronal integrity. However, contemporary MRS studies of the NAA levels in gray and white matter suggest equal levels in contrast to *in vitro* analyses showing 4:1 differences between gray and white matter. ¹H-NMR spectroscopy can reveal the relative concentrations of total NAA as well as phosphocreatine (PCr), creatine, phosphocholine, and lactate. ¹H-NMR offers improved signal to noise ratio and a drastic reduction in signal averaging time over ³¹P spectra.

In our study, cortical NAA was reduced by 19% in the calcarine area, 24.6% in the middle frontal gyrus, 28.6% in the superior temporal gyrus, and about 50% in the parahippocampal gyrus. A loss of neocortical neurons in AD has been documented by several investigators to be in similar ranges to the magnitude of the NAA changes which we detected.[107-112] Marked loss of neurons within the entorhinal cortex of the parahippocampal gyrus is reported in AD, although not quantitatively determined.[113] Finally, the degree of synaptic loss has recently been observed to be the major indicator of dementia severity in AD.[114] Since NAA is found in the neuronal somata as well as the nerve endings[115] and, more specifically in the synaptosomal subfractions,[116-118] it is not known if the reduced cortical NAA in AD represents the combined reduction of NAA present in the synaptosomal fractions and the soluble fractions in depleted neurons. In the study by Klunk et al.,[119] NAA was significantly reduced only in AD brains with high SP counts but not in those with low counts. It is believed that loss of synapses in the neocortex precedes neuronal reduction.[120,121] Thus, an association between cortical NAA reduction and decreased synaptic density may exist. A sequential loss of synaptosomal NAA and cellular NAA as the disease progresses is a hypothesis for further consideration. Though there has been some justification presented for the stability of NAA in post-mortem studies, our recent studies show major decreases in NAA concentrations with faster declines in white matter than gray matter. This argues for careful *in vivo* MRS studies with high resolution before valid conclusions can be made.

H. MYO-INOSITOL

Proton (¹H) MRS research[122] has indicated there is an elevation of myoinositol (MI) in patients with mild to moderate AD (Figure 11). This suggests that abnormalities in the inositol polyphosphate messenger pathway occur in the natural history of AD. The increase in MI, which amounted to approximately 1.5 mmol/kg (22% of normal concentration), was consistent with the observation of 50% reduction in phosphatidyl inositol and a marked but statistically nonsignificant elevation of MI in cadaveric brains of patients with AD.[123] The increase in MI suggests the most likely mechanism to be inhibition of the enzyme(s) responsible for conversion of MI to phosphatidyl inositol. The increase in MI has been linked to the phosphorylation state of cellular proteins or to changes in membrane structure caused by altered phospholipid metabolism. These data are from large volumes of mixed gray and white matter and CSF. Studies using spectroscopic volumes five times smaller are now possible and this observation will have further evaluations at other laboratories.

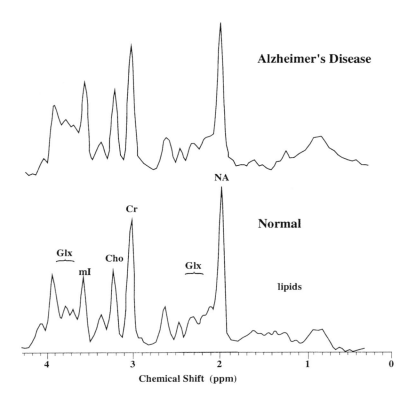

FIGURE 11 Proton (¹H) MRS sum of the spectra of eight patients with AD (top) and eight healthy patients (bottom). (From Miller et al., *Radiology,* 1993. With permission.)

VI. ELECTRICAL ACTIVITY MAPPING (EEG)

The multielectrode electroencephalograph (EEG) has been well documented as an aid in the diagnosis of AD.[124] The routine EEG is also useful in following the progression of AD. In a test-retest reliability study of EEG abnormalities, the routine EEG was superior to the computerized EEG in showing progression of slowing over time.[125] The degree of EEG abnormality shows a significant inverse association with clinical response to antidepressants in studies of depression, dementia, and dementia with depression.[126] With the advent of computerized EEG, it is now practical to obtain maps or images of spatial differences in the EEG frequencies. Quantitative analyses by topographic maps of the power in specific frequency bands from region to region on the EEG consistently show different patterns in AD relative to age-matched normal subjects.[7,127-132] Relative theta power has been found to be a sensitive classifier for differentiation of demented patients (vascular and AD) from normals[131] and, whereas the topographic map of relative alpha, theta, and delta power show global variation, there is not as consistent a regional pattern as in the parietal-temporal decrease of glucose metabolism seen in PET nor is there correspondence between the diffuse changes and the topography of SPECT hypoperfusion.[129] As severity of dementia increases there is an increase in delta and theta activity.[128] All of the reports in the past 10 years have emphasized the fact that the low-frequency delta and theta bands are of higher power in AD than in control subjects. A coherence analysis of each electrode with neighboring electrodes showed a low temporal coherence in AD relative to normal subjects and this could be interpreted as a loss of neocortical connection.[133] In addition to frequency ban analysis, other metrics have been proposed for the objective analysis of the multiple lead EEG. The student-t topographic map of significance of deviation from the normal has been proposed as a robust method for detection of patterns of abnormalities.[134] The fractal analysis method applied to the EEG wave patterns has been shown to give a nonlinear metric, fractal dimension, which is lower in AD than in the normal controls.[135] Discriminate analysis of the power in various frequency bands and their ratios has also been used to distinguish AD from non-AD subjects.[136]

Insofar as the changes noted by a number of investigators show a consistent increase in delta and theta activity and that these increases have some proportionality to the severity of the dementia, a simple topographic image representing a ratio of power in frequency bands might be an important and inexpensive adjunct to quantifying the severity and response to therapy in AD (Figure 6). A prominent example of the use of EEG to follow therapy is that of the first intracranial infusion of nerve growth factor.[137] The single patient report included the observation of a decrease in the low-frequency components of the EEG along with improvement in other aspects of brain physiology (i.e.,. blood flow and nicotine receptor concentration). Mody and co-workers[7] found that some of their quantitative encephalographic measures correlated well with the clinical degree of severity of dementia as measured by the Mini-Mental Status Exam (MMSE) score and the clinical dementia rating (CDR).

VII. FUNCTIONAL ACTIVATION IMAGING STUDIES

Three classes of studies to investigate the brain's response to cognitive or CO_2 challenges have been done using PET and SPECT. The incremental increase in glucose metabolism after a cognitive challenge is the same in AD as it is in normal subjects.[138] The relative change in flow as measured by $H_2^{15}O$ was also not less than expected from normal studies during a visual recognition test.[139]

During a Word Pain Learning and Recall test there was a significant increase of regional cerebral blood flow in 28 of 32 brain regions in AD as compared to increases in 13 of 32 regions in controls.[140] In those studies ^{133}Xe and SPECT were used.

VIII. INFLAMMATION AND IMMUNE SYSTEM

Imaging methods have a high potential for the investigation of tissue inflammatory and immunological characteristics of the AD brain *in vivo*. Though there is no strong evidence for inflammation as part of the pathophysiology of AD, we truly have not had the opportunities to examine the brain for abnormal accumulations of white cells or abnormal concentrations of cytokines. Neutrophils labeled with ^{11}C-PK 11195[141] will give 15 or more times improved sensitivity over conventional ^{99m}Tc-labeled neutrophils with SPECT. Perhaps of greater promise is the use of labeled probes for cytokines (e.g., TGFβ,[142] TNF,[143] IL1, IL2, IL8, etc.). Whereas labeled immunoglobins (IgG) will not cross the blood-brain barrier, labeled aptamers might be effective probes for cytokines in the brain.[144] Aptamers are short single strand DNA molecules which are specific for a given protein. Labeling technology for aptamers or oligonucleotides is under active development.

IX. NEAR FUTURE POSSIBILITIES

Noninvasive studies of human neurodegeneration depend on innovations in PET instrumentation and radiochemistry and improvements in magnetic resonance technologies. Specific approaches for characterizing brain neurochemistry and neuroanatomy are

- Development and implementation of more sophisticated techniques (mitochondrial, enzyme, neuroreceptor, and cellular probes) for charting the progress of neurodegeneration by the use of markers of mitochondrial brain function and neurochemical systems (Table 2).

- Development of three-dimensional quantitation of brain glucose metabolism in neocortical and limbic brain structures in patients with AD using registered high-resolution MRI and regional NAA to normalize very high resolution (2 mm) PET.
- Development of three-dimensional magnetic resonance microscopy of neocortical and limbic brain morphology at resolutions (100 μm or better), for applications to AD including development of an 8- to 10-T resource for detailed studies of the human cortex.
- Investigation of the chemical composition of the cortex of AD relative to normal controls using proton spectroscopy for choline compounds, creatine, *N*-acetylaspartate, glutamate, glutamine, GABA, myoinositol, and lactate (if present) (Table 1).
- Development of radiopharmaceutical tracers with specificity for neurochemistry and for cytokines which might be involved in the mechanisms of AD.
- Use PET and metabolic or neuroreceptor ligands for monitoring the consequences of chemical treatments, (e.g., Nerve growth factor (NGF) infusion, neural transplantation, and gene therapy.

Advances in the emerging field of gene therapy may lead to genetically modified neurons that are capable of synthesizing neurotrophic factors or missing neurotransmitters. The use of neural transplantation to replace nerve cells in neurodegenerative disorders such as Parkinson's disease has been proposed specifically for the dopamine system. Are we now in a position to perform neural transplantation in AD? If so, we can expect imaging techniques will provide the noninvasive method whereby the transplantation process can be monitored in animal and human studies. The model for this application of noninvasive techniques to modern molecular medicine is in the evaluation of the efficacy of tissue transplantation for treatment of Parkinson's disease wherein PET has effectively studied presynaptic dopamine activity using ^{18}F-dopa and ^{18}F-*m*-tyrosine.

ACKNOWLEDGMENT

I thank Dr. Kathleen M. Brennan for the extensive literature background material and the technical development of this chapter. This work was supported by the National Institute of Aging and the Office of Health and Environmental Research of DOE.

REFERENCES

1. Kuhl, D. E. and Edwards, R. Q., Image separation radioisotope scanning, *Radiology,* 80, 653, 1963.
2. Tsui, B. M., Zhao, X., Frey, E. C. and McCartney, W. H., Quantitative single-photon emission computed tomography: basics and clinical considerations, *Semin. Nuclear Med.,* 24, 38, 1994.
3. Budinger, T. F., Gullberg, G. T. and Huesman, R. H., Emission computed tomography, in *Topics in Applied Physics: Image Reconstruction from Projections: Implementation and Applications,* Herman, G. T., Springer-Verlag, Berlin, 1979, 147.
4. Budinger, T. F., Derenzo, S. E., Huesman, R. H., Jagust, W. J. and Valk, P. E., High resolution positron emission tomography for medical science studies, *Acta Radiol. Supple.,* 376, 15, 1991.
5. Moses, W. W., Derenzo, S. E. and Budinger, T. F., PET detector modules based on novel detector technologies, *Nuclear Instrum. Methods Phys. Res.,* A 353, 189, 1994.
6. Pettegrew, J. W., Panchalingam, K., Klunk, W. E., McClure, R. J. and Muenz, L. R., Alterations of cerebral metabolism in probable Alzheimer's disease: a preliminary study. Appendix, *Neurobiol. Aging,* 15, 117, 1994.
7. Mody, C. K., McIntyre, H. B., Miller, B. L., Altman, K., and Read, S., Computerized EEG frequency analysis and topographic brain mapping in Alzheimer's disease, *Ann. N.Y. Acad. Sci.,* 620, 45, 1991.
8. Huckman, M. S., Fox, J., and Topel, J., The validity of criteria for the evaluation of cerebral atrophy by computed tomography, *Radiology,* 116, 85, 1975.
9. de Leon, M. J., Ferris, S. H., George, A. E., Reisberg, B., Kricheff, I. I. and Gershon, S., Computed tomography evaluations of brain-behavior relationships in senile dementia of the Alzheimer's type, *Neurobiol. Aging,* 1, 69, 1980.
10. Jacoby, R. J. and Levy, R., Computed tomography in the elderly. II. Senile dementia: diagnosis and functional impairment, *Br. J. Psychiat.,* 136, 256, 1980.

11. Ford, C. V., and Winter, J., Computerized axial tomograms and dementia in elderly patients, *J Gerontol.,* 36, 164, 1981.

12. de Leon, M. J., Golomb, J., George, A. E., Convit, A., Tarshish, C. Y., McRae, T., De Santi, S., et al. The radiologic prediction of Alzheimer's disease: the atrophic hippocampal formation, *Am. J. Neuroradiol.,* 14, 897, 1993.

13. Seab, J. P., Jagust, W. J., Wong, S. T., Roos, M. S., Reed, B. R. and Budinger, T. F. Quantitative NMR measurements of hippocampal atrophy in Alzheimer's disease, *Magnet. Reson. Med.,* 200, 1988.

14. Lehericy, S., Baulac, M., Chiras, J., Pierot, L., Martin, N., Pillon, B., Deweer, B., et al. Amygdalohippocampal MR volume measurements in the early stages of Alzheimer's disease, *Am. J. Neuroradiol.,* 15, 929, 1994.

15. Killiany, R. J., Moss, M. B., Albert, M. S., Sandor, T., Tieman, J. and Jolesz, F. Temporal lobe regions on magnetic resonance imaging identify patients with early Alzheimer's disease, *Arch. Neurol.,* 50, 949, 1993.

16. Kesslak, J. P., Nalcioglu, O., and Cotman, C. W. Quantification of magnetic resonance scans for hippocampal and parahippocampal atrophy in Alzheimer's disease [see comments], *Neurology,* 41, 51, 1991.

17. Erkinjuntti, T., Lee, D. H., Gao, F., Steenhuis, R., Eliasziw, M., Fry, R., Merskey, H., et al. Temporal lobe atrophy on magnetic resonance imaging in the diagnosis of early Alzheimer's disease, *Arch. Neurol.;* 50, 305, 1993.

18. Jack, C. R. J., Petersen, R. C., O'Brien, P. C., and Tangalos, E. G., MR-based hippocampal volumetry in the diagnosis of Alzheimer's disease, *Neurology,* 42, 183, 1992.

19. Damasio, H., Kuljis, R. O., Yuh, W., van Hoesen, G. W. and Ehrhard, J., Magnetic resonance imaging of human intracortical structure *in vivo, Cerebral Cortex,* 1, 374, 1991.

20. Clark, V. P., Courchesne, E., and Grafe, M., *In vivo* myeloarchitectonic analysis of human striate and extrastriate cortex using magnetic resonance imaging, *Cerebral Cortex,* 2, 417, 1992.

21. Jagust, W. J., Eberling, J. L., Richardson, B. C., Reed, B. R., Baker, M. G., Nordahl, T. E., and Budinger, T., The cortical topography of temporal lobe hypometabolism in early Alzheimer's disease, *Brain Res.,* 629, 189, 1993.

22. Golomb, J., de Leon, M. J., Kluger, A., George, A. E., Tarshish, C., and Ferris, S. H., Hippocampal atrophy in normal aging. An association with recent memory impairment, *Arch. Neurol.,* 50, 967, 1993.

23. Katz, D., Taubenberger, J. K., Cannella, B., McFarlin, D. E., Raine, C. S., and McFarland, H. F., Correlation between magnetic resonance imaging findings and lesion development in chronic, active multiple sclerosis, *Ann. Neurol.,* 34, 661, 1993.

24. Kawai, M., Cras, P., and Perry, G., Serial reconstruction of beta-protein amyloid plaques: relationship to microvessels and size distribution, *Brain Res.,* 592, 278, 1992.

25. Budinger, T. F., Emerging nuclear magnetic resonance technologies. Health and safety, *Ann. N.Y. Acad. Sci.,* 649, 1, 1992.

26. Postiglione, A., Lassen, N. A., and Holman, B. L., Cerebral blood flow in patients with dementia of Alzheimer's type, *Aging,* 5, 19, 1993.

27. Kuwabara, Y., Ichiya, Y., Otsuka, M., Tahara, T., Fukumura, T., Gunasekera, R., Ichimiya, A., et al., Comparison of I-123 IMP and Tc-99m HMPAO SPECT studies with PET in dementia, *Ann. Nuclear Med.,* 4, 75, 1990.

28. Jagust, W. J., Budinger, T. F. and Reed, B. R., The diagnosis of dementia with single photon emission computed tomography, *Arch. Neurol.,* 44, 258, 1987.

29. Dekosky, S. T., Shih, W. J., Schmitt, F. A., Coupal, J., and Kirkpatrick, C., Assessing utility of single photon computed tomography (SPECT) scan in Alzheimer's Disease: correlation with cognitive severity, *Alzheimer's Dis. Assoc. Disord.,* 4, 14, 1990.

30. Kuhl, D. E., Barrio, J. R., Huang, S. C., Selin, C., Ackermann, R. F., Lear, J. L., Wu, J. L., et al., Quantifying local cerebral blood flow by *N*-isopropyl-p-[123I]iodoamphetamine (IMP) tomography, *J. Nuclear Med.,* 23, 196, 1982.

31. Hill, T. C., Holman, B. L., Lovett, R., O'Leary, D. H., Front, D., Magistretti, P., Zimmerman, R. E., et al., Initial experience with SPECT (single photon computerized tomography) of the brain using *n*-isopropyl I-123-*p*-iodoamphetamine, *J. Nuclear Med.,* 23, 191, 1982.

32. Holman, B. L., Johnson, K. A., Gerada, B., Carvalho, P. A. and Satlin, A., The scintigraphic appearance of Alzheimer's Disease: a prospective study using rtechnecium-99m-HMPAO SPECT. *J. Nuclear Med.,* 33: 181, 1992.

33. Perani, D., Di Piero, V., and Vallar, G., Technecium-99m HMPAO SPECT study of regional cerebral perfusion in early Alzheimer's disease, *J. Nuclear Med.,* 29, 1507, 1988.

34. Hellman, R. S., Collier, B. D., Tikofsky, R. S., Kilgore, D. P., Daniels, D. L., Haughton V.M., Walsh P.R., et al. Comparison of single-photon emission computed tomography with [123I]iodoamphetamine and xenon-enhanced computed tomography for assessing regional cerebral blood flow, *J. Cereb. Blood Flow Metab.,* 6, 747, 1986.

35. Bonte, F. J., Hom, J., Tinter, R., and Weiner, M. F., Single photon tomography in Alzheimer's disease and the dementias, *Semin. Nuclear Med.,* 20, 342, 1990.

36. Devous, M. D. S., Payne, J. K. and Lowe, J. L., Dual-isotope brain SPECT imaging with technetium-99m and iodine-123: clinical validation using xenon-133 SPECT, *J. Nuclear Med.,* 33, 1919, 1992.

37. Wilhelm, K. R., Schroder, J., Henningsen, H., Sauer, H., and Georgi, P., Preliminary results of 99mTc-HMPAO-SPECT studies in endogenous psychoses, *J. Nuclear Med.,* 28, 88, 1989.

38. Mayberg, H. S., Lewis, P. J., Regenold, W., and Wagner, H. N. J., Paralimbic hypoperfusion in unipolar depression, *J. Nuclear Med.,* 35, 929, 1994.

39. Messa, C., Perani, D., Lucignani, G., Zenorini, A., Zito, F., Rizzo, G., Grassi, F., et al., High resolution technecium-99m-HMPAO SPECT in patients with probable Alzheimer's disease: comparison with fluorine-18-FDG PET, *J. Nuclear Med.,* 35, 210, 1994.

40. Mielke, R., Pietrzyk, U., Jacobs, A., Fink, G. R., Ichimiya, A., Kessler, J., Herholz, K., et al., HMPAO SPECT and FDG PET in Alzheimer's disease and vascular dementia: comparison of perfusion and metabolic pattern, *Eur. J. Nuclear Med.,* 21, 1052, 1994.

41. Friedland, R. P., Budinger, T. F., and Jagust, W. J., Positron tomography and the differential diagnosis and pathophysiology of Alzheimer's disease, in *Senile Dementia of the Alzheimer's Type*, Traber, J. and Gispen, W. H., Eds., Springer-Verlag, Heidelberg, 1985.

42. Kuhl, D. E., Small, G. W., Riege, W. H., Fujikawa, D. G., Metter, E. J., Benson, D. F., Ashford, J. W., et al., Cerebral metabolic patterns before the diagnosis of probable Alzheimer's disease, *J. Cereb. Blood Flow Metab.,* 7(Suppl.), 406, 1987.

43. Shapiro, M. B., Pietrini, P., Grady, C. L., Ball, M. J., DeCarli, C., A. K., Kaye, J. A., et al., Reductions in parietal and temporal cerebral metabolic rates for glucose are not specific for Alzheimer's disease, *J. Neurol. Neurosurg. Psychiat.,* 56, 859, 1993.

44. Cutler, N. R., Haxby, J. V., Duara, R., Grady, C. L., Moore, A. M., Parisi, J. E., White J., et al. Brain metabolism as measured with positron emission tomography: serial assessment in a patient with familial Alzheimer's disease, *Neurology,* 35, 1556, 1985.

45. Jagust, W. J., Friedland, R. P., Budinger, T. F., Koss, E., and Ober, B., Longitudinal studies of regional cerebral metabolism in Alzheimer's disease, *Neurology,* 38, 909, 1988.

46. Kuhl, D. E., Metter, E. J., Riege, W. H. and Markham, C. H. Patterns of cerebral glucose utilization in Parkinson's disease and Huntington's disease, *Ann. Neurol.,* 15(Suppl.), 119, 1984.

47. Peppard, R. F., Martin, W. R., Carr, G. D., Grochowski, E., Schulzer, M., Guttman, M., McGeer, P. L., et al., Cerebral glucose metabolism in Parkinson's disease with and without dementia, *Arch. Neurol.,* 49, 1262, 1992.

48. VanBrocklin, H. F., Enas, J. D., Hanrahan, S. M., Brennan, K. M., O'Neil, J. P., and S.E.T. [F-18]Fluorodihydrororotrnone: synthesis and evaluation of a mitochondrial electron transport chain (ETC) complex I probe for PET, *J. Nuclear Med.,* 35, 73P, 1994.

49. Linnane, A. W., Baumer, A., Maxwell, R. J., Preston, H., Zhang, C. F., and Marzuki, S., Mitochondrial gene mutation: the ageing process and degenerative diseases, *Biochem. Int.,* 22, 1067, 1990.

50. Miquel, J., An integrated theory of aging as a result of mitochondrial-DNA mutation in differentiated cells, *Arch. Gerontol. Geriat.,* 12, 99, 1991.

51. Wallace, D. C., Mitochondrial genetics: a paradigm for aging and degenerative diseases? *Science,* 256, 628, 1992.

52. Linnane, A. W., Marzuki, S., Ozawa, T., and Tanaka, M., Mitochondrial DNA mutations as an important contributor to ageing and degenerative diseases, *Lancet,* 1, 642, 1989.

53. Mecocci, P., MacGarvey, U., Kaufman, A. E., Koontz, D., Shoffner, J. M., Wallace, D. W., and Beal, M. F., Oxidative damage to mitochondrial DNA shows marked age-dependent increases in human brain, *Ann. Neurol.,* 34, 609, 1993.

54. Arnheim, N., and Cortopassi, G., Deleterious mitochondrial DNA mutations accumulate in aging human tissues, *Mutat. Res.,* 275, 157, 1992.

55. Harmon, H. J., Nank, S., and R. A. F., Age-dependent changes in rat brain mitochondria of synaptic and non-synaptic origins, *Mechanisms Aging Dev.,* 38, 167, 1987.

56. Mathis, C. A., Taylor, S. E., Biegon, A., and Enas, J. D., [125I]5-iodo-6-nitroquipazine: a potent and selective ligand for the 5-hydroxytryptamine uptake complex. I. *In vitro* studies, *Brain Res.,* 619, 229, 1993.

57. Kuhl, D. E., Koeppe, R. A., Fessler, J. A., Minoshima, S., Ackermann, R. J., Carey, J. E., Gildersleeve, D. L., et al., *In vivo* mapping of cholinergic neurons in the human brain using SPECT and IBVM, *J. Nuclear Med.,* 35, 405, 1994.

58. Biegon, A., Mathis, C. A., and Budinger, T. F., Quantitative *in vitro* and *ex vivo* autoradiography of the alpha 2-adrenoceptor antagonist [3H]atipamezole, *Eur. J. Pharmacol.,* 224, 27, 1992.

59. Blusztajn J.K. and Wurtman R.J. Choline and cholinergic neurons, *Science,* 221, 614, 1983.

60. Miller, B. L., Moats, R. A., Shonk, T., Ernst, T., Woolley, S., and Ross, B. D. Alzheimer's disease: depiction of increased cerebral myo-inositol with proton MR spectroscopy, *Radiology,* 187, 433, 1993.

61. Dewey, S. L., MacGregor, R. R., Brodie, J. D., Bendriem, B., King, P. T., Volkow N.D., Schlyer D.J., et al. Mapping muscarinic receptors in human and baboon brain using [*N*-11C-methyl]-benztropine, *Synapse,* 5, 213, 1990.

62. Frey, K. A., Koeppe, R. A., Mulholland, G. K., Jewett, D., Hichwa, R., Ehrenkaufer, R. L., Carey, J. E., et al. *In vivo* muscarinic cholinergic receptor imaging in human brain with [11C]scopolamine and positron emission tomography, *J. Cereb. Blood Flow Metab.,* 12, 147, 1992.

63. Holman, B. L., Gibson, R. E., Hill, T. C., Eckelman, W. C., Albert, M. and Reba, R. C. Muscarinic acetylcholine receptors in Alzheimer's disease. *In vivo* imaging with iodine 123-labeled 3-quinuclidinyl-4-iodobenzilate and emission tomography, *JAMA,* 254, 3063, 1985.

64. Weinberger, D. R., Gibson, R. E., Coppola, R., Jones, D. W., Braun, A. R., Mann, U., Berman, K. F., et al. Distribution of muscarinic receptors in patients with dementia: A controlled study of 123I-QNB and SPECT, *J. Cereb. Blood Flow Metab.,* 9, 537(abstr.), 1989.

65. Weinberger, D. R., Jones, D., Reba, R. C., Mann, U., Coppola, R., Gibson, R., Gorey, J., et al. A comparison of FDG PET and IQNB SPECT in normal subjects and in patients with dementia, *J. Neuropsychiat. Clin. Neurosci.*, 4, 239, 1992.

66. Weinberger, D. R., Gibson, R., Coppola, R., Jones, D. W., Molchan, S., Sunderland, T., Berman, K. F., et al. The distribution of cerebral muscarinic acetylcholine receptors *in vivo* in patients with dementia. A controlled study with 123IQNB and single photon emission computed tomography [see comments], *Arch. Neurol.*, 48, 169, 1991.

67. Wyper, D., Teasdale, E., Patterson, J., Montaldi, D., Brown, D., Hunter, R., Graham, D., et al., Abnormalities in rCBF and computed tomography in patients with Alzheimer's disease and in controls, *Br. J. Radiol.*, 66, 23, 1993.

68. Zeeberg, B. R., Kim, H. J. and Reba, R. C., Pharmacokinetic simulations of SPECT quantitation of the M2 muscarinic neuroreceptor subtype in disease states using radioiodinated (R,R)-4IQNB, *Life Sci.*, 51, 661, 1992.

69. Blin, J., Baron, J. C., Dubois, B., Crouzel, C., Fiorelli, M., Attar-Levy, D., Pillon, B., et al., Loss of brain 5-HT2 receptors in Alzheimer's disease. *In vivo* assessment with positron emission tomography and [^{18}F]setoperone, *Brain.*, 116, 497, 1993.

70. Kung, H. F., Radiopharmaceuticals for CNS receptor imaging with SPECT, *Int. J. Radiat. Appl. Instrum. B*, 17, 85, 1990.

71. Jagust, W. J., Eberling, J. L., Roberts, J. A., Brennan, K. M., Hanrahan, S. M., VanBrocklin, H., Enas, J. D., et al. *In vivo* imaging of the 5-hydroxytryptamine reuptake site in primate brain using single photon emission computed tomography and [123I]5-iodo-6-nitroquipazine, *Eur. J. Pharmacol.*, 242, 189, 1993.

72. Hartvig, P., Lindner, K. J., Tedroff, J., Andersson, Y., Bjurling, P. and Langstrom, B., Brain kinetics of ^{11}C-labeled L-tryptophan and 5-hydroxy-L-tryptophan in the rhesus monkey. A study using positron emission tomography, *J. Neur. Transm.*, 88, 1, 1992.

73. Mach, R. H., Luedtke, R. R., Unsworth, C. D., Boundy, V. A., Nowak, P. A., Scripto, J. G., Elder, S. T., et al., 18F-labeled benzamides for studying the dopamine D2 receptor with positron emission tomography, *J. Med. Chem.*, 36, 3707, 1993.

74. Nordberg, A., Neuroreceptor changes in Alzheimer's disease, *Cerebrovasc. Brain Metab. Rev.*, 4, 303, 1992.

75. Nordberg, A., Hartvig, P., Lundqvist, H., Antoni, G., Ulin, J., and Langstrom, B., Uptake and regional distribution of (+)-(*R*)- and (−)-(*S*)-N-[methyl-^{11}C]-nicotine in the brains of rhesus monkey. An attempt to study nicotinic receptors *in vivo. J. Neur. Transm. Parkinsons Dis. Dementia Sect.*, 1, 195, 1989.

76. Nordberg, A., Hartvig, P., Lilja, A., Viitanen, M., Amberla, K., Lundqvist, H., Andersson, Y., et al., Decreased uptake and binding of 11C-nicotine in brain of Alzheimer patients as visualized by positron emission tomography, *J. Neur. Transm. Parkinsons Dis. Dementia Sect.*, 2, 215, 1990.

77. Bylund, D. B., Ray-Prenger, C., and Murphy, T. J., Alpha-2A and alpha-2B adrenergic receptor subtypes: antagonist binding in tissues and cell lines containing only one subtype, *J. Pharmacol. Exp. Ther.*, 245, 600, 1988.

78. Unnerstall, J. R., Kopajtic, T. A. and Kuhar, M. J., Distribution of alpha 2 agonist binding sites in the rat and human central nervous system: analysis of some functional, anatomic correlates of the pharmacologic effects of clonidine and related adrenergic agents, *Brain Res.*, 319, 69, 1984.

79. Asakura, M., Tsukamoto, T., Imafuku, J., Matsui, H., Ino, H., and Hasegawa, K., Quantitative analysis of rat alpha2 receptors discriminated by [^{3}H]clonidine and [^{3}H]rauwolscine, *Eur. J. Pharmacol.*, 106, 141, 1985.

80. Shimohama, S., Taniguchi, T., Fujiwara, M., and Kameyama, M., Biochemical characterization of alpha-adrenergic receptors in human brain and changes in Alzheimer-type dementia, *J. Neurochem.*, 47, 1295, 1986.

81. Pazos A., Gonzalez, A. M., Pascual, J., Meana, J. J., Barturen, F., and Garcia-Sevilla, J. A., Alpha 2-adrenoceptors in human forebrain: autoradiographic visualization and biochemical parameters using the agonist [^{3}H]UK-14304, *Brain Res.*, 475, 361, 1988.

82. Boyajian, C. L., Loughlin, S. E. and Leslie, F. M., Anatomical evidence for alpha-2 adrenoceptor heterogeneity: differential autoradiographic distributions of [3H]rauwolscine and [3H]idazoxan in rat brain, *J. Pharmacol. Exp. Ther.*, 241, 1079, 1987.

83. Kalaria, R. N., and Andorn, A. C., Adrenergic receptors in aging and Alzheimer's disease: decreased alpha 2-receptors demonstrated by [^{3}H]*p*-aminoclonidine binding in prefrontal cortex, *Neurobiol. Aging*, 12, 131, 1991.

84. Hudson, A. L., Mallard, N. J., Tyacke, R., and Nutt, D. J., [3H]RX1002: a highly selective ligand for identification of α-adrenoceptors in the rat brain, *Mol. Neuropharmacol.*, 1, 219, 1992.

85. Meana, J. J., Barturen, F., and Garcia-Sevilla, J. A., Characterization and regional distribution of alpha 2-adrenoceptors in post-mortem human brain using the full agonist [^{3}H]UK 14304, *J. Neurochem.*, 52, 1210, 1989.

86. Pascual, J., Grijalba, B., Garcia-Sevilla, J. A., Zarranz, J. J. and Pazos, A., Loss of high-affinity alpha 2-adrenoceptors in Alzheimer's disease: an autoradiographic study in frontal cortex and hippocampus, *Neurosci. Lett.*, 142, 36, 1992.

87. Adolfsson, R., Gottfries, C. G., Roos, B. E., and Winblad, B., Changes in the brain catecholamines in patients with dementia of Alzheimer type, *Br. J. Psychiat.*, 135, 216, 1979.

88. Marcyniuk, B., Mann, D. M., and Yates, P. O. The topography of cell loss from locus caeruleus in Alzheimer's disease, *J. Neurol. Sci.*, 76, 335, 1986.

89. Burke, W. J., Chung, H. D., Huang, J. S., Huang, S. S., Haring, J. H., Strong, R., Marshall, G. L., et al., Evidence for retrograde degeneration of epinephrine neurons in Alzheimer's disease, *Ann. Neurol.*, 24, 532, 1988.

90. Kalaria, R. N., Andorn, A. C. and Harik, S. I., Alterations in adrenergic receptors of frontal cortex and cerebral microvessels in Alzheimer's disease and aging, *Prog. Clin. Biol. Res.*, 317, 367, 1989.

91. Bondareff, W., Mountjoy, C. Q., and Roth, M., Loss of neurons of origin of the adrenergic projection to cerebral cortex (nucleus locus ceruleus) in senile dementia, *Neurology,* 32, 164, 1982.

92. Mann, D. M., Lincoln, J., Yates, P. O., Stamp, J. E., and Toper, S., Changes in the monoamine containing neurones of the human CNS in senile dementia, *Br. J. Psychiat.,* 136, 533, 1980.

93. Starke, K., Gothert, M., and Kilbinger, H., Modulation of neurotransmitter release by presynaptic autoreceptors, *Physiol. Rev.,* 69, 864, 1989.

94. Jones, E. G., and Hendry, S. H. C., GABAergic, substance P-immunoreactive neurons in the monkey cerebral cortex, *Soc. Neurosci. Abstr.,* 11, 145, 1985.

95. Auchus, A. P., Green, R. C., and Nemeroff, C. B., Cortical and subcortical neuropeptides in Alzheimer's disease *Neurobiol. Aging,* 15, 589, 1994.

96. Banks, W. A., Schally, A. V., Barrera, C. M., Fasold, M. B., Durham, D. A., Csernus V. J., Groot K., et al. Permeability of the murine blood-brain barrier to some octapeptide analogs of somatostatin, *Proc. Natl. Acad. Sci. U.S.A.,* 87, 6762, 1990.

97. Wurtman, R. J., and Bettiker, R. L., How to find a treatment for Alzheimer's disease, *Neurobiol. Aging,* 15(Suppl.), 179, 1994.

98. Mooradian, A. D., Blood-brain barrier transport of choline is reduced in the aged rat, *Brain Res.,* 440, 328, 1988.

99. Holmes, T. C., Nitsch, R. M., Erfurth, A., and Wurtman, R. J., Phospholipid and phospholipid metabolites in rat frontal cortex are decreased following nucleus basalis lesions, *Ann. N.Y. Acad. Sci.,* 695, 241, 1993.

100. Kanfer, J. N., Pettegrew, J. W., Moossy, J., and McCartney, D. G., Alterations of selected enzymes of phospholipid metabolism in Alzheimer's disease brain tissue as compared to non-Alzheimer's demented controls, *Neurochem. Res.,* 18, 331, 1993.

101. Gauthier, S., Diksic, M., Yamamoto, Y. L., Tyler, J. L., and Feindel, W., Positron emission tomography with 11C-choline in human subjects, *Can. J. Neurol. Sci.,* 12, 214(abstr.), 1985.

102. Rosen, M. A., Jones, R. M., Yano, Y. and Budinger, T. F., Carbon-11 choline: synthesis, purification, and brain uptake inhibition by 2-dimethylaminoethanol, *J. Nuclear Med.,* 26, 1424, 1985.

103. Jackson, D., Stachowiak, M. K., Bruno, J. P. and Zigmond, M. J., Inhibition of striatal acetylcholine release by endogenous serotonin, *Brain Res.,* 457, 259, 1988.

104. Gillet, G., Ammor, S. and Fillion, G., Serotonin inhibits acetylcholine release from rat striatum slices: evidence for a presynaptic receptor-mediated effect, *J. Neurochem.,* 45, 1687, 1985.

105. Dewey, S. L., Smith, G. S., Logan, J., and Brodie, J. D., Modulation of central cholinergic activity by GABA and serotonin: PET studies with 11C-benztropine in primates, *Neuropsychopharmacology,* 8, 371, 1993.

106. Tallan, H. H., Moore, S., and Stein, W. H., *N*-Acetyl-L-aspartic acid in brain, *J. Biol. Chem.,* 257, 1956.

107. Longo, R., Giorgini, A., Magnaldi, S., Pascazio, L., and Ricci, C., Alzheimer's disease histologically proven studied by MRI and MRS: two cases, *Magnet. Reson. Imag.,* 11, 1209, 1993.

108. Mann, D. M. A., Marcyniuk, B., Yates, P. O., Neary, D., and Snowden, J. S., The progression of the pathological changes of Alzheimer's disease in frontal and temporal neocortex examined both at biopsy and at autopsy, *Neuro-pathol. Appl. Neurobiol.,* 177, 1988.

109. Miyake, M., Kakimoto, Y., and Sorimachi, M., A gas chromatographic method for the determination of *N*-acetyl-L-aspartic acid, *N*-acetyl-α-aspartylglutamic acid and β-citryl-L-glutamic acid and their distributions in the brain and other organs of various species of animals, *J. Neurochem.,* 804, 1981.

110. Procter, W. A., Lowe, S. L. and Palmer, A. M., et al., Topographical distribution of neurochemical changes in Alzheimer's disease, *J. Neurol. Sci.,* 125, 1988.

111. Terry, R., Masliah, E., and Salmon, D., et al., Physical basis of cognitive alterations in Alzheimer's disease: synapse loss is the major correlation of cognitive impairment. *Ann. Neurol.,* 572, 1991.

112. Terry, R. D. and Hansen, L. A., Some morphometric aspects of Alzheimer's disease and of normal aging, in *Aging and the Brain*, Terry, R. D., Ed., Raven Press, New York, 1988, 109.

113. Hyman, B. T., Van Hoesen, G. W., Kromer, L. J. and Damasio, A. R., Perforant pathway changes and the memory impairment of Alzheimer's disease, *Ann. Neurol.,* 472, 1986.

114. Tanaka, C., Naruse, S., Horikawa, Y., Hirakawa, K., Yoshizaki, K. and Nishikawa, H., Proton nuclear magnetic resonance spectra of brain tumors, *Magnet. Reson. Imag.,* 503, 1986.

115. Fleming, M. C. and Lowry, O. H., The measurement of free and N-acetylated aspartic acids in the nervous system, *J. Neurochem.,* 779, 1966.

116. McIntosh, J. and Cooper, J., Studies on the function of *N*-acetyl aspartic acid in brain, *Nature,* 658, 1964.

117. Rasool, C., Rogers, J., and Drachman, D., Neuron and neurite loss in Alzheimer's disease, *Neurosci. Abstr.,* 273, 1984.

118. Tews, J. K., Carter, S. H., Roa, P. D. and Stone, W. E., Free amino acids and related compounds in dog brain: post-mortem and anoxic changes, effects of ammonium chloride infusion, and levels during seizures induced by picrotoxin and by pentylenetetrazol, *J. Neurochem.,* 641, 1963.

119. Klunk, W., Panchalingham, K., Moossy, J., McClure, R., and Pettegrew, J., *N*-Acetyl-L-Aspartate and other amino acid metabolites in Alzheimer's disease brain: a preliminary proton nuclear magnetic resonance study, *Neurology,* 1578, 1992.

120. Davies, C., Mann, D., PQ S. and PO Y., A quantitative morphometric analysis of the neuronal and synaptic content of the frontal and temporal neocortex in patients with Alzheimer's disease, *J. Neurol. Sci.,* 157, 1987.

121. Mann, D.M.A., Yates, P.O., and Marcyniuk, B., Correlation between senile plaque and neurofibrillary tangle counts in cerebral cortex and neuronal counts in cortex and subcortical structures in Alzheimer's disease, *Neurosci. Lett.,* 51, 1985.

122. Miller, B. L., A review of chemical issues in 1H NMR spectroscopy: *N*-acetyl-L-aspartate, creatine and choline, *NMR Biomed.,* 4, 47, 1991.

123. Stokes, C. E. and Hawthorne, J. N., Reduced phosphoinositide concentrations in anterior temporal cortex of Alzheimer-diseased brains, *J. Neurochem.,* 48, 1018, 1987.

124. Robinson, D. J., Merskey, H., Blume, W. T., Fry, R., Williamson, P. C. and Hachinski V. C. Electroencephalography as an aid in the exclusion of Alzheimer's disease, *Arch. Neurol.,* 51, 280, 1994.

125. Hooijer, C., Jonker, C., Posthuma, J., and Visser, S. L., Reliability, validity and follow-up of the EEG in senile dementia: sequelae of sequential measurement, 76, 400, 1990.

126. Brenner, R. P., Reynolds, C. F. D., and Ulrich, R. F., EEG findings in depressive pseudodementia and dementia with secondary depression, *JAMA,* 72, 298, 1989.

127. Szelies, B., Grond, M., Herholz, K., Kessler, J., Wullen, T., and Heiss, W. D., Quantitative EEG mapping and PET in Alzheimer's disease, *J. Neurol. Sci.,* 110, 46, 1992.

128. Miyauchi, T., Hagimoto, H., Ishii, M., Endo, S., Tanaka, K., Kajiwara, S., Endo, K., et al., Quantitative EEG in patients with presenile and senile dementia of the Alzheimer type, *Acta Neurol. Scand.,* 89, 56, 1994.

129. Gueguen, B., Ancri, D., Derouesne, C., Bourdel, M. C., Guillou, S. and Landre, E., Comparison of SPECT and quantified EEG features in Alzheimer's type dementia, *Neurophysiol., Clin.,* 21, 377, 1991.

130. Dierks, T., Perisic, I., Frolich, L., Ihl, R., and Maurer, K., Topography of the quantitative electroencephalogram in dementia of the Alzheimer type: relation to severity of dementia, *Psychiat. Res.,* 40, 181, 1991.

131. Szelies, B., Mielke, R., Herholz, K. and Heiss, W. D. Quantitative topographical EEG compared to FDG PET for classification of vascular and degenerative dementia, *Electroencephalog. Clin. Neurophysiol.,* 91, 131, 1994.

132. Schreiter-Gasser, U., Gasser, T., and Ziegler, P., Quantitative EEG analysis in early onset Alzheimer's disease: correlations with severity, clinical characteristics, visual EEG and CCT, *Electroencephalog. Clin. Neurophysiol.,* 90, 267, 1994.

133. Besthorn, C., Forstl, H., Geiger-Kabisch, C., Sattel, H., Gasser, T., and Schreiter-Gasser, U., EEG coherence in Alzheimer's disease, *Electroencephalog. Clin. Neurophysiol.,* 90, 242, 1994.

134. Hassainia, F., Petit, D., and Montplaisir, J., Significance probability mapping: the final touch in t-statistic mapping, *Brain Topog.,* 7, 3, 1994.

135. Woyshville, M. J. and Calabrese, J. R., Quantification of occipital EEG changes in Alzheimer's disease utilizing a new metric: the fractal dimension, *Biol. Psychiat.,* 35, 381, 1994.

136. Leuchter, A. F., Daly, K. A., Rosenberg-Thompson, S., and Abrams, M., Prevalence and significance of electroencephalographic abnormalities in patients with suspected organic mental syndromes, *J. Am. Geriat. Soc.,* 41, 605, 1993.

137. Seiger, A., Nordberg, A., von Holst, H., Backman, L., Ebendal, T., Alafuzoff, I., Amberla, K., et al., Intracranial infusion of purified nerve growth factor to an Alzheimer patient: the first attempt of a possible future treatment strategy, *Behav. Brain Res.,* 57, 255, 1993.

138. Duara, R., Barker, W. W., S. P., Loewenstein, D. A., and Booth, T., Behavioral activation PET studies in normal aging and Alzheimer's disease (AD), *J. Nuclear Med.,* 31, 730 (Abstr.), 1990.

139. Rapoport, S. I., and Grady, C. L., Parametric *in vivo* brain imaging during activation to examine pathological mechanisms of functional failure in Alzheimer's disease, *Int. J. Neurosci.,* 70, 39, 1993.

140. Mubrin, Z., Knezevic, S., Spilich, G., Risberg, J., Gubarev, N., Wannenmacher, W., and Vucinic, G., Normalization of rCBF pattern in senile dementia of the Alzheimer's type. *Psychiat. Res.,* 29, 303, 1989.

141. Schlumpf, M., Parmar, R., Schreiber, A., Ramseier, H. R., Butikofer, E., Abriel, H., Barth, M., et al., Nervous and immune systems as targets for developmental effects of benzodiazepines. A review of recent studies, *Dev. Pharmacol. Ther.,* 18, 145, 1992.

142. Border, W. A., and Ruoslahti, E., Transforming growth factor-beta in disease: the dark side of tissue repair, *J. Clin. Invest.,* 90, 1, 1992.

143. DeForge, L. E., Nguyen, D. T., Kunkel, S. L., and Remick, D. G., Regulation of the pathophysiology of tumor necrosis factor, *J. Lab. Clin. Med.,* 116, 429, 1990.

144. Budinger, T. F., New approaches to targeting arthritis with radiopharmaceuticals, *J. Rheumatol.,* 22, 1995.

CAUSE(S)

Chapter **14**

INTRINSIC BIOLOGICAL AGING AS UNDERLYING PATHOGENETIC MECHANISMS IN DEMENTIAS OF THE ALZHEIMER'S TYPE

George M. Martin

CONTENTS

0-8493-8997-6/97/$0.00+$.50
© 1996 by CRC Press, Inc.

I. INTRODUCTION

Plant biologists argue that aging begins at birth. They would use the term "senescence" to refer only to those changes in structure and function which develop near the end of the life span and which lead to organismal death. From the point of view of a geneticist, there is considerable merit in these arguments. Consider, for example, human subjects who have inherited a dominant point mutation in the structural gene coding for the beta amyloid precursor protein or individuals overexpressing that locus because of either a mosaic or constitutional form of trisomy 21, the chromosome carrying that gene. For both cases, the altered metabolism is expressed soon after birth, when the neuronal isoform of this differentially spliced gene message is expressed in connection with the development of the analage of the central nervous system. A number of investigators believe that metabolism of that precursor protein, via the gradual aggregation and deposition of a derivative peptide, β-amyloid, is of seminal importance in the pathogenesis of the most important neurodegenerative process of aging human subjects, Alzheimer's disease (AD), perhaps in connection with the generation of oxidative damage to neuronal cells. While it takes many decades for β-amyloidosis to reach a threshold of clinical expression, the process certainly initiates early enough so as to occur side by side with the normative processes of development. Most gerontologists, however, sharply differentiate between the processes of *development* and the processes of *aging* or *senescence*. (Mammalian gerontologists often use those latter two terms interchangeably.) Aging, they would argue, only begins after the organism has reached sexual maturation, peak physiological fitness, and (for most mammals) an adult size or stature. There then ensue slow, insidious, and progressive changes in the structure and function of molecules, cells, tissues, organs, and behavior, some of which are adaptive (presumably compensating for some physiological decline), but most of which are nonadaptive and lead to an increasing probability of death with chronological time. This is not to say that gerontologists are not aware of the importance of development in influencing different aspects of aging. Consider the metaphor of the organism as a factory designed to produce very large numbers of protein molecules. How one *builds* such a factory is of obvious importance to how long it lasts! We shall return to this metaphor later in this chapter to help us think about what might go wrong in our protein-synthesizing factories as we age. Once built, factories have to be properly *maintained*. This requires good mechanisms for *quality control* and *repair*.

II. THE SENESCENT PHENOTYPE

One can use this term to refer to the large array of alterations in structure and function that characterize senescing (or aging) organisms. At the level of the intact organism, for example, an essentially universal feature of the senescent phenotype is a decline in spontaneous motility. This is seen in organisms ranging from man to nematodes. At the level of cells, one typically observes, in certain terminally differentiated cell types within an equally wide range of organisms, aggregates of complex fluorescent pigments known as lipofuscins. These are presumed to be the result of lipid peroxidations and, as such, provide support for the theory that oxidative damage to macromolecules is a major mechanism of aging (the free radical theory of aging). At the level of molecules, declines in protein synthesis and protein turnover have been described in a number of organisms.

III. DISEASES ASSOCIATED WITH AGING

Can one age and die without developing diseases? Many gerontologists believe that this may occur, although for the case of both rodents and man, for which species there are substantial amounts of necropsy data, it is unusual not to find some type of characteristic age-related pathology. In the case of human autopsies, for example, one can essentially always document some degree of vascular pathology, as well as alterations in the regulation of cell proliferation in many other tissues. These

TABLE 1   Autopsy Findings in an 88-Year-Old Male with Alzheimer's Disease

  I. Alzheimer's disease with extensive involvement of hippocampus and neocortex (neuritic plaques, neurofibrillary tangles, granulovacuolar degeneration, and congophilic angiopathy)

 II. Bilateral patchy bronchopneumonia

     A. Mild to moderate centroacinar emphysema

     B. Congestion and mucopurulent exudate in upper airways

     C. Dense left pleural adhesions with obliteration of left pleural space

III. Congestive heart failure

     A. Bilateral ventricular hypertrophy

        1. Enlarged left atrium

        2. Dilated pulmonic and tricuspid valves and thickening and calcification of aortic and mitral valves

     B. Diffuse pulmonary congestion

     C. Right pleural effusion (500 cc)

     D. Pericardial effusion (100 cc)

     E. Marked venous congestion of liver and spleen

     F. Nonocclusive coronary artery atherosclerosis

IV. Atherosclerosis

     A. Severe atherosclerosis of aorta

        1. Atherosclerosis and dilatation of proximal ascending aorta and thoracic aorta

        2. Saccular aneurysm aorta and thoracic aorta with mural thrombus

     B. Nephrosclerosis

 V. Poorly differentiated prostate adenocarcinoma, metastatic to bladder wall, pelvic lymph nodes, and small bowel mesentery

     A. Status post bilateral orchiectomy

     B. Mild bladder hypertrophy

VI. Miscellaneous

     A. Regenerative epithelial hyperplasia in left pulmonary scar

     B. Healed granuloma at left pulmonary hilus

     C. Localized cluster of pancreatic islet cells

     D. Bilateral nodular adrenal cortical hyperplasia

     E. Follicular cysts of thyroid

     F. Sigmoid diverticuli with thickening of bowel wall and dense adhesions, consistent with previous diverticulitis

     G. Duodenal diverticulum (first portion)

     H. Gallstones

declines in "proliferative homeostasis" are associated with such disorders as atherosclerosis, osteoarthrosis, benign prostatic hyperplasia, adenomatous polyps of the colon, and basal cell papillomas of the skin. Paradoxically, these multifocal proliferations typically develop side by side with tissue atrophies. This raises the question of major aberrations in cell–cell interactions during aging.

More often than not, one can find a panorama of geriatric pathologies, as is illustrated by the autopsy report of a randomly selected case of AD from the files of the University of Washington Medical Center (Table 1). It is a challenge for the gerontologist to discover how underlying basic mechanisms of aging set the stage for the emergence of these numerous diseases of aging.

IV. INTRINSIC BIOLOGICAL AGING VS. CHRONOLOGICAL AGING

It is not easy to differentiate between processes that merely reflect the passage of chronological time and processes that reflect intrinsic biological aging. The latter could be defined as processes whose kinetics are appropriately correlated with the maximum life span potentials of taxonomically related groups of organisms, member species of which differ in their life-span potentials. An example of a molecular clock whose rate constants probably do not differ substantially among mammalian species is the racemization of certain optically active amino acids, such as aspartic acid, in homologous proteins with very low turnovers, such as dental enamel. For such proteins, there is a steady rate constant of transition from the L- to the D-enantiomer. By contrast, the rates of accumulation of carbonyl groups in various proteins probably do vary significantly among mammals, presumably reflecting differing susceptibilities to oxidative damage. This view is supported by evidence of intraspecific variations in the rates of accumulation of this marker for oxidative damage to proteins; cultured somatic cells from human subjects suffering from certain progeroid mutations (the Werner syndrome and the Hutchinson-Gilford syndrome) exhibit accelerated rates of such posttranslational alterations of their proteins.

V. NATURE VS. NURTURE IN THE PATHOGENESIS OF AGING AND DISEASE

Senescent phenotypes, like all phenotypes, result from interactions between one's inheritance ("nature") and one's environmental experiences ("nurture"). In rodent species, a single environmental manipulation, caloric restriction (but in the presence of an otherwise balanced nutrition), can lead to 50% increases in maximum life spans of typical experimental cohorts of around 100 animals. Such caloric restriction is associated with a dramatic postponement of the two major causes of mortality in typical laboratory rodent populations, neoplasia and glomerulosclerotic renal disease. A number of other phenotypes suggest that there is retention of youthfulness in calorically restricted animals during the latter part of the usual life span. This includes superior performances on certain tests of cognitive function.

Does caloric restriction postpone aging in man? There is currently no credible evidence that it can, although some small-scale experiments on nonhuman primates are under way. Moreover, there are theoretical arguments that such interventions are not likely to be successful in species such as higher primates that in contrast to rodents and other rapidly reproducing species, have evolved comparatively long life spans, undergo long periods of development, and have comparatively small numbers of progeny. The genetic endowment of an organism is of paramount importance in setting these differing life course strategies (although, as we shall see below, environmental pressures over evolutionary time were responsible for the ultimate emergence of the genetic bases for those parameters).

VI. EPIDEMIOLOGICAL EVIDENCE LINKING AGING AND ALZHEIMER'S DISEASE

There are two general conclusions from prevalence and incidence studies of AD in a variety of populations in developed societies: (1) age-specific incidence increases exponentially as a function of age and (2) prevalence and incidence rates can therefore be exceptionally high in that proportion of the population over the age of 85 years, with prevalence estimates ranging from about 28 to 47%. Such observations are consistent with the hypothesis that there is an intimate coupling of AD with some underlying process or processes of aging in our species. The fact that AD is not a *universal* concomitant of aging does not falsify that hypothesis, given the extraordinary genetic heterogeneity of *Homo sapiens*. Let us consider a "thought experiment" to address this issue. First of all, we know that in a subset of familial forms of AD, one can develop the disorder in middle age or late middle age on the basis of a heritable autosomal dominant mutation. Second, let us make the assumption that as is the case for Huntington's disease, comparable phenotypes can be observed in homozygotes (as would be expected for a true autosomal dominant trait, such as Huntington's disease). Now let us imagine that a very few individuals homozygous for identical mutations (but otherwise genetically heterogeneous) founded a colony on some remote island, that they successfully reproduced, and that their colony eventually developed a sizeable population, including some "home-grown" geriatricians. Such physicians would be amazed to discover, upon visiting the mother country, that there were actually sizable numbers of individuals who aged *without* developing AD! This anecdote underscores the fact that there can be no universal set of *standard* ways to age. That conclusion is supported by the evolutionary theory of aging.

VII. WHY WE AGE: THE EVOLUTIONARY BIOLOGICAL THEORY OF AGING

Evolutionary biologists believe that they understand *why* we age, although they emphasize that this understanding tells us little about *how* we age. Put in simple terms, aging of individuals in age-structured populations such as ours is inevitable because of the attenuation, with age, of the force of natural selection. There is no evidence that aging (or senescence) is adaptive for the species. This would require some mechanism of group selection, for which there is little support. Selection acts on the basis of the reproductive fitness of the individual. As species evolve, life history strategies are shaped by the external forces of predation, accidents, diseases, and malnutrition. There is little selective pressure for or against gene mutations or polymorphisms which reach some phenotypic threshold after the peak age of reproductive fitness, which is relatively early for the evolved life history strategy of a mouse, but relatively late for humans. Even for the case of phenotypes with middle or late-middle age onset, such as certain familial forms of AD, selection would be substantially attenuated compared to gene variations reaching phenotypic expression at say, age 19. Considering our remote ancestors, such late teenagers were far more likely to have contributed to our current gene pool. In theory, given many thousands of years of continuation of current secular trends, in some segments of our society, for postponement of reproduction, nature would indeed be given the opportunity to select for gene variations that would provide enhanced reproductive fitness later in the life course and, incidentally, provide longer life spans.

Two classes of gene action are thought to modulate patterns of aging. The first class, best enunciated by the late Peter Medawar, consists of constitutional mutations the phenotypic expressions of which may have been postponed to the late phases of the life span by changes of forms of genes at other genetic loci (suppressor mutations). The ultimate effects of the initial inherited mutations are ultimately inevitable, however, thus contributing to the complex senescent phenotype. We have already mentioned one possible example of such gene action, namely the gradual development of β-amyloidosis. We do not yet know which, if any, suppressor genes evolved to postpone such gene action. One possibility, however, is the currently prevalent epsilon 3 allelic form of the Apolipoprotein E gene in many human populations. The second class of gene action has come to be known as "antagonistic pleiotropy" or "negative pleiotropy". It was most clearly defined by George C. Williams in a classic 1957 paper. According to this idea, there are many allelic forms of genes that while having been selected because of their contributions to the enhancement of the reproductive fitness of the individual, paradoxically exhibit deleterious effects late in the life span, when such phenotypes can escape the force of natural selection. The example chosen by Professor Williams was the inadvertent incorporation of calcium into arteries via gene action selected because of the need for efficient incorporation of calcium into bones. While there is as yet no proof of that particular gene action, one can imagine many other possible examples. For instance, our bodies could "pay a price" for the evolution of biochemical systems for the generation of highly reactive chemical free radicals as one mechanism for the killing of pathogenetic microorganisms. Although such systems are confined to certain specialized white blood cell types (macrophages and neutrophiles), their activities could potentially lead to oxidative attacks upon "bystander" molecules in localized tissues. One such type of altered molecule could be an oxidized low-density lipoprotein in arterial tissue which in turn could contribute to the development of atherosclerosis. Oxidative damage is also thought to mediate various forms of neurodegeneration, including AD.

There are several interesting and important implications of the evolutionary theory of aging. First of all, the theory argues strongly against the notion that there is a genetic program designed to actively and deliberately produce aging. Aging (or senescence) is an innocent and inevitable by-product of gene action selected for entirely different purposes (reproduction). Second, one would expect that there are a large number of genes that can modulate different aspects of aging and that these would be members of different families of genes related to different ways (mechanisms) of aging. Third, since these mechanisms are not under direct, deterministic, and precisely timed genetic controls, one could anticipate that chance phenomena (stochastic mechanisms) will play a large role in how we age. Thus, it would not be surprising if identical twins developed AD, for example, at quite different ages. (This has in fact been observed.) Fourth, there is no reason to believe that all species must age in the same ways, even closely related species such as mammals. Consider, for example, how different the genes must be that regulate mating behavior in different species. Allelic forms of such genes are obviously under exceedingly strong selective pressure and thus would be good candidates for those that might paradoxically contribute to the senescent phenotype via "antagonistic pleiotropy". Related to this conclusion is the expectation that different patterns of aging are likely to be observed among individual members of a genetically heterogeneous species. Since our own species exhibits very substantial genetic heterogeneity, one might conclude that it would be difficult to decide upon an exact definition of "normal" aging. Many people do indeed appear to age in seemingly unusual ways because of both genetic and environmental factors. Should they be considered to be aging "abnormally"? A final implication of the evolutionary theory of aging is that the actual length of life should be relatively plastic, i.e., given sufficient genetic variability and changing environmental opportunities, the "maximum" life span of our species could change. For instance, if the present secular trend for individuals to postpone their ages of reproduction were to continue for millennia, allelic variants might be selected that resulted in significantly enhanced life spans. There is in fact experimental evidence, in fruit flies, that such a phenomenon is possible. There are likely to be limits to such enhanced life span, however, related to the basic design of the organism. It is not likely that the experimental selections in fruit flies, mentioned above, will result in flies living as long as mice, for example.

The evolutionary theory of aging also provides some improved understanding of why human beings are so susceptible to AD. One can consider that common ailment to be either the price we pay for some types of gene action that was selected ages ago because of enhanced reproductive fitness or which, because of the chance "fixation" of certain forms of genes among our ancestors ("genetic founder effects"), made us particularly vulnerable to this pattern of aging. The theory also provides optimism that once the details of gene action (including gene-gene interactions and gene-environmental interactions) are known, we may be able to phenotypically intervene ("phenotypic engineering").

VIII. GENE VARIATIONS IN MAN THAT AFFECT SPECIFIC ASPECTS OF AGING

As indicated above, we human beings are exceptionally heterogeneous from a genetic point of view. With the exception of identical twins (or some futuristic somatic cell cloning), one could state that no two individuals have ever been born or will ever be born who will be genetically identical. What can we learn from a study of how these genetic variations might influence patterns of aging? Such research is still in its infancy. One can tentatively make several important conclusions, however. First, it is clear that there does not exist a single genetic locus' mutation at which can accelerate all of the known features of aging. This is not surprising, given the above discussion of evolutionary aspects of aging. Second, there are gene mutations with profound and widespread effects upon patterns of aging in multiple organ systems but which appear to spare the central nervous system. A striking example is the Werner syndrome. It is sometimes referred to as "Progeria of the Adult" to distinguish it from "Progeria of Childhood" (the Hutchinson-Gilford syndrome or "Progeria"). The Werner syndrome is inherited as an autosomal recessive, whereas, the Hutchinson-Gilford syndrome is probably inherited as an autosomal dominant. They are likely be due to mutations at different genetic loci. There has been more progress for the case of the Werner syndrome, the mutation for which maps to the short arm of the number 8 chromosome. The responsible gene may code for an enzyme or for a transcription factor. Its deficiency leads to premature greying and thinning of the hair, atrophy of skin, regional atrophy of subcutaneous fat, ocular cataracts, insulin-resistant diabetes mellitus, osteoporosis, hypogonadism, various forms of arteriosclerosis, and various forms of benign and malignant neoplasms. The usual cause of death is a myocardial infarction due to atherosclerosis, and the second most common cause of death is cancer. The median age of death is 47. The patients appear to be normal at birth and during childhood, but fail to undergo the usual adolescent growth spurt. (They thus are quite short as adults.) Although there have been occasional reports of central nervous system pathologies, the great majority of patients age without signs or symptoms of accelerated aging within the brain. Autopsy examinations have failed to document any of the changes found in AD. One does not know if the mechanisms whereby patients with the Werner syndrome develop these various age-related abnormalities are comparable to what is operative in most individuals. The findings do demonstrate, however, an uncoupling of these peripheral types of pathologies from the most common type of age-related pathology in the brain, AD. Similarly, it is the case that there are several different genetic loci in man that can modulate one's susceptibility to AD, but which appear not to have any significant peripheral effects.

IX. HOW WE AGE

Returning to our metaphor of the organism as a protein-synthesizing factory, let us first consider issues related to the initial construction of this factory. We have already seen how the genetic blueprints can have a profound influence on the functioning of the enterprise many years after its construction. The details of the genetic blueprints are also of obvious importance to the quality of the construction. This is the domain of *development*. One principle that comes into play, for example, is that of the degree of redundancy of the basic building blocks. These consist of families of different classes of somatic cells. For some classes of cells, the adult organism maintains reserves of multipotent stem cells that are capable of generating entire lineages of highly specialized descendent cells. For the case of hematopoietic stem cells, most people and most strains of laboratory mice appear to have more than enough reserve cells to last for a usual life span and much more than a life span. (Transplantation experiments in mice have established that fact.) Intestinal cells are also capable of continual repopulations as are, to a lesser extent, hepatic parenchymal cells. Most people therefore do not appear to age because they run out of such cells or their precursors. We know much less about the replicative potentials of the family of central nervous system cells collectively referred to as glia. In fact, we do not even know how many different members make up this family of cell types. The term "glia" suggests that the main function of these cells is to provide physical support ("glue") for the brain tissue, but it is clear that they have a large number of additional and still poorly defined functions. During aging, there is some evidence that certain types of glial cells actually increase in numbers, at least regionally. This is certainly the case for certain of the lesions associated with AD and with many other neurodegenerative disorders. In such instances, they could be viewed as creating a sort of "scar tissue" in the brain. As noted earlier, there are many examples of the regional ("multifocal") overreplication of cell types in different organs of aging mammals, often in association with tissue atrophy. This loss of proliferative homeostasis is thus one of the cellular problems the aging organism faces in attempting to *maintain* a properly organized protein-synthesizing factory. In the brain, the atrophy involves subsets of neuronal cells. There is evidence that this is often manifested as a *shrinkage* of cells rather than a loss of cells, although the latter can also occur during aging and certainly occurs during the course of AD. Such cell loss cannot be compensated, as with the exception of certain olfactory epithelial cells in the posterior portions of the nose and some rare bona fide neuronal stem cells near the ependymal lining of the ventricles, neurons are terminally differentiated cells that have lost the ability to replicate their genetic material and to create daughter cells.

How do such terminally differentiated cells (and some slowly replicating cells) age? Our knowledge is still very incomplete, but a few generalizations are emerging related to damage to the macromolecules within and around such cells. Perhaps the best documented alterations involve the proteins. As we age, the rates of protein synthesis decline, as do the rates at which older proteins are broken down by enzymes. The result is an increase in the average "dwell time" of proteins. This is particularly significant for the case of particularly long-lived proteins, such as the very abundant collagens of our connective tissues and the crystallins of our ocular lenses. It is therefore not surprising that one can observe a large number of structural alterations of proteins in the aging organism. These are not the result of errors in the machinery with which the proteins are initially synthesized, but are the result of postsynthetic ("posttranslational") errors. The types of chemical modifications include those that are thought to result from oxidative attacks, such as the creation of carbonyl groups and sulfoxidations of the sulfur-containing amino acid methionine. This provides some support for what is currently the most popular theory of aging — the "free radical theory". According to this theory, aging is due to our inability to completely defend ourselves against the highly reactive chemical free radicals that are generated as a result of our metabolism. While nature did evolve a highly efficient mechanism (the cytochrome oxidase system) for reducing molecular oxygen four electrons at a time in the powerhouses of our cells (the mitochondria), there is a bit of "leakage" in that system, leading to the creation of highly reactive radicals, notably the hydroxyl radical. Nature has also done a good job of evolving a series of nonenzymatic and enzymatic scavengers of such dangerous radicals, but these defenses are not perfect.

In addition to the oxidative damage (and other types of damage) observed in proteins, there is also evidence of oxidative damage to fatty molecules of the cell membranes. Essentially all organisms that utilize oxygen as a means of generating energy, for example, gradually accumulate, in certain cell types, complex yellowish fluorescent pigments called "lipofuscins". These are also known as "wear and tear" pigments. It is thought that such pigments are the result of lipid peroxidations.

Finally, there is also evidence that the DNA of aging cells can also be oxidatively attacked. It is not surprising that mitochondrial DNA appears to be particularly vulnerable, as it occurs in close proximity to the machinery that generates a large proportion of the organism's free radicals. Moreover, the systems for the repair of this type of DNA appear to be much less efficient than those that evolved to repair damaged DNA within the nucleus. The result is that mutations accumulate in these circular DNA molecules with aging in postreplicative cells such as neurons, heart muscle cells, and the multinucleated myocytes of skeletal muscle. Very recently, and quite surprisingly, mutations have also been documented in a nuclear gene in aging neurons in a hypothalamic nucleus responsible for the synthesis of vasopressin, a neuropeptide that is important in controlling the reabsorption of water from urine and in the regulation of blood pressure.

Damage to proteins has also been shown to result from the action of reducing sugars such as glucose, the main source of fuel in our bodies, particularly in the brain. The sugar can combine with certain amino acids to alter the structure of the proteins bearing that amino acid. This process is nonenzymatic and is known as "glycation". Glycation can also alter DNA and in model systems, has been shown to result in mutations.

The reader will certainly appreciate the deficiencies of the above brief overview of current ideas concerning some dominating cellular and molecular mechanisms of aging. For instance, one might ask how it is that aging organisms exhibit declines in their rates of synthesis and turnover of proteins. If this is due to alterations in the neuroendocrine milieu of cells, what causes *those* changes? One could also express skepticism regarding the functional significance of the altered proteins that we have so strongly emphasized. After all, we know that the parents of patients with many different types of recessively inherited enzyme deficiencies typically appear to be perfectly normal, yet the levels of activity of the relevant enzyme is reduced by 50%. Perhaps alterations in proteins that are important for the regulation of the synthesis of other proteins are of particular importance (transcription factors, for example). Deficiencies in the rates of response of genes to various inducing paradigms have indeed been documented in aging mammals. Those interested in systems physiology should be rightly concerned about how little we know about the dynamics of complex interactive systems in aging mammals. Finally, at a more fundamental level, the picture of a multicausal, multigenic basis for aging that we have emphasized could be reasonably attacked by gerontologists who work with experimental models of caloric restriction. As noted above, a simple dietary intervention has been shown to enhance the life spans and delay the age-related disabilities of a wide range of relatively short lived animals, including small mammals. This raises the possibility that there could indeed be a single dominating mechanism of aging, perhaps oxidative stress. That theory would be compatible with the concept of polygenic modulation since one can draw up a very long list of genes that could play a role in the generation of free radicals, their scavenging, and the repair of the damage they produce. Tests of these theories could involve the creation of transgenic organisms in which the above parameters could be modified so as to reduce the rates of oxidative damage. One such approach in fruit flies has met with some success and a number of laboratories are now testing these ideas in laboratory mice. Since there are now transgenic mouse models that partially express the lesions of AD (as a result of overexpression of a human β-amyloid precursor protein), the role of oxidative stress in the generation of AD pathologies should be readily testable.

REFERENCES

Finch, C. E., *Longevity, Senescence and the Genome*, University of Chicago Press, Chicago, 1990.

Rose, M. R., *Evolutionary Biology of Aging*, Oxford University Press, New York, 1991.

Evans, D. A., van der Kleij, A. A., Sonnemans, M. A., Burbach, J. P., and van Leeuwen, F. W., Frameshift mutations at two hotspots in vasopressin transcripts in post-mitotic neurons, *Proc. Soc. Natl. Acad. Sci. U.S.A.* 91, 6059, 1994.

Esser, K., and Martin, G. M., Eds., *Molecular Aspects of Aging*, Dahlem Workshop Reports, Life Sciences Research Report 56, John Wiley & Sons, New York, 1995.

Masoro, E. J., Ed., *Handbook of Physiology, Section 11, Aging*, Oxford University Press, New York, 1995.

Chapter 15

CEREBRAL METABOLIC IMPAIRMENTS

John P. Blass

CONTENTS

0-8493-8997-6/97/$0.00+$.50

I. INTRODUCTION

A large body of evidence exists, and new evidence continues to accumulate, which indicates that impairments of oxidative metabolism in the nervous system occur in a variety of neurodegenerative disorders.[1-4] These disorders include not only Alzheimer's Disease (AD) but also Parkinson's disease, Huntington's disease, motor neuron disease/ALS, and hereditary ataxias including late-onset forms of multiple system disorder/olivopontocerebellar atrophy, a variety of inborn errors of metabolism,[4] and to some extent in "statistically normal" aging.[1,2] Increasing evidence is also accumulating that in some of these patients genetic abnormalities in components of oxidative metabolism occur and are at least contributory causes to the development of the clinical disability (Table 1). Furthermore, secondary impairments of cerebral oxidative metabolism, due to cerebrovascular disease, head injury, metabolic encephalopathies (deliria), and a number of other conditions, are the subject of a huge literature.[1,4]

TABLE 1   Neurodegenerative Diseases with Mitochondrial Involvement

Disorder	Abnormal Mitochondrial Component
MELAS	mtDNA*
MERRF	mtDNA*
Kearns-Sayre-Shy Syndrome	mtDNA*
SNE (Leigh's disease)	PDHC*; Complex IV
Spinocerebellar Ataxias	
Forms of multiple system degeneration	Glutamate Dehydrogenase
Friedreich ataxia phenocopies	PDHC
Huntington's disease	Complex I
Parkinson's disease	Complex I
Alzheimer's disease	KGDHC, PDHC, Complex IV

Note: See Reference 2 for more detailed discussion and original references. * indicates that the defect has been documented at the molecular (DNA) level. A striking common characteristic of these disorders is that they show *selective vulnerability.*[2] Neuropathologically, these disorders typically affect certain parts of the nervous system strikingly and spare other parts. The affected parts of the nervous system in each disease are therefore referred to as *selectively vulnerable.* Another striking characteristic of these disorders is that the areas which are selectively vulnerable differ among the specific conditions involved. Thus, at the level of pathophysiology and neuropathology, specific forms of mitochondrial damage which differ in detail from each other have neuropathological consequences, more or less specific for each type of mitochondrial disorder. Parkinson's and Alzheimer's diseases are typically disorders of the elderly; Huntington disease can strike at a wide variety of ages, but has been considered to be typically a disorder of middle life; the other conditions are typically pediatric disorders.

The following review concentrates on AD. Other disorders are discussed only to the extent that they illuminate points about AD. Because of considerations of space, relatively few primary data are presented. References are given to lead reviews as well as to publications presenting the primary observations.

A. CEREBRAL METABOLISM IN NORMAL BRAIN

In humans, the brain typically accounts for about 2% of body weight and 20% of the oxygen utilized, making the nervous system the "most oxidative" tissue in the body. (See Reference 5 for a detailed discussion of brain metabolism). The major and quantitatively only significant pathways for cerebral oxidative metabolism are *glycolysis* (glucose to pyruvate/lactate), *pyruvate dehydrogenase* (pyruvate to acetyl-coenzyme A), the *Krebs tricarboxylic acid cycle* (formation of CO_2 and reducing equivalents), and *electron transport* (oxidation of reducing equivalents to H_2O). *Glycolysis*

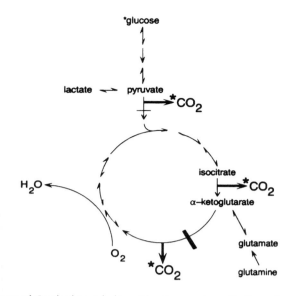

FIGURE 1 Major Pathways of Cerebral Metabolism. The figure *schematically* outlines the quantitatively major pathways of carbohydrate and oxidative metabolism in the brain. The pathway from glucose to pyruvate/lactate is *glycolysis*, and that indicated by the arrow from O_2 to H_2O is electron transport. The intraconversions of glutamine, glutamate, and α-ketoglutarate constitute part of the pathways of glutamate metabolism. Each of these pathways itself consists of a complex series of enzyme-catalyzed steps; each of these pathways is subject to complex control mechanisms. CO_2 from glucose (and therefore radioactive CO_2 from radioactive glucose) is generated at the three indicated steps, those catalyzed by PDHC, by isocitrate dehydrogenase (ICDH), and by KGDHC. The thin bar indicates a decrease in the activity of PDHC in Alzheimer brain; the thicker bar indicates the possibility of a functionally significant decrease in the activity of KGDHC in AD brain.

occurs in the cytosol, and the *tricarboxylic acid cycle* and *electron transport* in the inner mitochondrial compartment (Figure 1).

Other pathways can be quantitatively important under special circumstances, e.g., oxidation of amino acids or oxidation of ketone bodies after *prolonged* starvation or in infancy. However, even those pathways which bypass glycolysis use substrates whose oxidation requires the *tricarboxylic acid cycle* and *electron transport*. Quantitatively minor oxidative pathways in the brain are important for special activities such as the oxidation of aromatic amino acids to the neurotransmitters noradrenaline or 5-hydroxytryptamine. However, these pathways make a trivial contribution to overall oxygen consumption or to energy generation. Thus, a key point in discussing oxidative metabolism in brain is that there are *no* quantitatively significant redundant pathways to bypass the *tricarboxylic acid cycle* and the *electron transport system*. Therefore, *functional impairments in these pathways cannot be bypassed by other mechanisms in the brain.*

Oxidative metabolism is the only pathway important enough quantitatively to maintain the energy production necessary for the function of the brain. This energy is produced in the form of pyrophosphate bonds with a high free energy of hydrolysis, notably the γ-phosphate bond of ATP. Not surprisingly, the terms "energy metabolism" and "oxidative metabolism" have been used almost interchangeably. This usage can, however, be misleading if it obscures the other functions of oxidative metabolism. Fundamentally, *electron transport* generates an *electromotive force* across the inner mitochondrial membrane (Mitchell potential; proton gradient). This force can be used for a number of purposes. If the free intercellular calcium concentration reaches pathological levels, the *electromotive force* is used to sequester calcium. This function takes precedence over other functions, including ATP generation.[6,7] If the amount of calcium available is high enough, mitochondria will concentrate calcium until calcium phosphate crystallizes; the formation of such intramitochondrial crystals of hydroxyapatite occurs in pathological states such as ischemia. The *electromotive force* can also be coupled to the phosphorylation of ADP to ATP, in the process of *oxidative phosphorylation.* In healthy mitochondria, the molar ratio of H atoms oxidized to ATP molecules formed is almost 1:3. Such mitochondria are said to be *tightly coupled.* The *electromotive force* has also been hypothesized to be an important regulator of cellular functions.[8] An attractive aspect of this hypothesis is that information about the energy state of the cell would be communicated throughout the cell at physical speed rather than be limited by the rate of diffusion of messenger molecules.

Given the high rate of normal brain oxidative metabolism, the lack of redundancy in these pathways, and their important functions, it is not surprising that the brain has a second-to-second dependence on intact oxidative metabolism to maintain its function. The continuous requirement for intact oxidative metabolism for normal brain function has been extensively documented, notably in aviation medicine.[9] Cutting off oxygen to the brain for more than a few seconds leads to loss of consciousness. Partial reductions in oxidative metabolism lead to milder functional impairments. In humans, even relatively slight reductions in oxygen tension which do not lead to unconsciousness lead to impairments in memory and judgment. The changes in delerium due to hypoxia or other forms of metabolic encephalopathies resemble those which occur in dementia, except that in the metabolic encephopathies the impairments in cognitive function are reversible.[10]

As oxidative metabolism is reduced, tissues reduce their function to maintain activities critical to their structure.[11] The reduction can take the form of reduced biosynthetic activities. In the nervous system, it also takes the form of impaired neuronal activity.[9] The ability to maintain transysnaptic activities is particularly sensitive to partial impairment of oxidative metabolism.[12]

B. CEREBRAL METABOLISM IN NEUROLOGICAL DISEASES

As indicated in the first paragraph of this article, impaired oxidative metabolism has been well documented in a large variety of both common and rare diseases of the nervous system. These include not only AD, which is the focus of this article, but other typical neurodegenerative diseases such as Parkinson's disease, motor neuron disease,[1] and multiple system disease.[13] In AD, decreases in cerebral metabolism occur even in incipient AD, *before* major clinical changes are evident.[14-16] Although a minority of unusually healthy elderly people can be identified in whom cerebral oxidative metabolism is indistinguishable from the young adult population, cerebral metabolism declines with age in the elderly population as a whole and particularly in the large fraction of the population who have cardiovascular risk factors.[17] Indeed, conditions which are associated with decreased mentation are typically if not invariably associated with decreased cerebral oxidative metabolism.[5,8]

Therefore, the problem in discussing abnormalities in oxidative metabolism in relation to AD or other neurodegenerative disease is not whether or not they occur. They do. The question is whether or not elucidating their mechanisms and finding ways to ameliorate these abnormalities is likely to be of any value to the patients whom we try to serve. This issue is close to but not identical with the epistomolgic question of whether or not there is any use for patients with AD or other neurodegenerative disorders in trying to define a single "seminal" event or molecule in the pathogenesis of their clinical disability. AD is now recognized to be a heterogeneous syndrome,[2] at the molecular[18] as well as at the clinical[19] level, and it therefore seems unlikely that a single cause for it will be found. Since the brain shows a second-to-second dependence on quantitatively normal oxidative metabolism to maintain its functions including particularly cognition, it is difficult to imagine a functionally significant impairment in the quantitatively major, nonredundant pathways of oxidative metabolism which will not contribute to the impaired brain function in this disorder.

C. "LEAKY DEFICIENCIES" AND DISEASE

In the early studies of genetic diseases, workers concentrated on severe, usually recessive disorders which abolished the function of the particular gene product involved. They therefore tended to concentrate on severe diseases with onset in early childhood, the characteristic *"inborn errors of metabolism."*

However, as long ago as the early 1920s, Sir Archibald Garrod[20] pointed out that the more common contribution of genetics to clinical medicine was likely to be genetically determined partial deficiencies in specific gene products. Such partial deficiencies would impair the body's ability to respond to certain types of stressors and thus act as predisposing causes in the development of a specific illnesses. To use an older terminology, such a partial deficiency would act as a genetic site of least resistance (*locus minoris resistentius*).

With the growth of modern molecular genetics, it is now amply clear that "leaky mutations" can have deleterious effects on a variety of organisms and particularly the ability of organisms to respond to specific stressors. (Leaky mutations reduce but do not abolish the function of the product of a gene.) Among the organisms affected by leaky mutations are humans. One of the best worked-out examples of genetic predisposition in a human disease is type II hyper-β-lipoproteinemia.[21] Inheritance of two abnormal genes, one from each parent, leads to early death from the complications of atherosclerosis. Inheritance of one abnormal gene and one normal gene leads to a predisposition to develop atherosclerosis in later adult life. Other well worked-out examples include leaky forms of a number of recessive disorders including disorders which affect the nervous system.[22]

One of the mechanisms by which an abnormal gene product can interfere with the action of a normal gene product is *negative dominance*. In this situation, the abnormal gene product disrupts the structure and therefore function of a biological material containing the normal as well as the abnormal gene product. An example is a dimeric protein containing one normal and one abnormal monomer.[23] As discussed below, these precedents are directly relevant to molecular studies of the oxidative machinery in AD.

II. EVIDENCE FOR CEREBRAL METABOLIC IMPAIRMENTS IN ALZHEIMER'S DISEASE

The evidence for impairments of cerebral metabolism in AD covers a range from *in vivo* to molecular studies.

A. *IN VIVO* STUDIES

Reductions in cerebral metabolic rate in AD are incontrovertable. Data supporting this statement have been gathered since the late 1940s, by invasive methods, measurement of regional cerebral blood flow (rCBF), and more recently by positron emission tomography (PET), single photon emission computerized tomography (SPECT), and other more modern techniques.[2,3,5,17] The reduction affects glucose utilization, oxygen uptake, and cerebral blood flow. Indeed, the diminutions in glucose utilization (with positron-emitting fluorodeoxyglucose as label), or in oxygen uptake or cerebral blood flow, are commonly used to study *in vivo* the location and degree of brain impairment in AD.

The problem with these reductions in metabolism is not whether they occur. They do. The problem is what they mean. Specifically, do they simply reflect decreased brain mass and function or do they contribute to or cause brain dysfunction. The workers who originally described the deficiencies in brain metabolism in AD assumed implicitly that these reductions were functionally significant. That concensus view changed when it became clear that the venous blood draining from the AD brain still contained significant amounts of glucose and oxygen and that autoregulation of cerebral blood flow remained intact in AD.

However, the reduction in cerebral metabolic rate in moderate to severe AD is too great to be accounted for quantitatively by either tissue loss or decrease in activity. In moderate to severe AD, the reduction in cerebral metabolic rate is approximately 15 to 30%, i.e., to 70 to 85% of normal. This reduction cannot be attributed to loss of total brain substance, since measurements of metabolic rate are made *per unit mass of remaining brain*. It has also been proposed that the decrease is due to relatively selective loss of the more rapidly metabolizing neurons and nerve endings compared to glia. However, the relative gliosis in AD cannot explain quantitatively the reductions in cerebral metabolic rate in AD. Older studies suggested that rate of neuronal metabolism is as much as twice the rate of glial metabolism, but more recent studies suggest that the metabolic rates of glia and neurons are more or less comparable.[24] Even overestimating the relative rate of neuronal to glial metabolism as 2:1, reducing cerebral metabolic rate by removing neurons would require loss of at least 40% of the *total* population of cerebral neurons in order to account for the overall reduction of cerebral metabolism in severe AD. In fact, however, the loss of neurons in AD is regionally selective. While loss of 40% of neurons in affected areas is possible, rarely if ever does AD lead to a loss of 40% of the total neurons in the brain. The reduction in oxidative metabolism in AD brain cannot be accounted for quantitatively by the loss of neurons. Similar calculations can be made for nerve endings, i.e., neuropil.[5,25]

It has been suggested that the characteristic reduction in cerebral metabolism in AD is due to a decrease in cerebral activity accompanying the dementia. The problem is that neither electro-physiological nor clinical evidence supports that suggestion. The characteristic electroencephalo-graphic abnormality in AD is "nonspecific slowing". Patients with degrees of impairment of cerebral metabolism comparable to that seen in severe AD but from drug overdose or other exogenous impairment of cerebral metabolism are in coma, with essentially flat EEGs. Flat EEGs have not been described even in severe AD. Clinically, advanced AD patients can be hyperactive rather than inactive. There is no reason to conclude that their struggle to think despite the damaged wiring of their brains leads to reduced metabolism by their remaining brain tissue.

Thus, the available data from *in vivo* studies suggest that the reduction in cerebral metabolism characteristic of AD is due, at least in part, to constitutive impairments in the oxidative machinery of the AD brain.

B. *EX VIVO* STUDIES

The simplest way to study whether or not there are intrinsic impairments of cerebral oxidative metabolism in AD would appear to be to examine *in vitro* the rate of oxidative metabolism in pieces of brain from AD subjects. In autopsy brain, such studies are unfortunately not meaningful because of the rapid decay of oxidative metabolism *post-mortem*.[5] However, in the 1980s the availability in England of samples of diagnostic brain biopsies for AD made measurements on living AD brain possible.[26,27] The first study[26] showed that the conversion of [U-^{14}C]glucose to $^{14}CO_2$ was statistically significantly increased in AD brain; the conditions were such as to measure primarily the conversion of pyruvate to acetyl-coenzyme A by the pyruvate dehydrogenase complex.[28] (Under the conditions used, the bulk of the glucose carbons are "trapped" in glutamate.) The second study[27] showed that using pyruvate as substrate (specifically, the pyruvate-malate complex), O_2 uptake was increased in AD brain compared to normal in the absence of ADP and normal in the presence of ADP or of an uncoupler of oxidative phosphorylation. These studies both provide evidence against a func-tionally important impairment of *pyruvate dehydrogenase* or of *electron transport* in AD brain. They do *not* argue against the existence of a functional deficiency in the *Krebs tricarboxylic acid cycle*. Indeed, they can be interpreted as favoring the existence of such an abnormality, since increased rates in steps in a pathway preceding an enzymatic deficiency are frequently found in inborn errors of metabolism.[22,28] These observations also argue *for* an inherent abnormality in oxidative metabolism, since they suggest the existence of *mitochondrial uncoupling*.

Measurements of "high energy" phosphate levels in AD brain studied *ex vivo* are also difficult to interpret.[26] Levels of ATP were found to be reduced in biopsies of AD brain. The ratio of ATP to ADP and the *energy charge potential* were, however, normal. Levels of creatinine phosphate to creatinine were not measured in these brain samples, although these are a more sensitive indicator of an impairment in "*energy metabolism*" than are ATP/ADP ratios. Subsequent *in vivo* studies using magnetic resonance spectroscopy indicate that creatinine phosphate is reduced in AD brain early in the disease process.[29] Those *in vivo* observations support the significance of abnormalities in AD brain metabolism early in the illness. Furthermore, as pointed out in the Introduction, falls in ATP/ADP ratio cannot be assumed to be either the earliest or the only pathogenetically significant consequence of an impairment in cerebral oxidative metabolism.

C. AUTOPSY BRAIN: ENZYMOLOGY AND IMMUNOHISTOCHEMISTRY

Clearer results have come from studies of autopsy brain. Classical experiments in England in the 1970s documented that study of chemical constituents could be carried out meaningfully in human brain obtained at ordinary autopsy provided that the constituents being studied were stable *post-mortem* and, even more important, agonally.[30,31]

One of the stable constituents which can be studied in autopsy brain is the pyruvate dehydrogenase complex (PDHC), which catalyzes the first step in cereberal oxidative metabolism. Its activity is unequivocally decreased in AD brain, in reports from at least four laboratories,[32-35] with no contravening reports. Reductions to about 50% of normal activity are found in all parts of AD brain which have been examined, both pathologically abnormal and neuropathologically normal parts of AD brain such as caudate nucleus.[33] The reduction in PDHC activity in autopsy AD brain appears to be due to a reduction in the amount of an immunochemically normal complex.[36]

The α-ketoglutarate dehydrogenase complex (KGDHC) is a mitochondrial, *tricarboxylic acid cycle* component the activity of which is also reduced in AD brain. The reduction in KGDHC activity, to 50% or less of normal, has also been found in four laboratories without any contravening reports.[34,37-39] The reduction also occurs in all areas of AD brain studied, specifically including such neuropathologically normal areas as caudate. Unfortunately, KGDHC is not as stable as PDHC in autopsy tissues, so the interpretation of these robustly replicable measurements in autopsy AD brain is less straightforward than for PDHC.

Another mitochondrial component which has been reported to be deficient in AD brain is Complex IV of the *electron transport chain*.[40] Complex IV is also known as cytochrome oxidase or as cytochrome a/a_3. Reports of complex IV deficiency are not as robust as for PDHC or KGDHC, either among laboratories (DiMauro, personal communication) nor among areas of brain. Deficiencies are found in neuropathologically abnormal areas of AD brain, but not in pathoanatomically normal areas.[40] Other enzymes of carbohydrate metabolism have been reported to be decreased in AD brain. The activity of *transketolase* (TK), an enzyme of pentose phosphate metabolism, is reduced to about 85% of normal activity in AD brain.[41] The activities of two rate-limiting enzymes of *glycolysis*, namely *hexokinase* and *phosphofructokinase*, have been reported to be reduced in autopsy AD brain. *Hexokinase* activity was reduced in subcortical but not in cortical nuclei[42] and *phosphofructokinase* activity was found to be normal in biopsy AD brain.[43] The observations with these enzymes contrast with the consistent decreases in the activities of PDHC and KGDHC in all areas of AD brain examined.

An inherent problem in molecular studies of a diseased tissue, such as brain in AD, is the possibility that the molecular changes are primarily consequences of the anatomical change. (A classical example is the accumulation of glial protein and glial mRNA in regions of gliosis.) However, abnormality of the molecular component in tissue regions which are normal by the criteria of anatomic pathology argues that the molecular abnormality is not secondary to the pathological change. For instance, the reduction in KGDHC activity even in anatomically normal AD caudate nucleus argues that the decrease in KGDHC activity in AD brain is not due primarily to anatomic change.[2,44]

D. FIBROBLASTS AND OTHER NONNEURAL TISSUES

Even stronger evidence that the abnormalities in oxidative metabolism in AD are not due simply to tissue damage come from studies of clinically unaffected tissues. Indeed, such studies have clearly confirmed that inherent abnormalities in oxidative metabolism occur in AD tissues.[44,45]

Abnormalities which persist in serial tissue culture are of particular interest, since they cannot be attributed to such extraneous clinical variables as medications or nutrition or, if cells are cultured with appropriate care, to differences in biological age in culture of AD and non-AD control cells.[28,44,45] Cultured skin fibroblasts from AD patients show abnormal oxidative metabolism. When the oxidation of [U-^{14}C]glucose to $^{14}CO_2$ is studied under conditions which presumably reflect the activity of the whole *Krebs tricarboxylic acid cycle*, oxidation is reduced.[28,46] Under conditions which measure primarily the oxidation of glucose carbons across the step catalyzed by PDHC, oxidation appears increased in fibroblasts, as it is under similar conditions in brain.[28,47] Oxidation of $[U^{14}C]$glutamine to $^{14}CO_2$, which requires the step catalyzed by KGDHC, is replicably reduced in AD fibroblasts.[46,47] Furthermore, nonradioactive, mass measurements of O_2-uptake in cultured fibroblasts using endogenous substrate (presumably glutamine) show reduced rate in AD compared to non-AD cells.[47] Direct measurements in cultured fibroblasts of metabolic enzymes whose activity is reduced in AD brain show normal activity of PDHC.[48] They also show small reductions in the activity of transketolase, which are abolished by inclusion of protease inhibitors in the assay mixture.[37,49] In contrast, reductions to about 50% of normal activity in KGDHC have been found in cultured AD fibroblasts, approximating the reductions found in brain.[48] The reduction in KGDHC activity is not due to a soluble inhibitor or activator, since mixtures of normal and AD cell extracts have the activities expected from each of the extracts alone (Table 2). Reported reductions in the activity of complex IV (cytochrome oxidase) in AD platelets are not large[50] and have not proven robustly replicable across laboratories.[51,52]

TABLE 2   Ketoglutarate Dehydrogenase Complex (KGDHC) Activity in Alzheimer and Control Fibroblasts Extracts

Sample	Specific Activity[a]	
	Measured	Calculated
Alzheimer (AD)	1.02	
Control (Non-AD)	2.27	
Mixture[b]	1.74[c]	1.64

Note: Data for Alzheimer and control subjects shown in table is typical of AD and control values in that study.

[a]   Nanomoles/min/mg protein.
[b]   Equal mixture of AD and Control samples
[c]   106% of calculated value

From Sheu, K.-F. R., Cooper, A. J. L., Koike, K., Koike, M., Lindsay, J. G., and Blass, J. P., *Ann. Neurol.* 35, 312, 1994. With permission.

E.   MOLECULAR GENETICS (INCLUDING mtDNA)

Enzymatic abnormalities which persist in serial culture can be but do not have to be due to mutations in a gene coding for one of the components of the enzyme.[45] Deficiencies in mitochondrial enzyme activities in AD brain and in other tissues have led to studies of the genes coding for these enzymes. These have included both studies of the DNA which occurs in mitochondria (mtDNA) and of parts of the nuclear genome which code for mitochondrial constituents.

mtDNA is a circular DNA which has been fully sequenced in a number of species including humans.[53] In humans it is approximately 160 kb in length, varying somewhat among individuals. mtDNA codes for tRNAs and for gene products involved in electron transport. However, all of the complexes of *electron transport* contain proteins coded in the nuclear genome as well. Several uncommon inborn errors of metabolism are associated with inherited defects in mtDNA.[53] Since mitochondria are inherited from the mother (the ovum), these diseases show a pattern of maternal inheritance. Since mitochondria distribute among daughter cells in early stages of division, diseases due to primary errors of mtDNA often show mosaicism.

mtDNA is less protected against damage than is nuclear DNA. mtDNA is "naked" rather than closely complexed with histones and other nuclear proteins. Mitochondria lack the panoply of DNA repair enzymes which exist in nuclei, and the location of mtDNA within the mitochondrion places it close to a major generator of oxygen free radicals, in *electron transport*. Accumulation of damage in mtDNA appears to be a frequent concomitant of chronological aging. A number of workers have tested for abnormalities in mtDNA characteristic of AD or of subgroups of AD, but reports of abnormalities specific to AD have generally not been robust across laboratories, at least as yet.[53-55] Whether or not there are "hot spots" in mtDNA which tend to somatic mutation during lifetime and thus contribute to the mitochondrial lesion in AD remains an open question.[54]

The studies described above, in brain and fibroblasts, made the KGDHC complex an attractive candidate for a genetic alteration in AD. Specifically, the activity of KGDHC was reduced in *both* AD brain and in AD fibroblasts in serial culture, and a funtionally significant deficiency in KGDHC activity can explain the metabolic findings in AD brain biopsies studied *ex vivo*. In contrast, the studies in AD brain *ex vivo* suggested that both *PDHC* and *electron transport* can function at normal rates in AD brain. Enzyme assays in cultured fibroblasts also argue against a genetically determined aberration in *PDHC* in AD tissues.[48] Since uncoupling of oxidative phosphorylation is a nonspecific and sensitive indicator of mitochondrial damage, its occurrence in AD fibroblasts does not provide evidence on the location of the mitochondrial lesion in AD.

KGDHC consists of a complex array of three proteins: E1k, E2k, and E3. Human E1k is on chromsome 7p11.2-p13;[56] human E3 is on chromosome 7q31-q32.[57] The human gene coding for E2k (the DLST gene), is on chromosome 14q24.3 (Table 3), in the region closely linked to the most common form of familial, early onset AD.[58,59] A pseudogene is on chromosome 1 (Figure 2). In a collaboration between Tanzi and co-workers and our group, E2k has been found to be within 3.2 Mb of the FAD locus on 14q24.3; there are no crossovers. Further studies, including studies of the DLST gene in relation to later onset, apparently sporadic AD are under way. At the time of this writing, the combination of chromosomal location, enzymatic deficiency, and pathophysiological plausability make the DLST (E2k) gene an excellent candidate gene for at least some forms of AD.

At the present time, no other good candidate mitochondrial gene for AD has been identified. However, it seems possible that in this heterogeneous disease, already linked to a number of different genes, a number of different mitochondrial genes will be found to contribute to the syndrome.

III. CEREBRAL METABOLIC IMPAIRMENTS IN THE PATHOPHYSIOLOGY OF ALZHEIMER'S DISEASE

As noted above, mitochondrial oxidative metabolism is critical for the function of the nervous system, on a second-to-second basis. There is no quantitatively significant redundancy to these pathways in the adult brain. Impairment of these pathways has prompt effects on almost all aspects of cerebral function, including specifically those relevant to AD. Of particular interest is that even partial impairment of cerebral oxidative metabolism, such as those described in AD brain, can lead to abnormalities similar to those seen characteristically in AD. The following discussion describes some of the effects most interesting for the pathophysiologically of AD, and then summarizes the possible role of the impairments of oxidative metabolism in the context of other abnormalities in AD.

A. NEUROPSYCHOLOGICAL DEFICITS

The neuropsychologic deficits which accompany impaired cerebral oxidative metabolism have been exhaustively described, notably in the aviation literature of the 1930s to the 1950s in regard to pure hypoxia.[9] The pattern of development of deficits in progressive hypoxia resembles the pattern of deficits seen in progressive AD (Figure 3). These data indicate that impairment of cerebral mitochondrial oxidative metabolism *can of itself cause* impaired mentation similar to that seen in AD and other dementias.

TABLE 3 Hybrid Cell Panel Analysis for Chromosomal Mapping of the E2k Gene

Chromosome	% Discordance	
	DNA (a–c)	DNA (d)
1	44	**0**
2	44	22
3	28	39
4	39	28
5	44	44
6	28	39
7	22	33
8	44	33
9	72	28
10	50	17
11	61	50
12	33	56
13	39	17
14	**0**	44
15	44	22
16	72	28
17	17	61
18	33	22
19	33	11
20	22	33
21	44	56
22	28	33
X	72	28

DNA from 28 human-mouse hybrid lines was digested with *Hind*III and blot hybridized with the human E2k cDNA.[59] Each cell was scored for the absence/presence of specific hybridizing bands. See Reference 59 for details. For evidence that the chromosome 1 site is a pseudogene, see Figure 3 and Reference 99.

```
779  ACTC[A]GATGCCACCAGTGCCCTCGCCCTCACAACCTCCTTCTAGCAAACCTGTGTCTGCAGTAAAACCC
181  T  Q   M  P  P  V  P  S  P  S  Q  P  P  S  S  K  P   V  S  A  V  K  P
     T  A   C  H  Q  C  P  R  P  H  N  L  L  L  A  N  L   C  L  Q      *


848  ACTGCTGTCCCACCACTAGCTGAGCCAGGAGCTGGCAAAGGTCTGCATTCAGAACATCGGGAGAAAATGAAC
204  T  A  V  P  P  L  A  E  P  G  A  G  K  G  L  H  S  E  H  R  E  K  M  N
                                             →
                                            (A)
920  AGGATGCGGCAGTGCATTGCTCAGCGTCTGAAGGAGGCCCAGAATACT GTGCCAATGCTGACAATT...
228  R  M  R  Q  C  I  A  Q  R  L  K  E  A  Q  N  T   V  P  M  L  T  I
```

FIGURE 2 Effects of decreasing oxygen tension on mentation. See References 9, 100, and 101 for more detailed discussion. (From Plum, F. and Posner, J. B., *The Diagnosis of Stupor and Coma*, F. A. Davis, Philadelphia, 1980. With permission[99].)

B. NEUROTRANSMITTER DEFECTS

The modern era of study of AD was ushered in by the discovery in the mid-1970s of prominent deficits in the cholinergic system in AD.[30,31] Other experiments at that time indicated that the cholinergic system is exquisitely sensitive to conditions which impair oxidative metabolism, and specifically the oxidation of pyruvate to acetyl-coenzyme A.[60] *PDHC*, which carries out this

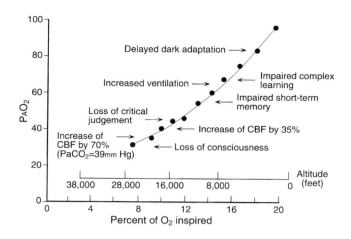

FIGURE 3 Partial sequence of the chromsome 1p31 pseudogene for E2k. The relevant portion of the sequence of the pseudogene on chromosome 1 is shown.[99] Deletion of the [A] indicated in brackets from the cDNA sequence leads to a frame shift and the presence of three stop codons, each of three stop codons (shaded). Subsequent insertion of an adenine nucleotide (A) reestablishes the original codon sequence. For other evidence that this site is a pseudogene, see reference.

reaction, is concentrated in cholinergic neurons including neurons of the nucleus basalis complex,[61] leading to "compartmentation" of pyruvate metabolism with respect to acetylcholine synthesis from acetyl-coenzyme A.[60] The decrease in acetylcholine synthesis appears to be linked to a deficit in calcium-dependent release.[6] In contrast, the release of other, potentially toxic neurotransmitters such as glutamate and L-dopa appears to be enhanced by impairments of oxidative metabolism.[62] The possible role of these neurotransmitters in cell death in AD and other neurodegenerative diseases is discussed elsewhere in this book (see Chapter 22). Thus, impairments of oxidative metabolism can *cause* abnormalities in neurotransmitter metabolism similar to those reported to occur in AD.

C. AMYLOID

The formation and effects of the amyloid which accumulates in characteristic plaques and in cerebral blood vessels in AD has become a major area of research (see Chapter 22). Debate is intense about whether or not amyloid accumulation is a central, "seminal" event in the pathogenesis of AD.[63,64]

Recent studies have shown that increased accumulation of Alzheimer amyloid precursor protein occurs in response to a number of injuries, including specifically impairments of oxidative metabolism.[65-68] Impairing mitochondrial function either by blocking *electron transport* with azide or uncoupling oxidative phosphorylation with the hydrazone CCCP has been reported to lead to alternate metabolism of APP into an "amyloidogenic" pathway, i.e., a pathway that favors the production of βA4.[69] Our group has found similar results (Gandy et al., unpublished). While further studies are clearly necessary, these results raise the possibility that impairment of mitochondrial oxidative pathways can *cause* accumulation of amyloid precursor protein and even of dense βA4.[70]

D. CYTOSKELETAL DERANGEMENTS

Abnormalities of the neuronal cytoskeleton are so prominent in AD that it has been described as a "cytoskeletal disorder" (see Chapter 3). The most characteristic of these abnormalities are neurofibrillary tangles (NFT), formed in large part from paired helical filaments (PHF). The major components of PHF are microtubule-associated tau proteins. These tau proteins have an abnormal secondary structure, in that they are not dephosphorylated post-mortem, are not broken down by the ubiquitin which is covalently linked to them, and may be hyperphosphorylated *in vivo*. The bases for these posttranslational modifications are an object of intense study.

Impairment of oxidation leads to collapse of the cytoskeleton.[71,72] Treatment of cultured human cells with the uncoupler CCCP has been reported to lead to the appearance of epitopes which cross-react with epitopes characteristic of tau proteins, even though tau proteins themselves have not been found in significant quantitites in cultured skin fibroblasts.[73] Ingram and colleagues[74] have reported the existence of a kinase which is activated by reduction in the concentration (more precisely, the thermodynamic activity) of ATP, and leads to the phosphorylation of epitopes on tau proteins which are characteristic of PHF. Impairments of oxidative metabolism lead to dysregulation of second messenger systems,[75] and therefore to dysregulation of the activities of a number of kinases and phosphatases. The abnormalities in second messengers are comparable to abnormalities found in AD cells.[76,77] However, direct evidence that impairment of oxidative metabolism contributes to the formation of NFT/PHF is lacking.

E. FREE RADICALS

Free radicals have again become a subject of great interest in regard to aging, neurodegenerative diseases, and specifically AD.[78-80] The discussion here focuses on the role of abnormalities in oxidative metabolism in the generation of free radicals.

It is widely accepted that impairments of mitochondrial oxidative metabolism lead to increased production of oxygen free radicals, by "spill" of electrons in monoelectron reactions with molecular oxygen. However, direct evidence on this point is surprisingly scanty.[81-84] It would obviously be desirable to know, in quantitative terms, how much damage to what step(s) in oxidative metabolism lead to the accumulation of which free radicals and in what amounts. The popular hypothesis that abnormalities in the mitochondrial apparatus of oxidative metabolism — including *electron transport* or *tricarboxylic acid cycle* enzymes such as KGDHC — lead to excess accumulation of oxygen free radicals is reasonable and not new,[78,79] and it deserves more complete experimental examination.

F. APOPTOSIS

Apoptosis refers to a series of programmed events which lead to cell death. Apopotosis has been proposed to be an important mechanism in AD and other neurodegenerative diseases.[85,86] Although "programmed cell death" is an extremely interesting process, particularly from the viewpoint of molding of the nervous system in development, apoptosis is only one of a number of mechanisms which can lead cells to die.

Recent studies indicate that one of the triggers for apoptosis is excess influx of calcium due to overstimulation of NMDA receptors. Impairments of oxidative metabolism lead to impairments of cellular calcium homeostasis,[6] and cellular calcium homeostasis is impaired in AD.[46,87] Intracellular calcium exists in pharmacologically definable pools, and AD cells have an exaggerated bradykinin-insensitive, A23187-sensitive calcium pool.[88] As discussed above, in pathological situations mitochondria act as important "sinks" to take up excess calcium from the cytoplasm, and it is reasonable to propose that impairments of mitochondrial oxidative metabolism might therefore sensitize cells to damage from influx of excess calcium. *In vitro* experiments with cultured AD cells are consistent with this proposal, but direct demonstration of it in neurons in autopsy brain is difficult.[89,90]

G. SELECTIVE CELL DEATH

Impairment of mitochondrial oxidative metabolism is such a classical cause of premature cell death as to hardly need documentation. What is less widely recognized is that impairments of oxidative metabolism can lead to selective cell death and within the nervous system to selective neuronal death. Indeed, well-documented examples exist both experimentally and clinically.[2]

Experimentally, the standard current model of selective neuronal cell death is the four-vessel occlusion stroke model.[19] In this model, a controlled period of total hypoxia/ischemia leads to death of specific populations of neurons and sparing of others. For instance, CA1 neurons of the hippocampus die within 48 hours, but CA2 neurons do not die — exquisitely selective vulnerability due to a controlled impairment in brain oxidative metabolism. Experimental thiamine deficiency is a classic model for selective vulnerability in the nervous system. Recent studies implicate the impairment of oxidative metabolism, specifically of the activity of mitochondrial *KGDHC*, in mediating the action of thiamine deficiency.[67] MPP is toxin which causes selective vulnerability of dopaminergic neurons and whose action is mediated by mitochondria.[92] It is important to note that each of these conditions, although mediated by impairment of mitochondrial function, leads to a *distinct pattern of selective vulnerability*.

Clinically, a number of neurological disorders are known to affect mitochondrial oxidative metabolism and to show selective vulnerability at neuropathology (Table 1). These clinical examples document that impairments of mitochondrial oxidative metabolism can lead to brain damage in specific patterns of selective neuropathological vulnerability, in naturally occurring human diseases. Thus, both firm experimental and firm clinical data document.

- That mitochondrial lesions can lead to characteristic forms of brain damage
- That these disorders display different and distinctive patterns of selective vulnerability, depending on the precise nature of the mitochondrial lesion

H. IMPAIRMENT OF ADAPTATION

The deficiencies in oxidative metabolism in AD may contribute to the development of the disease in part by limiting the ability of brain cells to increase their metabolism in response to metabolic demand. The residual activity of KGDHC and other mitochondrial components may be enough to maintain function under normal circumstances, but not in the face of increased need for energy when neural tissues are placed under physiological or pathological stress (Figure 4).

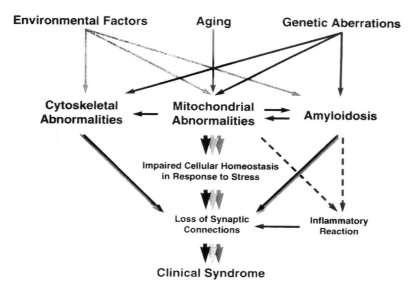

FIGURE 4 Possible role of mitochondrial abnormalities in AD. The diagram illustrates a role for the mitochondrial lesion in AD as one of the determinants of the pathophysiology. The model is discussed at greater length in Reference 2, in which this diagram originally appeared. The model conceptualizes AD as a form of characteristic scarring of the brain, with the clinical manifestations of the disease becoming apparent when the damage to the brain becomes extensive enough to prevent the patient from functioning satisfactorily in the environment in which the patient lives. From this viewpoint, any combination of genetic and nongenetic factors which lead to the scarring are then "causes" of AD. The disorder is therefore conceptualized as a syndrome rather than as a disease entity with a single, dominant, "seminal" cause. A major role of the mitochondrial lesion is a limitation on the ability of the cells to adapt to challenges which require the mobilization of increased energy metabolism to maintain cellular homeostasis, as discussed in Reference 2. (From Blass, J. P., *Neurology,* 43(Suppl.), 25, 1993. With permission.)

Basic science evidence which supports this possibillity includes well-documented mechanisms which increase the rate of oxidative metabolism when demands on cells increase.[11] These mechanisms allow cells to increase the production of available metabolic energy, in the forms of pyrophosphate bonds with high energy of hydrolysis, when the cell needs energy to reestablish concentration gradients (e.g., of ions), repair damaged constituents, or to excrete toxic accumulations. Among the best known of these mechanisms are the *coupling* of oxygen uptake to the phosphorylation of ADP to ATP in healthy, "well-coupled" mitochondria. These mechanisms exist in brain.[5] Indeed, the rate of oxygen uptake by neurons is linearly related to their rate of depolarization, i.e., their "firing rate".[12,60]

A number of direct studies indicate that cell damage and death can be caused by the combination of an impairment of oxidative metabolism not of itself severe enough to cause significant cell damage and a stressor not of itself severe enough to cause significant cell damage. For instance, cultured neurons have been reported to survive when deprived of glucose or when incubated with a low dose of the excitotoxic amino acid glutamate but not when subjected to both together.[89] Glucose deprivation has been reported to act synergystically with toxic fragments of amyloid on neurons in tissue culture.[93,94] Sapolsky and co-workers[95] have emphasized the synergisim of impairment of carbohydrate metabolism and adrenal steroid toxicity on the death of hippocampal cells *in vitro* and *in vivo*. Indeed, classical studies of experimental seizures in animals have shown that neurons die in that model when they "outrun their metabolism".[96]

These data suggest that the impairments of oxidative metabolism in general and in KGDHC in particular contribute to the pathogenesis of AD by impairing the ability of the clinically affected cells to mobilize the energy needed to respond effectively to a variety of intracurrent stressors which occur during life and accumulate in older age.[2] This formulation suggests an interaction of the deficiencies in oxidative metabolism with other abnormalities in the causation of AD.

I.   ALZHEIMER'S DISEASE AS A CONVERGENCE SYNDROME [2]

In a number of degenerative diseases of aging, a specific and well-characterized type of anatomical scarring occurs, which when it exceeds a certain tissue burden or occurs in a particular area leads to tissue dysfunction and clinical illness. This effect is not unique to brain. Indeed, it is instructive to draw the parallels between atherosclerosis and AD. In atherosclerosis, a specific form of scarring (i.e., atheromata) accumulates in a particular tissue (i.e., blood vessels); in AD, specific forms of scarring (i.e., plaques and tangles) accumulate in the brain. In atherosclerosis, which is relatively well understood, a number of mechanistic risk factors, genetic and environmental, have been identified which can combine to lead to the formation of the typical lesions. In AD, a variety of mechanisms have been implicated which have been proposed to contribute to the characteristic brain damage. This reasoning by analogy suggests that any factor or combination of factors which lead to the accumulation of an adequate density of the characteristic scarring in appropriate parts of the brain are "causes" of AD (Figures 4 and 5). Indeed, studies demonstrating genetic heterogeneity in AD indicate strongly that the disease is heterogeneous biologically as well as clinically and can therefore have a number of "causes".[18,19] While a number of these mechanisms may well be part of a common cascade of events leading to the formation of the typical AD scar tissue, there is no obvious heuristic benefit in naming one of these events as more "seminal" than the others. The well-documented abnormalities in AD in oxidative metabolism in general and in KGDHC activity in particular may, therefore, be one of a number of "contributory causes" which converge to cause clinical AD (Figure 5). One can easily develop such scenarios in more detail. For instance, the combination of an otherwise clinically silent partial deficiency in KGDHC activity combined with an otherwise clinically silent accumulation of defects in mtDNA may impair a neuron from metabolizing amyloid or other materials normally, when faced with a concurrent insult such as an otherwise clinically silent episode of inflammation.

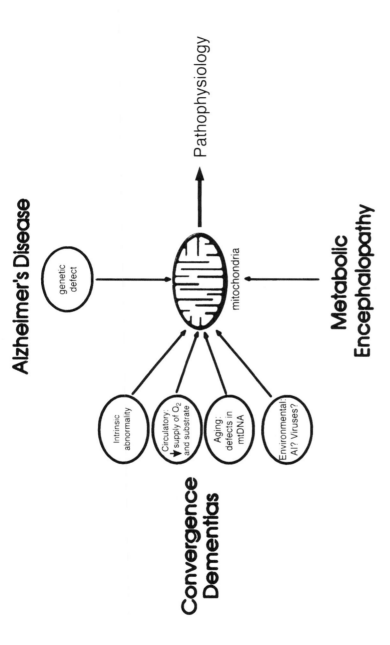

FIGURE 5   Origins of impairments of mitochondrial function in AD. The hypothesis illustrated by the diagram is that the causes of mitochondrial dysfunction in AD can be grouped into several categories, correlating roughly with different forms of AD. In *early onset* FAD, a genetic abnormality leads directly or indirectly to mitochondrial dysfunction, with consequences for pathophysiology illustrated in Figure 4 and discussed in the text and in Reference 2. In *later onset* AD, a variety of abnormalities may contribute to the mitochondrial dysfunction. These may include a genetic predisposition, which may or may not be allelic with an abnormal gene in FAD; an impairment in the supply of substrate and oxygen to the brain, due to cardiovascular/cerebrovascular disease; accumulation with age of errors in mtDNA; and exposure during the relatively long lives of these characteristically elderly patients to toxins, viruses, or other injurious agents. Although the origins of mitochondrial impairment in this situation are multifactorial, the consequences in terms of pathophysiology of AD are similar to those from a more discrete genetic cause. In *delerium* (metabolic encaphalopathy), a coexistent medical disease (for instance, excess of a drug or toxin) leads characteristically to impairment of mitochondrial oxidative metabolism[10,99] and to confusion similar to that seen chronically in Alzheimer dementia.[10] The pathophysiological mechanisms downstream of the mitochondrial impairment are again similar to those due to the mitochondrial impairment in early onset or later onset AD. This formulation helps to explain the similar clinical manifestations in early and late onset AD and in delerium. It also helps to explain why susceptibility to metabolic encephalopathy may be an early manifestation of AD, even before significant cerebral atrophy is evident by CT or MRI scan.

J. ALZHEIMER'S DISEASE AND CEREBROVASCULAR DISEASE

Of particular interest is the potential interaction between an inherent abnormality of cellular oxidative machinery (e.g., in KGDHC) and an abnormality in cerebral circulation. The original descriptions of AD posited an interaction between an "inherent susceptibility" and an abnormality of circulation,[97] and recent studies have again suggested that impaired circulation may be an independent risk factor for neuropathologically confirmed AD.[98] A cell whose mitochondria are already limited in their capacity to utilize oxygen and substrate because of a deficiency in a critical enzyme such as KGDHC might be expected to be particularly sensitive to otherwise clinically silent impairments of the supply of oxygen and substrate through the circulation. Indeed, such synergism at a *mechanistic* level may explain some of the current difficulties in trying to separate clearly the syndromes of "vascular dementia" from AD in patients who also have cardiovascular disease (Figure 5).

The formulation of AD as a convergence syndrome has both scientific and therapeutic implications. Scientifically, it supports the validity of examining mechanisms demonstrated to occur in AD including the abnormalities in oxidative metabolism, without a need to assume primacy in the pathogenesis for one or the other. In terms of therapeutics, this formulation suggests that, for AD as for other complex degenerative diseases of aging, a number of mechanisms including oxidative metabolism may provide sites to which appropriate medications can be directed to help the patients and their families.

IV. SUMMARY

In his Croonian lecture of 1923, Sir Archibald Garrod[20] pointed out that the main contribution of genetics to the causation of disease may not be rare inborn errors but instead otherwise silent genetic variants which impair the ability of the body to respond adequately to environmental stressors. The well-documented abnormalities in oxidative metabolism in AD including those in KGDHC may fit within Garrod's proposal.

REFERENCES

1. Luft, R., The development of mitochondrial medicine, *Proc. Natl. Acad. Sci. U.S.A.*, 91: 8731, 1994.
2. Blass, J. P., Pathophysiology of the Alzheimer syndrome, *Neurology*, 43(Suppl.), 25, 1993.
3. Blass, J. P. and Gibson, G. E., The role of oxidative abnormalities in the pathophysiology of Alzheimer's Disease, *Rev. Neurol*, 147, 513, 1991.
4. Blass, J. P., Sheu, K-F. R., and Cederbaum, J. M., Energy metabolism in disorders of the nervous system, *Rev. Neurol*, 144, 543, 1988.
5. Clarke, D. D. and Sokoloff, L., Circulation and energy metabolism in the brain, in *Basic Neurochemistry* 5th ed., Siegel, G. J., Agranoff, B. W., Albers, R. W., and Molinoff, P. B, Eds, Raven Press, New York, 645.
6. Carroll, J. M., Toral-Barza, L., and Gibson, G., Cytosolic free calcium and gene expression during chemical hypoxia, *J. Neurochem.*, 59, 1836, 1992.
7. Orrenius, S., Burkitt, M. J., Kass, G. E., Dypbukt, J. M., and Nicotera, P., Calcium ions and oxidative cell injury, *Ann. Neurol.*, 32(Suppl.), 33, 1992.
8. Blass, J. P. and Gibson, G. E., Consequences of mild, graded hypoxia, *Ann. Neurol.*, 18, 229, 1979.
9. Gibson, G. E., Pulsinelli, W. A., and Blass, J. P., Brain dysfunction in mild to moderate hypoxia, *Am. J. Med.*, 70, 1247, 1981.
10. Blass, J. P., Nolan, K. A., Black, R. S., and Kurita, A., Delirium: phenomenology and diagnosis — a neurobiological view, *Int. Psychogeriat*, 3, 121, 1992.
11. Atkinson, D., *Cellular Energy Metabolism and its Regulation*. Academic Press, 1977, New York.
12. Blass, J. P. and Gibson, G. E., Consequences of mild, graded hypoxia, *Adv. Neurol.* 229, 1979.
13. Sorbi, S. and Blass, J. P., Mitochondrial abnormalities in hereditary ataxias. In *Cerebellar Degenerations: Clinical Neurobiology*, Pliatakis, A, Ed., Kluwer Academic, Boston, 1992, 391.
14. Hoyer, S., Abnormalities of glucose metabolism in Alzheimer's disease, *Ann. N.Y. Acad. Sci.*, 640, 53, 1991.
15. Mielke, R., Herholz, K., Grond, M., Kessler, J., and Heiss, W. D., Differences of regional cerebral glucose metabolism between presenile and senile dementia of the Alzheimer type, *Neurobiol. Aging*, 13, 93, 1992.

16. Hoyer, S., Sporadic dementia of the Alzheimer type: Role of amyloid in etiology is challenged, *J. Neural. Transm.,* 6, 159, 1993.
17. Jagust, W. J., Friedland, P. R., and Budinger, T. F., Longitudinal studies of cerebral glucose metabolism in Alzheimer's disease, *Neurology,* 38, 909, 1988.
18. Tanzi, R., Gaston, S., Bush, A., Romano, D., Pettingell, W., Pepercorn, J., Paradis, M., Gurubhagavatula, S., Jenkins, B., and Wasco, W., Genetic heterogeneity of gene defects responsible for Alzheimer's disease, *Genetica,* 91, 255, 1993.
19. Ritchie, K. and Touchon, J., Heterogeneity in senile dementia of the Alzheimer type: individual differences, progressive deterioration, or clinical sub-types?, *J. Clin. Epidemiol.,* 45, 1391, 1992.
20. Garrod, A. E., *Inborn Errors of Metabolism,* Oxford Press, London, 1923.
21. Brown, M. S. and Goldstein, J. L., Familial hypercholesterolemia: model for genetic receptor disease, *Harvey Lecture Ser.,* 73, 163, 1979.
22. Stanbury, J. B., Wyngaarden, J. B., Fredrickson, D. S., Goldstein, J. L., and Brown, M. S., Eds., *The Metabolic Basis of Inherited Disease,* 5th ed., McGraw-Hill, 1983, New York.
23. Sahin-Toth, M., Lawrence, M. C., and Kaback, H. R., Properties of permease dimer, a fusion protein containing two lactose permease molecules from Escherichia coli, *Proc. Natl. Acad. Sci. U.S.A.,* 91, 5421, 1994.
24. Westergaard, N., Varming, T., Peng, L., Sonnewald, U., Hertz, L., and Schousboe, A., Uptake, release, and metabolism of alanine in neurons and astrocytes in primary cultures, *J. Neurosci. Res.,* 35, 540, 1993.
25. Terry, R. D., Masliah, E., and Salmon D. P., Physical basis of cognitive loss in Alzheimer's disease: synapse loss is the major correlate of cognitive impairment, *Ann. Neurol.,* 30, 572, 1991.
26. Sims, N. R., Bowen, D. M., Neary, D., and Davison, N. M., Metabolic process in Alzheimer's disease: adenine nucleotide content and production of $^{14}CO_2$ from [U-^{14}C]glucose *in vitro* in human neocortex, *J. Neurochem.,* 41, 1329, 1983.
27. Sims, N. R., Finegan, J. M., Blass, J. P., Bowen, D. M., and Neary, D., Mitochondrial function in brain in primary degenerative dementia, *Brain Res.,* 436, 30, 1987.
28. Blass, J. P., Metabolic alterations common to neural and non-neural cells in Alzheimer's disease, *Hippocampus,* 3, 45, 1993
29. Pettegrew, J. W., Panchalinam, K., Klunk, W. E., McClure, R. J., and Muenz, L. R., Alterations of cerebral metabolism in probable Alzheimer's disease: A preliminary study, *Neurobiol Aging,* 15, 117, 1994.
30. Bowen, D. M., Smith, C. B., White, P., and Davison, A. N., Neurotransmitter-related enzymes and indices of hypoxia in senile dementia and other abiotrophies, *Brain* 99, 459, 1976.
31. Davies, P. and Maloney, A. J. F., Selective loss of central cholinergic neurons in Alzheimer's disease, *Lancet,* 2, 1403.
32. Perry, E. K., Perry, R. H., Tomlinson, B. E., Blessed, G., and Gibson, P. H., Coenzyme-A acetylating-enzymes in Alzheimer's disease: possible cholinergic "compartment" of pyruvate dehydrogenase, *Neurosci. Lett.,* 18, 105, 1980.
33. Sorbi, S., Bird, E. D., and Blass, J. P., Decreased pyruvate dehydrogenase activity in Huntington and Alzheimer brain, *Ann. Neurol.,* 13, 72, 1983.
34. Butterworth, R. M. and Besnard, A. M., Thiamin-dependent enzyme changes in temporal cortex of patients with Alzheimer's disease, *Metab. Brain Dis.* 4, 179, 1990.
35. Yates, C. M., Butterworth, J., Tennant, M. C., and Gordon, A., Enzyme activities in relation to pH and lactate in post-mortem brain in Alzheimer and other dementias, *J. Neurochem.,* 55, 1624, 1991.
36. Sheu, K-F. R., Kim, Y-Y., Blass, J. P., and Weksler, M.E., An immunochemical study on the deficit of pyruvate dehydrogenase in Alzheimer's disease, *Ann. Neurol.* 17 444, 1985.
37. Gibson, G. E., Sheu, K-F. R., Blass, J. P., Baker, A., Carlson, K. C., Harding, B., and Perrino, P., Reduced activities of thiamin-dependent enzymes in the brains and peripheral tissues of patients with Alzheimer's disease, *Arch. Neurol.,* 35, 312, 1988.
38. Mastrogiacomo, F., Bergeron, C., and Kish, S. J., Brain α-ketoglutarate dehydrogenase complex activity in Alzheimer's disease, *J. Neurochem.,* 61, 2007, 1993.
39. Terwel, D., Bothmer, J., Meng, F., Wolf, E., Markerink, M., and Jolles, J., Reduced enzyme activities in Alzheimer's disease are sensitive to hypoxia, *Neurobiol. Aging,* 15(Suppl.), 120, 1994.
40. Kish, S. J., Bergeron, C., Rajput, A., Dozic, S., Mastrogiacomo, F., et al., Brain cytochrome c oxidase in Alzheimer's disease, *J. Neurochem.,* 59, 776, 1992.
41. Jung, E. H., Sheu, K-F. R., and Blass, J. P., An enzymatic and immunochemical analysis of transketolase in fibroblasts from the Wernicke-Korsakoff syndrome, *J. Neurol. Sci.,* 114, 123.
42. Liguri, G., Taddei, N., Nassi, P., Latorraca, S., Nediani, C., and Sorbi, S., Changes in Na$^+$,K$^+$-ATPase, Ca^{2+}-ATPase and some soluble enzymes related to energy metabolism in brains of patients with Alzheimer's disease, *Neurosci. Lett.,* 112, 338, 1990.
43. Sims, N. R., Blass, J. P., Murphy, C., Bowen, D. M., and Neary, D., Phosphofructokinase activity in the brain in Alzheimer's disease, *Ann. Neurol.,* 21, 509, 1987.
44. Blass, J. P. and Gibson, G. E., Non-neural markers in Alzheimer's disease, *Alz. Dis. Assoc. Dis.,* 6, 205, 1993.
45. Blass, J. P., The fibroblast model for studying neurodegenerative disorders, *J. Neural. Trans.,* 44, 87, 1994.
46. Peterson, C. and Goldman, J. E., Alterations in calcium content and biochemical processes in cultured fibroblasts from Alzheimer and aged donors, *Proc. Natl. Acad. Sci. U.S.A.,* 83, 2758, 1986.

47. Sims, N. R., Finegan, J. M., and Blass, J. P, Altered metabolic properties of cultured skin fibroblasts in Alzheimer's disease, *Ann. Neurol.*, 21, 451, 1987.

48. Sheu, K.-F. R., Cooper, A. J. L., Koike, K., Koike, M., Lindsay, J. G., and Blass, J. P., Abnormality of the α-ketoglutarate dehydrogenase complex in fibroblasts from familial Alzheimer's disease, *Ann. Neurol.*, 35, 312, 1994.

49. Paoletti, F. and Mocalli, A., Enhanced proteolytic activities in cultured fibroblasts of Alzheimer patients are revealed by peculiar transketolase alterations, *J. Neurol. Sci.*, 105, 211, 1991.

50. Parker, W. D., Mahr, N. J., Filley, C. M., Parks, J. K., Hughes, D., Young, D. A., and Cullum, C. M., Reduced platelet cytochrome c oxidase activity in Alzheimer's disease, *Neurology,* 44, 1086, 1994.

51. Van Zuylen, A. J., Bosman, G.J., Ruitenbeek, W., Van Kalmthout, P.J., and De Grip, W.J., No evidence found for reduced thrombocyte cytochrome oxidase activity in Alzheimer's disease, *Neurology,* 42, 1246, 1992.

52. Bothmer, J., Markerink, M., Coppens, R., and Jolles, J., Platelet phosphatidyl kinase activity is not altered in Alzheimer's disease, *Mol. Chem. Neuropathol.*, 19, 249, 1993.

53. Wallace, D. C., Mitochondrial DNA sequence variation in human evolution and disease, *Proc. Natl. Acad. Sci. U.S.A.,* 91, 8739, 1994.

54. Schoffner, J. M., Brown, M. D., Torroni, A., Lott, M. T., Cabell, M. F., et al., Mitochondrial DNA variants observed in Alzheimer's disease and Parkinson disease patients, *Genomics,* 17, 171, 1993.

55. Kosel, S., Egensperger, R., Mehraein, P., and Graeber, M. B., No association of mutations at nucleotide 5460 of mitochondrial NADH dehydrogenase with Alzheimer's disease, *Biochem. Biophys. Res. Commun.,* 203, 745, 1994.

56. Szabo, P., Cai, X., Ali, G., and Blass, J. P., Localization of the gene (OGDH) coding for the E1k component of the α-ketoglutarate dehydrogenase complex to chromosome 7p13-p11.2, *Genomics,* 20, 324, 1994.

57. Scherer, S. W., Otulakowski, G., Robinson, B. H., and Tsui, L. C., Localization of the human dihydrolipoamide dehydrogenase gene (DLD) to 7q31-q32, *Cytogenet. Cell Genet.*, 56, 176, 1991.

58. Nakano, K., Matsuda, S., Sakamoto, T., Takese, C., Nakagawa, S., Ohto, S., Ariyama, T., Inazawa, J., Abe, T., Miyata, T., Human dihydrolipoamide succinyltransferase. cDNA cloning and localization on chromosome 14q24.2-q24.3, *Biochim Biophys Acta,* 1216, 360, 1993.

59. Ali, G., Wasco, W., Cai, X., Szabo, P., Sheu, K-F. R., Cooper, A. J. L., Gaston, S. M., Gusella, J. F., Tanzi, R. E., and Blass, J. P., Isolation, characterization, and mapping of the dihydrolipoyl succcinyltransferase (E2k) gene of the human α-ketoglutarate dehydrogenase complex, *Somat. Cell Mol. Genet.*, 20, 99, 1994.

60. Gibson, G. E. and Blass, J. P., Metabolism and neurotransmission, in *Handbook of Neurochemistry*, Vol. 3, 2nd ed., Lajtha, A., Ed, Plenum Press, New York, 1983, 633.

61. Millner, T. A., Aoki, C., Sheu, K-F. R., Blass, J. P., and Pickel, V. M., Light microscopic immunocytochemical localization of pyruvate dehydrogenase in rat brain: topographical distribution and relation to cholinergic and catecholaminergic nuclei, *J. Neurosci.*, 7, 3171, 1987.

62. Gibson, G. E., Peterson, C., and Freeman, G., Alterations in neurotransmitter metabolism and calcium homeostasis during aging and Alzheimer's disease, *Banbury Rep.*, 27, 89.

63. Selkoe, D. J., Alzheimer's disease: a central role for amyloid, *J. Neurol. Neurosurg. Psychiat.*, 53, 438, 1994.

64. Roses, A., Apolipoprotein E affects the rate of Alzheimer's disease expression: β-amyloid burden is a secondary consequence dependent on APOE genotype and duration of disease, *J. Neurol. Neurosurg. Psychiat.*, 53, 429, 1994.

65. Kalaria, R. N., Bhatti, S. U., Lust, W. D., and Perry, G., The amyloid precursor protein in ischemic brain injury and chronic hypoperfusion, *Ann. N.Y. Acad. Sci.*, 695, 190, 1993.

66. Saido, T. C., Yokot, M., Maruyama, K., Yamao-Harigaya, W., Tani, E., Ihara, K., and Kawashima, S., Spatial resolution of the primary β-amyloidogenic process induced in postischemic hippocampus, *J. Biol. Chem.*, 269, 15253, 1994.

67. Calignasan, N. Y., Gandy, S. E., Baker, H., Kim, K. S., Wisniewski, H. M., Sheu, K-F. R., and Gibson, G. E., Accumulation of amyloid precursor protein in rat brain in response to impaired oxidation induced by thiamin deficiency, *Brain Res*, in press.

68. Tomimoto, H., Wakita, H., Akiguchi, I., Nakamura, S., and Kimura, J., Temporal profiles of accumulation of amyloid β/A4 protein precursor in the gerbil after graded ischemic stress, *J. Cereb. Blood Flow Metab.*, 14, 563, 1994.

69. Gabudza, D., Busciglio, J., Chen, L. B., Matsudaira, P., and Yankner, B. A., Inhibition of energy metabolism alters the processing of amyloid precursor protein and induces a potentially amyloidogenic derivative, *J. Biol. Chem.*, 269, 13623, 1994.

70. Meier-Ruge, W., Iwangoff, P., and Bertoni-Freddari, C., What is primary and what is secondary for amyloid deposition in Alzheimer's disease, *Ann. N.Y. Acad. Sci.*, 719, 230, 1994.

71. Maro, B. and Bornens, M., Reorganization of HeLa cell cytoskeleton induced by an uncoupler of oxidative phosphorylation, *Nature,* 295, 334, 1982.

72. Klymkowsky, M. W., Metabolic inhibitors and intermediate filament organization in human fibroblasts, *Exp. Cell Res.*, 174, 282, 1988.

73. Blass, J. P., Baker, A. C., Ko, L., and Black, R. S., Induction of Alzheimer antigens by an uncoupler of oxidative phosphorylation, *Arch. Neurol.*, 28, 111, 1990.

74. Blanchard, B. J., devi Raghunandan, R., Roder, H. M., and Ingram, V. M., Hyperphosphorylation of human tau by brain kinase PK40erk beyond phosphorylation by cAMPdependent PKA: relation to Alzheimer's disease, *Biochem. Biophys. Res. Commun.* 200, 187, 1994.

75. Huang, H.-M. and Gibson, G. E., Effects of *in vitro* hypoxia on depolarization-stimulated accumulation of inositol phosphates in synaptosomes, *Life Sci.,* 45, 1443, 1989.
76. Huang, H.-M. and Gibson, G. E., Altered β-adrenergic receptor-stimulated cAMP formation in cultured skin fibroblasts from Alzheimer donors, *J. Biol. Chem.,* 268, 14616, 1993.
77. Huang, H.-M., Lin, T-A., Sun, G. Y., and Gibson, G. E., Increased inositol 1,4,5-triphosphate accumulation correlates with an up-regulation of bradykinin receptors in Alzheimer's disease, *J. Neurochem.,* 64, 761, 1995.
78. Halliwell, B., Oxidants and the central nervous system: some fundamental questions. Is oxidant damage relevant to Parkinson's disease, Alzheimer's disease, traumatic injury, or stroke?, *Acta Neurol. Scand.,* 166(Suppl.), 23, 1989.
79. Allen, R. G., Role of free radicals in senescence, *Annu. Rev. Gerontol. Geriat.,* 10, 198, 1990.
80. Volicer, L. and Crino, P. B., Involvement of free radicals in dementia of the Alzheimer type: a hypothesis, *Neurobiol. Aging,* 11, 567, 1990.
81. Boveris, A. and Chance, B., The mitochondrial generation of hydrogen peroxide, *Biochem. J.,* 134, 707, 1973.
82. Benzi, G., Pastoris, Q., Marzatico, F., Villa, R.F., Dagani, F., and Curti, D., The mitochondrial electron transfer alteration as a factor involved in brain aging, *Neurobiol. Aging,* 13, 361, 1992.
83. McCord, J. M., Human disease, free radicals, and the oxidant/antioxidant balance, *Clin. Biochem.,* 26, 351, 1993.
84. Makar, T. K., Nedergaard, M., Preuss, A., Gelbard, A. S., Peruman, A. S., and Cooper, A. J. L., Vitamin E, ascorbate, glutathione, glutathione disulfide, and enzymes of glutathione metabolism in cultures of chick astrocytes and neurons: Evidence that astrocytes play an important role in autoxidative processes in the brain, *J. Neurochem.,* 62, 45, 1994.
85. Franklin, J. L. and Johnson, E. M., Suppression of programmed neuronal death by sustained elevation of cytoplasmic calcium, *Trends Neurosci.,* 15, 501, 1994.
86. Loo, D. T., Copani, A., Pike, C. J., Whittemore, E. R., Walencewicz, A. J., and Cotman, C. W., Apoptosis is induced by β-amyloid in cultured central nervous system neurons, *Proc. Natl. Acad. Sci. U.S.A.,* 90, 7951, 1993.
87. Peterson, C., Gibson, G. E., and Blass, J. P., Altered calcium homeostasis in fibroblasts from Alzheimer patients, *N. Eng. J. Med.,* 312, 1063.
88. Gibson, G. E. and Toral-Barza, L., Characterization of internal calcium stores in cultured skin fibroblasts from Alzheimer and control subjects, *Mol. Biol. Cell,* 3, 145a, 1995.
89. Henneberry, R. C., The role of neuronal energy in the neurotoxicity of amino acids, *Neurobiol. Aging,* 10, 611, 1989.
90. Beal, F. M., Does impairment of energy metabolism result in excitotoxic death in neurodegenerative illnesses?, *Ann. Neurol.,* 31, 119, 1992.
91. Sims, N. R. and Pulsinelli, W. A., Altered mitochondrial respiration in selectively vulnerable brain subregions following transient forebrain ischemia in the rat, *J. Neurochem.,* 49, 1367, 1987.
92. Gluck, M. R., Youngster, S. K., Ramsay, R. R., Singer, T. P., and Nicklas, W. J., Studies on the characterization of the inhibitory mechanisms of 4′-alkylated 1-methyl-4-pyridinium and phenylpyridine analogues in mitochondria and electron transport particles, *J. Neurochem.,* 63, 655, 1994.
93. Copani, A., Koh, J. Y., and Cotman, C. W., β-Amyloid increases neuronal susceptibility to injury by glucose deprivation, *Neuroreport,* 2, 763, 1991.
94. Cotman, C. W., Pike, C. J., and Copani, A., β-Amyloid neurotoxicity: a discussion of *in vitro* findings, *Neurobiol. Aging,* 13, 587, 1992.
95. Lawrence, M. S. and Sapolsky, R. M., Glucocorticoids accelerate ATP loss following metabolic insults in cultured hippocampal neurons, *Brain Res,* 646, 303, 1992.
96. Meldrum, B., Epileptic seizures, in *Basic Neurochemistry*, 5th Ed, Siegel, G. J., Agranoff, B. W., Albers, R. A., and Molinoff, P. B., Eds, Raven Press, New York, 1993, 885.
97. Bick, K., Amaducci, L., and Pepeu, G., *The Early Story of Alzheimer's Disease*, Lavinia Press, Padua, 1987.
98. Sparks, D. L., Hunsaker, J. C., Scheff, S. W., Kryscio, R. J., Henson, J. L., and Markesbery, W. R., Cortical senile plaques in coronary artery disease, aging, and Alzheimer's disease, *Neurobiol. Aging,* 11, 601.
99. Plum, F. and Posner, J. B., *The Diagnosis of Stupor and Coma*, F.A. Davis, Philadelphia, 1980.
100. Cai, X. and Blass, J. P., A pseudogene of dihydolipoyl succinyltransferase (E2k) found by PCR amplification and direct sequencing of rodent-human hybrid DNAs. *Somat. Cell Mol. Genet.,* in press.

Chapter 16

THE METABOLISM OF APOLIPOPROTEIN E AND THE ALZHEIMER'S DISEASES*

Allen D. Roses

CONTENTS

---

* Reprinted from *Experimental Neurology*. With permission.

I. THE DISEASES

Alzheimer's disease was "officially" defined by clinical and neuropathologic criteria more than a decade ago.[1,2] There are several different genetic etiologies that lead to a disease meeting these criteria.[3] In this perspective I have used the term "Alzheimer's diseases" to imply that there can be multiple genetic etiologies for the same phenotype. "Alzheimer's syndrome" would be another choice. The Alzheimer's diseases are characterized by dementia, a global impairment of higher cortical functions that usually starts selectively and gradually. Progression is usually obvious to family members, especially in younger patients. The disease progresses gradually, usually lasting 3 to 20 years, until functional incapacity and death. Impairment of recent memory is usually an early symptom, with increasing difficulties in performing activities of daily living, making supervision a constant concern. Recent memory loss can be potentially dangerous. Cooking a meal and forgetting to turn off the oven is an example of a common, potentially hazardous behavior problem. Wandering is another.

The early-onset autosomal dominant Alzheimer's diseases (mean 40- to 60-year old age of onset) are caused by the inheritance of one of at least three different gene mutations and account for less than 5% of the prevalence.[3] Late-onset disease is usually defined operationally as onset after 60 years and constitutes more than 95% of prevalent disease. Most often there is no family history fitting an autosomal dominant pattern, so that such cases are labeled "sporadic". In larger families, clusters or familial aggregations of patients may be observed. In general the duration of the disease is related to the age of onset, with younger patients (<60-year age of onset) living longer with disease than older patients. Therefore, the long-term care of middle-aged (50 to 80 years) patients is a serious social problem and accounts for enormous long-term health care costs to families and to society. It is estimated that there are 3 to 4 million patients in the U.S. today, and that number is expected to triple in the next 20 years unless the disease can be prevented.[4,5]

II. GENETIC HETEROGENEITY

Table 1 illustrates a current classification of the genetics of the Alzheimer's diseases. There are at least six genetic loci that cause an identical clinical disease, albeit crudely differentiated by the average age of onset. The most common form of the disease, probably accounting for 50 to 75% of cases is late-onset disease (>55 years) associated with the inheritance of various apolipoprotein E (APOE, gene; apoE, protein) genotypes.[6-9] The allele frequency (i.e., proportion of all chromosomes) of APOE4 is approximately 15% in the U.S. Therefore, approximately 31% of the population carry at least one APOE4 allele. Because of the high gene frequency of the APOE4 allele relative to Mendelian inherited diseases, the analyses of older age familial Alzheimer's disease (>75 years) require complex statistical methods that also factor in their APOE alleles in order to test for other susceptibility genes.

TABLE 1　Genetic Classification of the Alzheimer's Diseases

Type	Chromosome	Gene	Age	%
I. Late-onset familial and sporadic APOE allele associated	19	APOE	>55	50–75
II. Late-onset familial and sporadic Not APOE associated	UNK	UNK	>75	10–30
III. Early-onset familial autosomal dominant inheritance	14	PS1	Mean 40s 28–60+	≪1 <200 families
IV. Early-onset familial autosomal dominant inheritance	21	APP	Mean 50s 39–68	<20 families
V. Early-onset familial autosomal dominant inhertitance	1	PS2	Mean 50s	Volga-German founder
VI. Other				

All of the early-onset forms of autosomal dominant Alzheimer's disease are rare. The most common, representing more than 80% of this rare group, due to missense mutations of a gene named Presenilin 1 (PS1). This gene is associated with intracellular membranes.[10-11a] There are less than 20 families worldwide with mutations of the amyloid precursor protein (APP).[12-15] Several specific APP mutations segregate with clinical onset in the 40- to -60 year range. There appears to be an interaction with the inheritance of APOE genotypes in these families. Just as in late-onset Alzheimer's disease, APOE4 alleles may be associated with earlier onset and APOE2 with later onset.[9,16,17] A third locus is inherited in a group of families of Volga-German origin.[18] Missense mutations of Presenilin 2 (PS2) on chromosome 1 cause disease in the Volga-German and two Italian families. Although it is possible that some sporadic early-onset cases may carry either the chromosome 14 or the Volga-German mutation, about half of the Alzheimer patients presenting between ages 50 to 60 years may be associated with APOE4 inheritance.[19,20] It is certainly expected that other susceptibility genes exist.

III. THEORIES OF PATHOGENESIS BASED ON NEUROPATHOLOGY

The criteria defined by convention to diagnose definite Alzheimer's disease require the presence of neuritic plaque counts per high-power field modified for the age of the patient. Neuritic plaques are "spherical accumulations of argyrophilic dystrophic neurites supplemented by centrally located microglial cells and peripherally arranged astrocytes. In addition, diffuse deposits and/or condensed cores of amyloid are frequently but not consistently occurring components."[21] More than 20 other proteins have been localized to these neuritic plaques, including apoE, low-density lipoprotein-related receptor, very low-density lipoprotein receptor, anti-chymotrypsin, as well as the β-amyloid peptide (Aβ) of APP.[22] All definite Alzheimer's disease patients have neuritic plaques by definition; most of these plaques also contain Aβ aggregates.[2,23] It is frequently ignored in the literature that many cognitively intact elderly have senile plaques and Aβ deposition meeting the criteria sufficient for conventional diagnosis of Alzheimer's disease if dementia had been present.[24,25,25a] These nondemented individuals with plaques did not suffer from Alzheimer's disease, emphasizing that the conventional pathological criteria *do not define Alzheimer's disease in the absence of signs and symptoms*. Similarly, in most series of probable Alzheimer's disease patients who have autopsies, up to 10 to 20% of clinical patients who would be expected to have Alzheimer pathology do not meet the pathological criteria. As the genetic data are applied, it is becoming clear that increased Aβ deposition may be associated with individuals carrying one or two APOE4 alleles. Very old, probable Alzheimer's disease patients who may have little Aβ deposition are more likely to carry the APOE2/3 or APOE3/3 genotype. As more data are developed from large pathological series, consideration of revised diagnostic criteria may be appropriate.[25,25a]

These data impact on the amyloid theory of pathogenesis, a common viewpoint for the past decade summarized as "the central pathological event in Alzheimer's disease is the deposition of Aβ as amyloid fibrils within the senile plaques and cerebral blood vessels."[26-28] The pathological data relating the geography of amyloid deposition to Alzheimer's disease is poor.[29] Extensive pathological examination of a very large series of autopsies from individuals of all ages support the view that intracellular neurofibrillary tangles (NFTs) may develop many years before clinical disease and amyloid-containing neuritic plaques.[21] NFT counts after many years of disease may exhibit a ceiling effect because ghost tangles from dead cells may be reabsorbed. The neuroanatomical localization of NFTs more closely approximates the areas of the brain affected by Alzheimer's disease.[21,29]

The NFTs are made up of tau, one of the microtubule-associated proteins in neurons.[30,31] Tau binds to β-tubulin and functions to stabilize microtubules. NFTs are composed primarily of aggregated paired helical filaments (PHF) of highly phosphorylated tau. The presence of NFTs within the cytoplasm of neurons, particularly in the entorhinal and transentorhinal regions of the ambient and anterior parahippocampal gyri, appears to be associated with impaired cognitive functions in several degenerative diseases.[21] The prominence of NFTs in Alzheimer's disease contributes to the "tau" hypothesis. There has been considerable effort in studying the properties of PHF-tau, especially the role of protein kinases in tau phosphorylation.[32]

The basic difference between the amyloid and tau/NFT hypotheses is that the former begins the cascade with *extracellular* events, while the latter originates within affected neurons. In the former, amyloid deposition is said to be the necessary toxic event in the cascade; in the latter, PHF formation leading to NFT kills cells. From an anatomical point of view, NFTs are observed in the most relevant areas. The association of the APOE4 allele as a major risk factor for the earlier development of Alzheimer's disease led to experiments showing that apoE interacted with Aβ in an isoform-specific manner.[33,34] The role of apoE in the production and processing of APP and fibril formation with Aβ peptide became the immediate area for active research.[35-37] APOE mRNA is not known to be expressed in neurons, so it was deduced by most investigators that apoE was located outside of neuronal cells and that tau was found inside.[28] Based on this untested assumption, the reported apoE isoform-specific binding to tau was suspected to be an *in vitro* experimental artifact.[28]

The early-onset families with inherited APP mutations are usually put forward as the major support of the amyloid theory.[28,38] However, even in families with APP717 mutations, or in the single family with the APP670-671 mutation, the neuropathologic data do not support a direct relationship between Aβ plaque formation and clinical disease.[25,39] The arguments and literature supporting and questioning the amyloid theory have recently been summarized in a point/counterpoint context.[25,28]

Games et al. reported a transgenic mouse that formed amyloid plaques.[40] The transgene was a modified APP717 cDNA that contains the introns involved in alternative splicing of APP isoforms. This gene was highly overexpressed, and formation of amyloid plaques was illustrated. This appears to be an excellent model for amyloid deposition, yet the evidence that this model produces significant neuronal damage was limited to confocal microscopy that demonstrated decreased MAP2 and synaptophysin staining in an 11-month-old animal. These same changes occur in APOE-deficient mice (see below), but without amyloid plaques.[41,42] Additional studies of this transgenic model will no doubt be forthcoming, but several initial questions can be asked. It is now possible to demonstrate that a modified human gene in a mouse background can form amyloid plaques. It is probable, although unpublished, that these plaques are immunoreactive with apoE antibodies. Crossing the APP717 transgenic animals with APOE-deficient mice could provide some fascinating insight into what is necessary and specific for synaptic simplification. One prediction would be that amyloid plaques would not be produced, but the characteristic decreased MAP2 and synaptophysin changes characteristic of APOE-deficient animals would occur.[41,42] Similarly, crossing the APP717 mice with mice containing each of the human APOE genes on an APOE-deficient background may mimic the gradation of amyloid plaques related to APOE genotypes in humans. Another explanation is that the APP717 transgene may be necessary for plaques and sufficient for dendritic simplification, modeling the APP mutation form of Alzheimer's disease. It is clear that these mice will provide tools to determine what is necessary and sufficient for a model of the Alzheimer's diseases.

The original report of the genetic association of APOE4 and Alzheimer's disease contained photomicrographs that confirmed an earlier report of apoE immunostaining of plaques and tangles.[6,41-43] It was additionally noted, however, that there was prominent apoE staining of some *neurons that did not contain NFTs*. These data were subsequently examined more extensively and apoE-like immunoreactivity could be demonstrated in hippocampal granule cells in 30 Alzheimer's disease patients, several other neurodegenerative diseases, and several cognitively normal, elderly controls.[44] ApoE-like immunoreactivity was localized to the cytoplasm of neurons from the cerebral cortex of brain biopsies of nondemented patients using immunoelectron microscopy[45] (Figure 1).

There are important biological implications for the demonstration of intraneuronal, cytoplasmic apoE that go beyond the study of Alzheimer's disease. There are no data to demonstrate that APOE mRNA is expressed in neurons. Whether apoE is made in neurons or enters the cytoplasm through

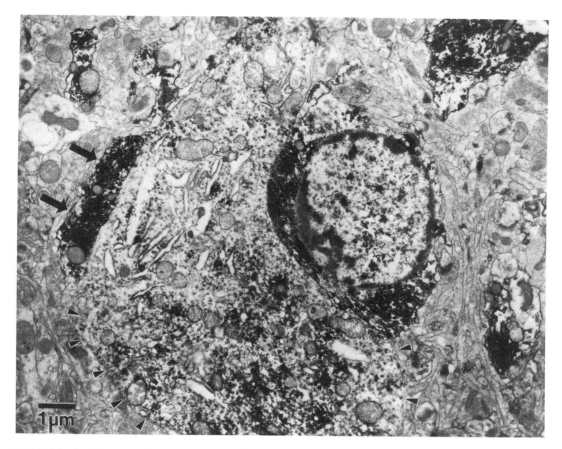

FIGURE 1 ApoE immunoelectron microscopic localization in neuronal cytoplasm. Electron microscopic analysis of immunoreacted vibratome section from a surgical specimen of lateral temporal lobe from a young (<30 years old) epilepsy patient. Fixation 2% paraformaldehyde/0.2% glutaraldehyde. Anti-apoE immunoreactivity is represented by peroxidase-positive, black staining. The densely immunoreactive cell in right center with relatively condensed nuclear chromatin is assumed to represent a satellite glial cell due to its close apposition to a large, less strongly immunoreactive region (arrowheads indicate border) filling much of the photograph. This region represents a proximal dendrite or perinuclear soma of a large cortical neuron given the size and shape of this process and the intensity of immunoreaction. ApoE immunoreactivity is present in the cytoplasm as well as small organelles including peroxisomes. On the left side of this lightly immunoreactive cell is a strongly immunoreactive process (arrows) which is also apposed to the presumed neuron. The overall appearance suggests the combined profile of satellite glial cells and a neuronal cell body. (From Han et al., 1994, with permission.)

undescribed biological mechanisms remains to be proven. Prior to the association of APOE with Alzheimer's disease, there was no scientific reason to carefully localize apoE in neurons. It is becoming clear that the known lipid transport functions of apoE are intimately related to the metabolism of apoE in neurons.[46,47] The mechanisms for apoE entry into neurons, whether through traditional endosomal pathways or by other modes, are currently being investigated in many laboratories. The low-density lipoprotein receptor-related (LRP) has been localized to neuronal cells.[48-53] There are already other known examples of peptides that enter cells by binding to specific regions of the LRP. Most of these studies have been performed in macrophages which also contain LRP.[54] Recently lactoferrin has been shown to cross the nuclear membrane without a canonical nuclear localization sequence, but with a binding region resembling the argenine-rich, receptor-binding sequence of apoE.[55] ApoE transfer within neurons may not be limited to the endosomal-lysosomal system proposed by its binding to LDL receptors in other cells.

Neuronal cells need to sustain themselves for 10 decades without dividing. There is ample precedent for entertaining the view that neurons have unique metabolic systems for maintainence and responses to stress. Neuron-specific metabolic pathways may also be anticipated from the large number of unique mRNAs known to be made in the brain.

The most striking data supporting a major role for apoE in brain comes from recent studies of APOE knock-out mice.[41,42] These mice are excellent models for studying atherosclerosis but little effort was made to study the brains of these animals. Masliah et al. have reported the age-related diminution of synapses in brains of homozygous APOE knock-out mice (Figure 2a, b, and e).[42] The differences are not present at birth, but become progressively more significant as the animals age over the 1st year. Earlier, by 4 to 8 months, vacuolization of dendrites with disruption of the endomembrane system and fragmentation of microtubular elements are observed using electron microscopic techniques (Figure 2c and d). Knocking out APOE, which codes for a protein that may function as a necessary cofactor protecting the microtubule-binding sites of molecules involved in stabilizing microtubules, produces extensive dendritic damage.[39] Thus, the *in vitro* molecular data leading to the hypothesis that apoE protects microtubule-associated proteins are supported by the anatomical location and initial electron microscopy in APOE knock-out mice.[41,42,45,56] Future studies of the APOE knock-out mouse will be of major interest, possibly providing an animal model for mechanisms of cell death and synaptic simplification involving mechanisms similar to the Alzheimer's diseases.

IV. PERSPECTIVE ON THE NEXT FEW YEARS

It is dangerous to speculate on the future of Alzheimer's disease research, especially with new surprising genetic mechanisms, such as trinucleotide repeats and genomic duplications, arising each year. There are, however, several obvious experiments to reconcile a common phenotype of diminished synapses, neuronal cell death, and loss of brain mass, with at least two genotypes: APP717 transgenic and APOE-deficient mice Figure 2. One set of experiments might lead to the design of a mouse model that has either normal or mutated human APP, human apoE isoforms, and human tau-replacing mouse genes. Perhaps such a model could recapitulate the expected phenotypic pathology of Alzheimer's disease with plaques, tangles, and apoE isoform-specific effects. Adding to the experimental foundation are the discovery of the PS1 and PS2 mutations.[11a,18a] Other late-onset Alzheimer's disease susceptibility genes are being actively sought. It is clear that hypotheses and experiments to explain the effects of relevant genetic variations on the pathogenesis of the Alzheimer's disease phenotype will also provide new insights into the basic metabolism of neurons and glia.

Perhaps, in the final analysis, the localization of apoE within the cytoplasm and peroxisomes of neurons will have a greater general impact than determining the isoform-specific metabolism leading to Alzheimer's disease.[45] Wide interest in potential mechanisms for the trafficking of ApoE will be cautious until the electron microscopy data are confirmed. With confirmation, the interaction of apoE with the LRP receptors on the neuronal surface will no doubt receive more experimental interest. The macrophage also expresses the LRP and provides an accessible model for studying apoE metabolism outside of the nervous system. Use of neuronal culture models, particularly primary neuronal tissue cultures derived from transgenic mouse models, will no doubt be useful in studying apoE metabolism. Finally, the role of apoE in lipid peroxidation and oxygen metabolism, associated with its peroxisomal localization, may provide important new insights into the relationships of other neurodegenerative disease.

The rapid confirmation of the genetic association of APOE alleles with the distribution of age of Alzheimer's disease expression have energized and diversified the field. Protagonists of either amyloid deposition theories or tau/NFT hypotheses are attempting to reconcile their theories with

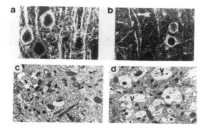

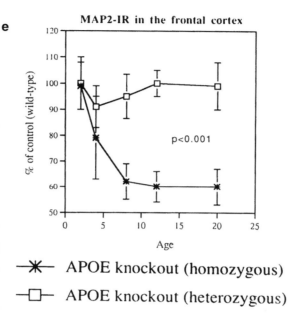

FIGURE 2   Comparison of APOE knock-out mice with controls. Neocortex of mice visualized with laser scanning confocal microscopy in sections immunolabeled with antibodies against MAP2. In control mice, MAP2-IR was associated with neuronal cell bodies and dendrites (a). In apoE deficient homozygous mice, the MAP2-IR dendritic processes displayed abundant vacuolization and distortion of their morphology (arrow, b) (790 ×). Electron microscopic characterization of dendritic alterations in apoE-deficient mice at 4 months of age. In wild-type mice, the dendritic and synaptic elements displayed normal organization (c), while in apoE deficient mice there was extensive vacuolization (V) and distortion of the dendrites (d). (5000 ×). Computer-aided quantitative analysis of the percent area occupied by MAP2-IR dendrites in the frontal cortex. Homozygous apoE deficient mice displayed a time-related decrease in dendritic MAP2-IR, decreasing to approximately 60% of wild-type by 12 months. Each group represents five to eight mice, with less mice in oldest groups due to death from early atherosclerotic complications.

a role for apoE. Others, with no prior experience in Alzheimer's disease research but great expertise in apoE and lipid metabolism or cell biology, are entering the field without prior biases of disease causation.[57] Starting with apoE isoform-specific differences, new mechanisms of neuronal biochemistry and physiology are being examined. The surprising localization of dendritic pathology in adult APOE knock-out mice provides support for pathogenic hypotheses involving proximal microtubule metabolism. We can expect great progress in the coming years in our understanding of brain mechanisms of homeostasis, response to stress, handling of nutrients such as glucose and oxygen, and mechanisms of neuronal degeneration. We can also expect drugs designed to correct apoE isoform-specific metabolic difficulties to be developed and tested in the APOE knock-out mouse models and patients with Alzheimer's disease.

ACKNOWLEDGMENTS

Supported by a National Institutes of Health Leadership and Excellence Award 5R35 AG-07922, National Institutes of Health Alzheimer's Disease Research Center 5P50 AG-05128, and numerous contributions to the Joseph and Kathleen Bryan Alzheimer's Disease Research Center. I wish to thank all my colleagues, collaborators, ADRC staff, and family members who provided me the opportunity and research experience to make a contribution and to provide a change in perspective.

REFERENCES

1. McKhann, G., Drachman, D., Folstein, M., Katzman, R., Price, D., and Stadlan, E. M., Clinical diagnosis of Alzheimer's disease: report of the NINCDS-ADRDA Work Group under the auspices of Department of Health and Human Services Task Force on Alzheimer's Disease, *Neurology,* 34(7), 939, 1984.
2. Khachaturian, Z. S., Diagnosis of Alzheimer's disease, *Arch. Neurol.,* 42, 1097, 1985.
3. Roses, A. D., The Alzheimer diseases, in *Current Neurology,* Appel, S. H., Ed., Mosby-Year Book, Chicago, 1994, 111.
4. Beckett, L. A. and Evans, D. A., Estimating prevalence and incidence of chronic conditions in the elderly: design and sampling issues, *Alzheimer Dis. Assoc. Disord.,* 1994.
5. Bennett, D. A. and Evans, D. A., Alzheimer's disease (review), *Dis. Mon.,* 38(1), 1, 1992.
6. Strittmatter, W. J., Saunders, A. M., Schmechel, D., Pericak, V. M., Enghild, J., Salvesen, G. S., et al., Apolipoprotein E: high-avidity binding to beta-amyloid and increased frequency of type 4 allele in late-onset familial Alzheimer disease, *Proc. Natl. Acad. Sci. U.S.A.,* 90(5), 1977, 1993.
7. Saunders, A.M. Strittmatter, W. J., Schmechel, D., St. George-Hyslop, P. H., P. V., M. A., Joo, S. H., et al., Association of apolipoprotein E allele epsilon 4 with late-onset familial and sporadic Alzheimer's disease, *Neurology,* 43(8), 1467, 1993.
8. Corder, E. H., Saunders, A. M., Strittmatter, W. J., Schmechel, D. E., Gaskell, P. C., Small, G. W., et al., Gene dose of apolipoprotein E type 4 allele and the risk of Alzheimer's disease in late onset families, *Science,* 261(5123), 921, 1993.
9. Corder, E. H., Saunders, A. M., Risch, N. J., Strittmatter, W. J., Schmechel, D. E., Gaskell, P. J., et al., Protective effect of apolipoprotein E type 2 allele for late onset Alzheimer disease, *Nat. Genet.,* 7(2), 180, 1994.
10. Schellenberg, G. D., Bird, T. D., Wijsman, E. M., Orr, H. T., Anderson, L., Nemens, E., et al., Genetic linkage evidence for a familial Alzheimer's disease locus on chromosome 14, *Science,* 258(5082), 668, 1992.
11. St. George-Hyslop, P., Haines, J., Rogaev, E., et al., Genetic evidence for a novel familial Alzheimer's disease locus on chromosome 14, *Nat. Genet.,* 2, 330, 1992.
11a. Sherrington, R., Rogaev, E. I., Liang, Y., Rogaeya, E. A., Levesque, G., Ikeda, M., et al., Cloning of a gene bearing missense mutations in early-onset familial Alzheimer's disease, *Nature (London),* 375, 754, 1995.
12. Goate, A., Chartier, H.M., Mullan, M., Brown, J., Crawford, F., Fidani, L., et al., Segregation of a missense mutation in the amyloid precursor protein gene with familial Alzheimer's disease (see comments), *Nature,* 349(6311), 704, 1991.
13. Murrell, J., Farlow, M., Ghetti, B., and Benson, M. D., A mutation in the amyloid precursor protein associated with hereditary Alzheimer's disease, *Science,* 254(5028), 97, 1991.
14. Chartier, H. M., Crawford, F., Houlden, H., Warren, A., Hughes, D., Fidani, L., et al., Early-onset Alzheimer's disease caused by mutations at codon 717 of the beta-amyloid precursor protein gene, *Nature,* 353(6347), 844, 1991.
15. Hendriks. L., Van, D. C., Cras, P., Cruts, M., Van, H. W., Van, H. F., et al., Presenile dementia and cerebral haemorrhage linked to a mutation at codon 692 of the beta-amyloid precursor protein gene, *Nat. Genet.,* 1(3), 218, 1992.
16. St. George-Hyslop, P., McLachlan, D. C., Tsuda, T., Rogaev, E., Karlinsky, H., Lippa, C. F., et al., Alzheimer's disease and possible gene interaction (letter) (Published erratum appears in *Science,* 263(5149), 904, 1994), *Science,* 263(5146), 1994.
17. Alzheimer's Disease Collaborative Group, Apolipoprotein E genotype and Alzheimer's disease (letter), *Lancet,* 342(8873), p. 737, 1993.
18. Bird, T. D., Lampe, T. H., Nemens, E. J., Miner, G. W., Sumi, S. M., and Schellenberg, G. D., Familial Alzheimer's disease in American descendants of the Volga Germans: probable genetic founder effect, *Ann. Neurol.,* 23(1), 25, 1988.
18a. Levy-Lehad, E., Wasco, W., Poorkaj, P., Romano, D. M., Oshima, J., Pettingell, W. H., et al., Candidate gene for the chromosome 1 familial Alzheimer's disease locus, *Science,* 269, 973, 1995.
19. van Duijn, C. M., de Knijff, P., Cruts, M., Wehnert, A., Havekes, L. M., Hofman, A., et al., Apolipoprotein E4 allele in a population-based study of early-onset Alzheimer's disease, *Nat. Genet.* 7, 74, 1994.
20. Okuizumi, K., Onodera, O., Tanaka, H., Kobayashi, H., Tsuji, S., Takahashi, H., et al., ApoE-epsilon 4 and early-onset Alzheimer's (letter), *Nat. Genet.,* 7(1), 10, 1994.

21. Braak, H. and Braak, E., The human entorhinal cortex: normal morphology and lamina-specific pathology in various diseases, *Neurosci. Res.*, 15, 6, 1992.

22. Beyreuther, K. and Masters, C. L., Amyloid precursor protein and βA4 amyloid in the etiology of Alzheimer's disease: precursor-product relationships in the derangement of neuronal function, *Brain Pathol.*, 1, 241, 1991.

23. Mirra, S. S., Heyman, A., McKeel, D., Sumi, S. M., Crain, B. J., Brownlee, L. M., et al., The Consortium to Establish a Registry for Alzheimer's Disease (CERAD). II. Standardization of the neuropathologic assessment of Alzheimer's disease, *Neurology*, 41(4), 479, 1991.

24. Terry, R. D., Neuropathological changes in Alzheimer disease (review), *Prog. Brain Res.*, 101(383), 383, 1994.

25. Roses, A. D., Apolipoprotein E affects the rate of Alzheimer disease espression: beta-amyloid burden is a secondary consequence dependent on APOE genotype and duration of disease, *J. Neuropathol. Exp. Neurol.*, 53(5), 429, 1994.

25a. Polvikoski, T., Sulkava, R., Haltia, M., Kainulainen, K., Vuorio, A., Verkkoneimi, A., et al., Apolipoprotein, dementia, and cortical deposition of beta-amyloid protein, *N. Eng. J. Med.*, 333(19), 1242, 1995.

26. Hardy, J., and Allsop, D., Amyloid deposition as the central event in the aetiology of Alzheimer's disease (review), *Trends Pharmacol. Sci.*, 12(10), 383, 1991.

27. Beyreuther, K., Pollwein, P., Multhaup, G., Monning, U., Konig, G., Dyrks, T., et al., Regulation and expression of the Alzheimer's beta/A4 amyloid protein precursor in health, disease, and Down's syndrome, (review), *Ann. N.Y. Acad. Sci.*, 695(91), 91, 1993.

28. Selkoe, D. J., Alzheimer's disease: a central role for amyloid, (review), *J. Neuropathol. Exp. Neurol.*, 53(5), 438, 1994.

29. Arnold, S. E., Hyman, B. T., Flory, J., Damasio, A. R., and Van, H. G., The topographical and neuroanatomical distribution of neurofibrillary tangles and neuritic plaques in the cerebral cortex of patients with Alzheimer's disease, *Cereb Cortex*, 1(1), 103, 1991.

30. Goedert, M., Wischik, C. M., Crowther, R. A., Walker, J. E., and Klug, A., Cloning and sequencing of the cDNA encoding a core protein of the paired helical filament of Alzheimer disease: identification as the microtubule-associated protein tau, *Proc. Natl. Acad. Sci. U.S.A.*, 85(11), 4051, 1988.

31. Lee, V. M., Balin, B. J., Otvos, L. J., and Trojanowski, J. Q., A68: a major subunit of paired helical filaments and derivatized forms of normal tau, *Science*, 251(4994), 675, 1991.

32. Goedert, M., Spillantini, M. G., Cairns, N. J., and Crowther, R. A., Tau proteins of Alzheimer paired helical filaments: abnormal phosphorylation of all six brain isoforms, *Neuron*, 8(1), 159, 1992.

33. Schmechel, D. E., Saunders, A. M., Strittmatter, W. J., Crain, B. J., Hulette, C. M., Joo, S. H., et al., Increased amyloid beta-peptide deposition in cerebral cortex as a consequence of apolipoprotein E genotype in late-onset Alzheimer disease, *Proc. Natl. Acad. Sci. U.S.A.*, 90(20), 9649, 1993.

34. Strittmatter, W. J., Weisgraber, K. H., Huang, D. Y., Dong, L. M., Salvesen, G. S., Pericak, V. M., et al., Binding of human apolipoprotein E to synthetic amyloid beta peptide: isoform-specific effects and implications for late-onset Alzheimer disease, *Proc. Natl. Acad. Sci. U.S.A.*, 90(17), 8098, 1993.

35. Wisniewski, T., Castano, E. M., Golabek, A., Vogel, T., and Frangione, B., Acceleration of Alzheimer's fibril formation by apolipoprotein E in vitro, *Am. J. Pathol.*, 145(5) 1030, 1994.

36. Sanan, D. A., Weisgraber, K. H., Russell, S. J., Mahley, R. W., Huang, D., and Saunders, A., et al., Apolipoprotein E associates with beta amyloid peptide of Alzheimer's disease to form novel monofibrils. Isoform apoE4 associates more efficiently than apoE3, *J. Clin. Invest.*, 94(2), 860, 1994.

37. Ma, J., Yee, A., Brewer, H. J., Das, S., and Potter, H., Amyloid-associated proteins alpha 1-antichymotrypsin and apolipoprotein E promote assembly of Alzheimer beta-protein into filaments (see comments), *Nature*, 372(6501), 92, 1994.

38. Selkoe, D. J., Alzheimer's disease. In the beginning… (news; comment), *Nature*, 354(6353), 432, 1991.

39. Strittmatter, W. J., Weisgraber, K. H., Goedert, M., Saunders, A. M., Huang, D., Corder, E. H., et al., Hypothesis: microtubule instability and paired helical filament formation in the Alzheimer's disease brain are related to apolipoprotein E genotype, (review), *Exp. Neurol.*, 125(2), 163, 1994.

40. Games, D., Adams, D., Alessandrini, R., Barbour, R., Carr, T., Clemens, J., et al., Alzheimer-type neuropathology in transgenic mice overexpressing V717F β-amyloid precursor protein, *Nature*, 373, 523, 1995.

41. Roses, A.D., Einstein, E., Gilbert, J., Goedert, M., Han, S.-H., Huang, D., et al., Morphological, biochemical, and genetic support for an apolipoprotein E effect on microtubular metabolism, *Ann. N.Y. Acad. Sci.*, in press.

42. Masliah, E., Mallory, M., Ge, N., Alford, M., Veinbergs, I., and Roses, A. D., Neurodegeneration in the central nervous system of apoE-deficient mice, *Exp. Neurol.*, 136(2), 107, 1995.

43. Namba, Y., Tomonaga, M., Kawasaki, H., Otomo, E., and Ikeda, K., Apolipoprotein E immunoreactivity in cerebral amyloid deposits and neurofibrillary tangles in Alzheimer's disease and kuru plaque amyloid in Creutzfeldt-Jakob disease, *Brain Res*, 541(1), 163, 1991.

44. Han, S. H., Hulette, C., Saunders, A. M., Einstein, G., Pericak, V. M., Strittmatter, W. J., et al., Apolipoprotein E is present in hippocampal neurons without neurofibrillary tangles in Alzheimer's disease and in age-matched controls, *Exp. Neurol.*, 128(1), 13, 1994.

45. Han, S. H., Einstein, G., Weisgraber, K. H., Strittmatter, W. J., Saunders, A. M., Pericak, V. M., et al., Apolipoprotein E is localized to the cytoplasm of human cortical neurons: a light and electron microscopic study, *J. Neuropathol. Exp. Neurol.*, 53(5), 535, 1994.

46. Weisgraber, K. H., Apolipoprotein E: structure-function relationships, (Review), *Adv. Protein Chem.*, 45(249), 249, 1994.

47. Weisgraber, K. H., Roses, A. D., and Strittmatter, W. J., The role of apolipoprotein E in the nervous system (review), *Curr. Opin. Lipidol.*, 5(2), 110, 1994.

48. Bu, G., Maksymovitch, E.A., Geuze, H., and Schwartz, A.L., Subcellular localization and endocytic function of low density lipoprotein receptor-related protein in human glioblastoma cells, *J. Biol. Chem.*, 269(47), 29874, 1994.

49. Bu, G., Maksymovitch, E. A., Nerbonne, J. M., and Schwartz, A. L., Expression and function of the low density lipoprotein receptor-related protein (LRP) in mammalian central neurons, *J. Biol. Chem.*, 269(28), 18521, 1994.

50. Lopes, M. B., Bogaev, C. A., Gonias, S. L., and VandenBerg, S. R., Expression of alpha 2-macroglobulin receptor/low density lipoprotein receptor-related protein is increased in reactive and neoplastic glial cells, *FEBS Lett.*, 338(3), 301, 1994.

51. Rebeck, G. W., Reiter, J. S., Strickland, D. K., and Hyman, B. T., Apolipoprotein E in sporadic Alzheimer's disease: allelic variation and receptor interactions, *Neuron*, 11(4), 575, 1993.

52. Wolf, B. B., Lopes, M. B., VandenBerg, S. R., and Gonias, S.L., Characterization and immunohistochemical localization of alpha 2-macroglobulin receptor (low-density lipoprotein receptor-related protein) in human brain, *Am. J. Pathol.,*, 141(1), 37, 1992.

53. Moestrup, S. K., Gliemann, J., and Pallesen, G., Distribution of the alpha 2-macroglobulin receptor/low density lipoprotein receptor-related protein in human tissues, *Cell. Tissue Res.*, 269(3), 375, 1992.

54. Krieger, M. and Herz, J., Structures and functions of multiligand lipoprotein receptors: macrophage scavenger receptors and LDL receptor-related protein (LRP) (Review), *Annu. Rev. Biochem.*, 63(601), 601, 1994.

55. He, J. and Furmanski, P., Sequence specificity and transcriptional activation in the binding of lactoferrin to DNA, *Nature*, 373, 721, 1995.

56. Strittmatter, W. J., Saunders, A. M., Goedert, M., Weisgraber, K. H., Dong, L.-M., Jakes, R., et al., Isoform-specific interactions of apolipoprotein E with microtubule-associated protein tau: implications for Alzheimer disease, *Proc. Natl. Acad. Sci. U.S.A.*, 91, 11183, 1994.

57. Nathan, B. P., Bellosta, S., Sanan, D. A., Weisgraber, K. H., Mahley, R. W., and Pitas, R. E., Differential effects of apolipoproteins E3 and E4 on neuronal growth *in vitro, Science*, 264(5160), 850, 1994.

Chapter 17

NEUROIMMUNE MECHANISMS IN THE PATHOGENESIS OF ALZHEIMER'S DISEASE

Patrick L. McGeer
Edith G. McGeer

CONTENTS

I. INTRODUCTION

It has often been suggested that the brain is immunologically privileged. The existence of the blood-brain barrier, the absence of conventional lymphatic drainage, and the unusual tolerance of the brain to transplanted tissue have reinforced the idea that brain is somehow isolated from immunological processes. However, recent evidence derived from the modern techniques of immunohistochemistry and molecular biology indicates that the brain is neither immunologically privileged nor immunologically isolated. In fact, it appears to be immunologically vulnerable, due to the fragility of neurons and their complex interconnections. The immune system is intended to be injurious to invading organisms. Any response to an immunological challenge places host tissue at risk. Neurons are postmitotic cells, with no ability to divide, and little ability to recover from injury. Therefore, processes that would have little effect on many organs of the body could have serious consequences for brain.

This chapter describes briefly evidence that there is a prominent immune response in Alzheimer's disease. Particular attention is paid to the autodestructive forces that are inherent to such a response and the potential harm they can cause. The possibility of ameliorating such damage through the use of antiinflammatory drugs is discussed. Detailed references to much of the original literature may be found in recent reviews.[1,2] Although the emphasis here is on Alzheimer's disease, there is some evidence that similar immune responses may play a role in a number of other chronic neurodegenerative disorders.[3]

At the outset it is necessary for us to define what is meant by an endogenous immune response of brain, as opposed to a general immune response where blood-borne elements reinforce a local reaction. Any immune response commences with inflammation, but this term also needs some definition. Celsus, in the first century A.D., described what were long believed to be the fundamental characteristics of inflammation: calor (heat), rubor (redness), tumor (swelling), and dolor (pain). Cohnheim in 1877 recognized that these signs were related to vascular changes which increased the blood supply and permitted exudation of serum and leukocytes into tissue. However, it was the great Metchnikoff, in his classic *Comparative Pathology of Inflammation,* published in 1892, who revealed that this was not the core process. He showed that the true reaction was one associated with wandering mesodermal cells acting against specific irritants. Metchnikoff named these mesodermal cells phagocytes. In brain, these cells are the microglia.

In this review, we use the descriptive term "inflammation" as appropriate for the core process perceived by Metchnikoff, i.e., a strictly local reaction to an injurious agent. A more precise term would be intrinsic inflammation to distinguish such an endogenous process from one that is reinforced from the blood stream. A reinforcing process must be carefully controlled for the brain, making it a special, although not a privileged, organ. The brain lies within a tight-fitting bony box, the skull. It relies on the blood-brain barrier to protect it from the lethal consequences of typical inflammatory swelling. Moreover, dolor (pain) is absent since brain tissue lacks pain fibers, and calor (temperature) cannot be externally measured. Thus, the process of inflammation of brain should appropriately be defined by the primary reactions of brain cells themselves and not by the secondary reactions that are commonly considered to define it for the periphery.

II. THE MICROGLIAL CELL

A. ROLE IN IMMUNE REACTIONS

The pivotal cell in local immune reactions is the tissue macrophage which, in the case of brain, is the microglial cell. Microglial cells can be activated by a myriad of processes. The precise signaling agents have yet to be identified. Presumably inflammatory cytokines are prominently involved. Upon activation, the microglial cell changes its morphology, with its cytoplasm enlarging, and its ramified processes retracting and thickening. It begins to express high levels of a variety

TABLE 1   Some Microglial Receptors and Their Immune System Ligands

Microglial Receptors[a]	Immune System Ligands
MHC class II glycoproteins	T8 receptors
MHC class I glycoproteins	T4 receptors
Leukocyte common antigen	Protein tyrosine phosphatase activators
LFA-1 (CD11a)[b]	ICAM-1, ICAM-II
Complement receptor 3 (CD11b)[b]	C3bi, C4b?
Complement receptor 4 (CD11c)[b]	C3bi, C4b?
Vitronectin receptor	Vitronectin
Fc-γ receptors (FcγRI and FcγRII)	Immunoglobulins
Thrombin receptor	Thrombin
CSF-1 receptor	Colony stimulating factor (CSF)

[a]   All are upregulated when microglia become activated.
[b]   Integrins.

TABLE 2   Some Inflammatory Cytokines Produced by Microglia, Astrocytes, and T Cells

Microglia	Astrocytes	T Cells
IL-1α	IL-1α	IL-2
IL-1β	IL-1β	γ-INF
IL-3	IL-3	TNF-β
IL-6	IL-6	
CSF-1	CSF-1	
TNF-α	TNF-α	

of surface receptors which have as their ligands immune system proteins. Table 1 lists some of these receptor-ligand inflammatory pairs. Many more will undoubtedly be discovered in the future. They illustrate the commonality of genotype between microglial cells and monocytes, in addition to the types of surface reactions these cells undergo.

Table 2 lists the inflammatory cytokines so far found to be produced by glial cells in culture. It is interesting that the profile is identical between astrocytes and microglia, indicating that astrocytes can play a significant role in stimulating an immune response. Included in the table are some inflammatory cytokines produced by T cells that are not produced by glial cells. Interleukin-2, γ-interferon, and TNF-β are powerful inflammatory stimulants, so that the small number of T cells seen in the vicinity of a lesion (Figure 1A) may be contributing significantly to an immune response even if they are not cloned to recognize a particular peptide.

B. APPEARANCE OF MICROGLIA IN THE HUMAN BRAIN

Microglia are estimated to make up about 10% of all brain glia. They can be easily detected immunohistochemically by staining for leukocyte common antigen (LCA) or for the FcγRI receptor (Figure 1B). LCA is a surface glycoprotein expressed by all cells of leukocyte origin, while the FcγRI receptor, which recognizes the Fc chain of immunoglobulins when there is a conformational change due to antigen binding, is expressed at high levels only by cells of the monocytic lines. Such staining is enhanced in activated microglia (Figure 1C).

Reactive microglia show altered morphology and an upregulation of many proteins (Table 1). Immunohistochemical staining for the MHC glycoprotein, HLA-DR, is a particularly sensitive method of detecting reactive microglia. Staining for HLA-DR of a section of normal tissue adjacent to that in Figure 1A is illustrated in Figure 1D. Only one cell in this field of many microglial cells

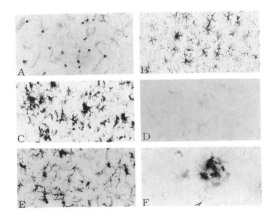

FIGURE 1 (A) Staining of Alzheimer's precentral gyrus for collagen (light brown staining of capillaries) and CD8, a marker of T8 cells (dark, purple on original slide). T8 and T4 cells accumulate in capillaries in lesioned areas and some penetrate into the tissue matrix. (B and C) Staining of brain microglia for the immunoglobulin receptor (FcγRI) in the temporal cortex from a neurologically normal aged control (B) and an Alzheimer case (C). (D) Staining for HLA-DR in a control section adjacent to that shown in (B); all microglia stain for FCγRI (1B) but only an occasional one stains for HLA-DR in controls. (E) Staining for HLA-DR in a section of temporal cortex from an Alzheimer's case. (F) Dark staining (purple on slide) of aggregates of HLA-DR positive microglia on senile plaque stained by an antibody to BAP (light staining, brown on original slide).

is positively stained for HLA-DR. This particular section was taken from a normal aged adult, and the appearance of HLA-DR-positive cells might be even less in a young adult.

Staining of white matter for HLA-DR is generally more intense in Alzheimer's disease and other neurologically diseased brains than in age-matched control brains. It is in gray matter, however, that the greatest contrast is noted. A profusion of microglia displaying the enlarged cytoplasm and shorter, thickened processes characteristic of the reactive form is seen in senile plaque areas. Such microglia are intensely positive for HLA-DR (Figure 1E), as well as for many other proteins characteristic of the reactive state (Table 1). The HLA-DR-positive cells on senile plaques tend to aggregate in a cap surrounding a central core known as the amyloid star (Figure 1F). Those in contact with the star contain amyloid fibrils which appear to be streaming between the cell and the star. Whether the amyloid fibers are moving in or out of the microglia is unclear. It is possible that the fibrils are formed within the microglia and extruded into the star early in senile plaque formation when the microglial load is high. They may subsequently be ingested from the star into the microglia when the phagocytic load is low.

Reactive microglia cluster around end stage debris and presumably phagocytose it over time. This debris consists of the amyloid star, which persists after the plaques have been denuded of dystrophic neurites. They also cluster around ghost tangles, which remain after tangled neurons have degenerated.

III. THE COMPLEMENT SYSTEM

The complement system is one of the most powerful ways of amplifying an immune response. It is often thought of as a system generated from serum in response to an antigen-antibody reaction. However, complement proteins can be produced by tissue cells, and the system can be activated by many factors other than an antibody reacting with an antigen.

There are two separate pathways, the classical and the alternative, but only proteins of the classical pathway (Figure 2) have been detected in Alzheimer's disease brain. For more details on the complement system, short[4] or more comprehensive[5] reviews are available.

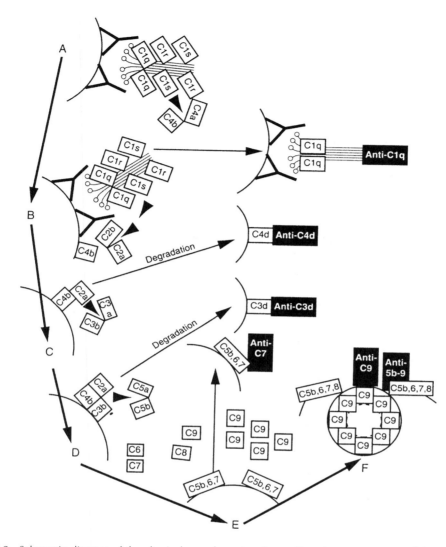

FIGURE 2 Schematic diagram of the classical complement pathway. Complement proteins and their fragments are shown as open rectangles or circles containing the appropriate designation. The antibodies used are indicated by the filled rectangles (see text for details).

A. THE CLASSICAL COMPLEMENT PATHWAY

When activated, this pathway generates a cascade of potent protein fragments, some of which attach chemically to target tissues, some of which are anaphylotoxins which stimulate further response, and some generate the membrane attack complex (MAC) to lyse cells. The intention is to destroy bacteria and viruses, but bystander lysis of host cells can occur.

The classical pathway is activated when C1q binds to a target (Figure 2). This releases the serine protease C1r which acts on C1s, which then cleaves C2 and C4 into a and b fragments. C2a and C4b combine, exposing a thiol ester bond on C4b. The thiol ester reacts with a free amino or hydroxyl group on tissue near the C1q binding site to form an ester or amide bond. This chemical attachment of complement proteins to tissue marked for phagocytosis secures identification of the site and amplifies the signal. The opsonization sequence is completed when the chemically bound C4b2a complex cleaves C3 into a and b fragments, with C3b also chemically attaching to tissue by the same mechanism as C4b and complexing with C4b2a. C4b and C3b gradually degrade, leaving as residues C4d and C3d, still chemically bound to tissue.

The complement cascade terminates by assembly of the MAC. The C4b2a3b trimolecular complex formed on an opsonized surface is a C5 protease. C5a, in common with the less powerful C3a, acts as an anaphylatoxin, stimulating enhanced immune cell activity, including stimulation of the respiratory burst apparatus of microglia. C5b combines with C6, followed by the addition of C7. The C5b67 complex is highly lipophilic and attaches to available cell membranes. Once attached, it attracts C8 molecules to form parallel C5b678 arrays. The parallel arrays can now add multiple molecules of C9, which disrupt the integrity of the membrane. This causes cell lysis.

B. STAINING OF HUMAN BRAIN FOR COMPLEMENT PROTEINS

Alzheimer lesions are richly decorated with complement. C1q, C3d, and C4d have all been found to colocalize with β-amyloid peptide (BAP), whether in the benign form of diffuse deposits or in the consolidated form found in senile plaques. Thus, complement opsonization of extracellular BAP must occur as the extracellular BAP is deposited but, since this occurs also in diffuse deposits which are devoid of neuronal damage, the opsonizing process cannot by itself be neurotoxic. It is probably beneficial by assisting in the removal of early BAP deposits. The staining of plaques and ghost tangles of Alzheimer's disease by antibodies to C3d and C4d (Figure 3A) is very sensitive and, since there is also almost no staining of control tissue (Figure 3B), it is an excellent method of revealing classical pathology.

The staining for the MAC is negative in control tissue and more limited in Alzheimer's disease brain than is the staining for C3d or C4d. There is, however, heavy labeling of dystrophic neurites in senile plaques, neuropil threads in the surrounding area, as well as some tangled neurons, indicating the possibility of bystander lysis (Figure 3C). Thus, in these areas, autodestruction of neurons or their processes may be taking place.

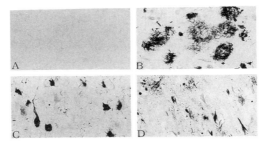

FIGURE 3   Complement staining of human brain tissue. (A and B) Staining for C4d in the entorhinal cortex of a case of Alzheimer's disease (A) and an aged control (B). Amyloid deposits and neurofibrillary tangles are intensely stained. (C) Staining for C5b-9 (the MAC) in Alzheimer's disease hippocampus. Strongly positive dendritic neurons and intracellular tangles can be seen; amyloid deposits are not stained. (D) Staining for protectin (MIRL) in Alzheimer's disease hippocampus. Staining is found on tangled neurons.

C. HOW IS THE COMPLEMENT CASCADE ACTIVATED IN ALZHEIMER'S DISEASE BRAIN?

It is not known what molecule or molecules activate the complement pathway in Alzheimer's disease, but it is clearly of fundamental importance to acquire that information. Although specific immunoglobulin antibodies are the best known activators of complement, their presence in BAP deposits has not been confirmed. Nevertheless, there have been several reports of autoantibody production in Alzheimer's disease, so immunoglobulins may be one source of complement activation.

Other more likely candidates are those known to occur in senile plaques which are also capable of activating the complement cascade in vitro. Among these are BAP, amyloid P, C-1 reactive protein, and the Hageman factor.[6] The most obvious molecule is BAP. It strongly binds to C1q *in vitro* and powerfully activates the classical complement pathway.[7] It is possible that multiple molecules, but particularly BAP, are functioning as complement activators. BAP has also been shown to be capable of stimulating the respiratory burst of macrophages[8] so that is may contribute in more than one fashion to the activation of the immune system.

D. COMPLEMENT INHIBITORS

Inhibitors exist for almost every step in the complement cascade. Thus, the system is normally kept under firm control. To date, only a few of the known complement inhibitors have been studied in Alzheimer's disease, but the results are interesting. C1 inhibitor has been shown to be present in brain and to be upregulated in Alzheimer's disease.[9] Inhibitors of the membrane attack complex are, however, of greater relevance since they presumably exist to protect against bystander lysis. Clusterin and vitronectin are secreted molecules which bind to C5b-9 as it forms and convert it from a lipophilic to a lipophobic macromolecule. Protectin (also called CD 59, the membrane inhibitor of reactive lysis or MIRL) is a third. It seems to be bound loosely to and to patrol the external surface of the host cell to be protected, intercepting the membrane attack complex as it approaches the cell. All of these inhibitors are upregulated in the AD brain and have localizations rather similar to those of the MAC (Figure 3D). Although these inhibitors may also act in the AD brain in ways other than as a defense mechanism against the MAC,[10] the most obvious interpretation is that they are being called upon in an attempt to limit the extent of bystander lysis.

E. SOURCES OF COMPLEMENT PROTEINS AND THEIR RECEPTORS

The most probable source of complement proteins is endogenous brain cells since the mRNAs for C1, C3, and C4 have been identified from bulk RNA extracts of brain tissue, with levels being raised severalfold above normal in Alzheimer disease. Serum is a possibility, but this would require permeability of the blood brain barrier, in which case a wide spectrum of serum proteins should appear in Alzheimer disease tissue. Such a spectrum has not been observed. Thus, the evidence is that brain generates its own complement proteins, possibly on a continuous basis at a very low level. Under pathological circumstances, such as in Alzheimer's disease, this production is upregulated. There is evidence that microglial cells, astrocytes, and neuroblastoma cells can produce various complement proteins in culture, suggesting a variety of sources *in vivo* (Table 3).

TABLE 3   Generation of Complement messenger RNAs by Various Cell Lines in Culture

Cell Type (line)	Complement Proteins
Astrocytoma (U373MG)	C3,C4,C9
Neuroblastoma	
(IMR32)	C4
(SK-SH)	C3,C4
(SK-MC)	C3,C4,C9
Microglia	C1q,C3

The cells which make receptors for complement have been more clearly defined. They are the microglia, which constitutively express all beta-2 integrins (Table 1). The β-2 integrin family includes complement receptors 3 and 4. These β-2 integrins are sharply upregulated when microglia become activated, as is the case with AD lesions. Thus, it appears possible that microglia send out their own identifiers in the form of opsonizing complement proteins, and, when those fragments that are receptor ligands become fixed to tissue, the microglia utilize their complement receptors to lock onto their phagocytic targets.

IV. IMPLICATIONS FOR THERAPY

The accumulating evidence of a chronic endogenous inflammatory reaction in the AD brain, and particularly the abundance of the MAC, has led to the hypothesis that immune system attack is responsible for much of the neuronal destruction in Alzheimer's disease. Based on this hypothesis, it has been suggested that chronic treatment with antiinflammatory agents might slow the progress of Alzheimer's disease or retard its onset.[11]

One group that routinely takes such antiinflammatory drugs, often of the nonsteroidal type (NSAIDs), are arthritics, and studies of the incidence of dementia in elderly persons with arthritis have generally shown a much lower prevalence than found in the age-matched general population (Figure 4). Another group that chronically take drugs of a different type, also having antiinflammatory actions, are sufferers from leprosy. Dapsone is the classic antileprosy drug. It has antiinflammatory properties and also appears to inhibit the deposition of amyloid, even in the brain. A study of the incidence of dementia in all Japanese leprosy cases over the age of 65 indicated that those remaining on dapsone, or its close relative promin, had a significantly lower incidence of dementia than those who had been taken off treatment for at least 5 years.[12] Support for the hypothesis has come from the work of Breitner et al.[13] who studied elderly twins discordant for dementia. The only factor they found of significance in analyzing the environmental and medical histories of these twins was that the chronic use of antiinflammatory agents appeared to have a sparing effect.

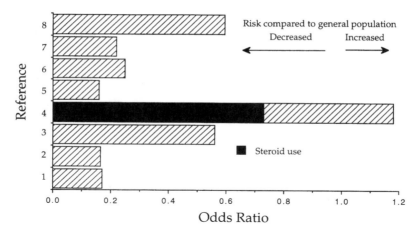

FIGURE 4 Published epidemiological studies on the frequency of clinically diagnosed Alzheimer's disease in persons with arthritis (columns 2 to 5 and 7) or those taking antiinflammatory drugs (6 and 8) divided by the frequency in age-matched control groups. Column 1 shows the frequency of arthritis in an Alzheimer's disease population divided by that in controls. A frequency of Alzheimer's disease of 2.5% in the general population over the age of 65 is assumed for the calculation of the odds ratio for column 2. (The data are taken from [column 1] Jenkinson et al., *Br. J. Rheumatol.*, 28, 86, 1989; [column 2] McGeer et al., *Lancet*, 335, 1037, 1990; [column 3] Broe et al., *Neurology*, 40, 1698, 1990; [column 4] Graves et al., *Ann. Neurol.*, 28, 766, 1990; [column 5] Li et al., *Neurology*, 42, 1481, 1992; [column 6] Breitner et al., *Neurology*, 44, 227, 1994; [column 7] Myllykangas-Luosujarvi and Isomaki, *Br. J. Rheumatol.*, 33, 501, 1994; [column 8] Beard et al., *Neurobiol. Aging*, 15, 545, 1994.)

Proof of the hypothesis must, however, await large-scale clinical trials. A pilot study has been done using indomethacin, an NSAID that crosses the blood/brain barrier.[14] In this small, but double-blind and placebo-controlled trial, the patients on 100 to 150 mg/day of indomethacin held their own over the 6-month period on a battery of cognitive tests, while the placebo-treated group showed the expected significant decline. Searches for new types of drugs capable of selective modulation of brain immune responses may lead to important new therapies for Alzheimer's disease and possibly other neurodegenerative diseases.

ACKNOWLEDGMENTS

This research was supported by grants from the Alzheimer Society of British Columbia and the Jack Brown and Family Alzheimer Disease Research Fund, as well as donations from individual British Columbians.

REFERENCES

1. McGeer, P. L., Rogers, J., and McGeer, E. G., Neuroimmune mechanisms in Alzheimer disease pathogenesis, *Alz. Dis. Assocd. Disord.,* 8, 149, 1994.
2. Aisen, P. S. and Davis, K. L., Inflammatory mechanisms in Alzheimer's disease: implications for therapy, *Am. J. Psychiatry,* 151, 1105, 1994.
3. McGeer, E. G. and McGeer, P. L., Neurodegeneration and the immune system, in *Neurodegenerative Disorders,* Calne, D. B., Ed., W.B. Saunders & Co., Philadelphia, 1994, chap. 18.
4. Cooper, N. R., The complement system, in *Basic and Clinical Immunology,* Sites, D. P., Stobo, J. D., and Wells, J. V., Eds., Appleton & Lange, Norwalk, CT, 1987, chap. 10.
5. Rother, K. and Till, G. O., Eds., *The Complement System,* Springer-Verlag, Berlin, Heidelberg, 1988.
6. Yasuhara, O., Walker, D. G., and McGeer, P. L., Hageman factor and its binding sites are present in senile plaques of Alzheimer's disease, *Brain Res.,* 654, 234, 1994.
7. Schultz, J., Schaller, J., McKinley, M., Bradt, B., Cooper, N., May, P., and Rogers, J., Enhanced cytotoxicity of amyloid β-peptide by a complement dependent mechanism, *Neurosci. Lett.,* 175, 99, 1994.
8. Klegeris, A., Walker, D. G., and McGeer, P. L., Activation of macrophages by Alzheimer β-amyloid peptide, *Biochem. Biophys. Res. Commun.,* 199, 984, 1994.
9. Walker, D. G. and McGeer, P. L., unpublished data, 1994.
10. Zhan, S.-S., Veerhuis, R., Janssen, I., Kamphorst, W., and Eikelenboom, P., Immunohistochemical distribution of the inhibitors of the terminal complement complex in Alzheimer's disease, *Neurodegeneration,* 3, 111, 1994.
11. McGeer, P. L. and Rogers, J., Anti-inflammatory agents as a therapeutic approach to Alzheimer's disease, *Neurology,* 42, 447, 1992.
12. McGeer, P. L., Harada, N., Kimura, H., McGeer, E. G., and Schulzer, M., Prevalence of dementia amongst elderly Japanese with leprosy: apparent effect of chronic drug therapy, *Dementia,* 3, 146, 1992.
13. Breitner, J. C. S., Gau, B. A., Welsh, K. A., Plassman, B. L., McDonald, W. M., Helms, M. J., and Anthony, J. C., Inverse association of anti-inflammatory treatments and Alzheimer's disease: initial results of a co-twin control study, *Neurology,* 44, 227, 1994.
14. Rogers, J., Kirby, L. C., Hempelman, S. R., Berry, D. L., McGeer, P. L., Kaszniak, A. W., Zalinski, J., Cofield, M., Mansukhani, L., Willson, P., and Kogan, F., Clinical trial of indomethacin in Alzheimer's disease, *Neurology,* 43, 1609, 1993.

Chapter 18

CAUSES OF ALZHEIMER'S DISEASE

———————————————————————————— Anne B. Young

CONTENTS

I. EXOGENOUS AND ENDOGENOUS TOXINS

A. GENERAL CONCEPTS

Neurons are postmitotic and do not divide once the brain has reached maturity. Although neurons do have substantial ability to form new processes and terminals in response to growth factors, synaptic activity, and injury, they cannot replace themselves in the same manner as do skin, liver, and intestinal cells. Toxic substances, therefore, affect neurons quite differently from the way they affect other cells in the body. Toxins can be either immediately lethal, thereby causing irrevocable damage, or they can cause sublethal changes within the neuron that lead to more sustained dysfunction.

At first glance, one might conclude that toxic exposure should put all neurons in jeopardy because the entire brain would presumably have been exposed to the circulating substance. The notion, however, that toxic substances can cause selective damage to certain subsets of brain neurons has been clearly verified in acute animal models of substantia nigra, striatal, cerebellar, and hippocampal damage. Whether such phenomena play a role in chronic, progressive neurodegenerative disorders remains controversial. Toxic substances might render some neurons less capable of compensating for normal stresses or reduce their capacity for synaptic plasticity. Since neurons do not turnover on a regular basis, their cellular machinery accumulates defects that impair function on a long-term basis.

Since certain of the genetic defects associated with Alzheimer's disease are risk factors and not absolute determinants, the possibility that disease onset and progression may also be influenced by endogenous and exogenous environmental factors must be carefully explored. For any therapeutic strategy to be effective, a clear understanding of such factors is required.

B. SELECTIVE VULNERABILITY

Certain neurons appear to be more vulnerable to toxins than others. Features of this selective vulnerability are readily understandable whereas other features are not. For instance, particular types of neurons may have special chemical properties that make them uniquely vulnerable to a toxin. A prime example of this type of toxicity is the selective vulnerability of dopamine neurons to 6-hydroxy-dopamine. Dopamine neurons have transporters on their plasma membrane that are selective for dopamine and its analogs. 6-Hydroxy-dopamine is selectively accumulated in dopamine neurons where it causes free radical formation and irreversible neuronal damage. Neurons that do not possess these transporters are spared.

Another example is the vulnerability of neurons to systemic kainic acid, a toxic substance derived from seaweed. Those neurons that possess high densities of membrane receptors for kainic acid die after systemic exposure to the compound. When injected directly into the brain, kainic acid is toxic to most neurons because most neurons have a few kainate receptors, and the compound is extremely toxic.

Other toxins cause selective neuronal damage by unknown mechanisms. The globus pallidus is especially vulnerable to carbon monoxide poisoning. The striatum is most vulnerable to 3-nitro-propionic acid, a succinate dehydrogenase inhibitor that is found in certain molds. In such situations, the entire brain is exposed to the toxins, yet only some neurons are damaged. The nature of the special requirements of these neurons that make them susceptible is unknown.

C. ENDOGENOUS TOXINS
1. Primary Toxins

The simple dicarboxylic amino acid glutamate is the putative neurotransmitter of the majority of synaptic contacts in the nervous system. Glutamate acts through four different families of receptors, three composed of ligand-gated ion channels, and a fourth consisting of g protein-linked receptors affecting second messenger systems. The three ligand-gated ion channels are named after the agonists that selectively activate them, *N*-methyl-D-aspartate (NMDA), D,L-α-amino-3-hydroxy-5-methyl-4-isoxazolepropionic acid (AMPA), and kainate. Activation of each of these receptors results in depolarization of the neuronal membrane. Kainate and AMPA receptors activate channels permeable to sodium; NMDA receptors activate channels permeable to calcium. Under certain conditions, AMPA receptors are also permeable to calcium. Metabotropic glutamate receptors stimulate inositol phospholipid metabolism through one set of receptors and inhibition of forskolin-stimulated cAMP formation through another set of receptors.

In the 1960s, John Olney observed that glutamate and aspartate produced hypothalamic damage when given systemically in the neonatal period.[1] Subsequent studies demonstrated the toxicity of these compounds when injected into brain. These ion channel agonists caused axon- and glia-sparing lesions. They appeared to inflict the damage by causing excessive membrane depolarization and the uncontrolled influx of sodium (which causes cell swelling) and calcium (which activates proteases, lipases, and kinases).[2] Different brain regions were differentially vulnerable to glutamate agonist damage based in part on the selective distribution of certain receptor subtypes.

Under normal circumstances, glutamate acts to activate neurons in response to internal and external stimuli (a normal function). When the neuron, however, is compromised due to lack of oxygen or due to cellular damage, resulting in impaired metabolism, glutamate becomes dramatically toxic.[3] Concentrations of glutamate that are completely tolerated in normal tissue are extremely destructive in compromised tissue. Thus, the endogenous neurotransmitter glutamate stands in a position to aggravate tissue damage due to other genetic or environmental factors.

In mammalian brain, additional naturally occurring compounds have been identified that cause neuronal damage. Two byproducts of serotonin metabolism, kynurenic acid and quinolinic acid, have interesting properties in this regard. Quinolinic acid was isolated as a toxic substance in 1983 by Schwarcz et al.[4] Subsequently, other members of this pathway were identified, and kynurenic acid was found to block the toxic effects of quinolinic acid. Quinolinic acid's toxic effects were mediated through its activation of the NMDA receptor and kynurenic acid as well as conventional NMDA antagonists blocked quinolinic acid's toxic effects.

Quinolinic acid has been examined in AD, but found to be normal.[5] In contrast, quinolinic acid levels are massively increased in AIDS brains and possibly in other disorders.[6] Whether other toxic substances are naturally present in brain and potentially accelerate neuronal degeneration when the subject is exposed to biochemical or metabolic stresses is unknown.

In Alzheimer's disease, prominent pathology is seen in pyramidal neurons of hippocampus and cerebral cortex. These neurons use glutamate as a neurotransmitter and also contain high densities of AMPA and NMDA receptors. They receive extensive excitatory inputs from other areas of cerebral cortex and subcortical areas. These neurons are therefore positioned to be particularly vulnerable to excitotoxic damage. Their vulnerability has been demonstrated in models of hypoxia-ischemia and epilepsy. In post-mortem brain from AD patients, NMDA receptors are preferentially decreased consistent with the notion that the cells that die in AD hippocampus, and cerebral cortex have a relatively greater abundance of NMDA receptors than their neighbors.[7-9]

2. Secondary Risk Factors

a. Oxidative Stress and Free Radicals

A popular theory in cardiac disease, brain disease, and cancer is that any mechanism that leads to free radical accumulation will likely contribute to the cause of certain forms of pathology in these organ systems.[10] What are free radicals? They are oxygen or nitric oxide-containing molecules with an unpaired electron that makes them very reactive. These free radicals react with amino acids and nucleotides on proteins, lipids, and DNA causing damage that results in malfunction of the protein, lipid, and DNA. There are repair mechanisms that can correct some of the damage, but if the free radical production is too great, the cell cannot keep up and the damage accumulates. In organs with rapid cell turnover, this mechanism of long-term damage is inconsequential and does not influence organ function because cells are rapidly replaced. For muscle and brain, however, the consequences are very significant since the cell may die or malfunction and cannot be replaced.

Nuclear DNA damage may be a factor, but damage to mitochondrial DNA (mtDNA) has been clearly demonstrated to occur with aging.[11] There are no repair mechanisms for mtDNA. In postmitotic cells, the mitochondria continue to replicate. When mtDNA is damaged, faulty replication occurs and deletions in mtDNA accumulate. The faulty mtDNA leads to mitochondrial dysfunction, inefficient energy metabolism, and consequent additional accumulation of free radicals. The process therefore becomes a vicious cycle. If the mitochondria are not functioning normally, neurons may have difficulty maintaining normal resting membrane potential and thus become susceptible to excitotoxic effects of normal excitatory amino acid inputs.

Mitochondrial toxins such as 3-nitro-propionic acid and cyanide cause focal neuronal damage in brain.[11] 3-Nitro-propionic acid is found in certain fungi that grow on grass and sugar cane. Cases of 3-nitro-propionic acid ingestion in cows and humans have been reported. The cows and humans develop an acute motor disorder characterized by dystonia and athetosis. Imaging studies and pathologic examination of the brain shows severe neuronal damage in the caudate nucleus and putamen, two areas involved in motor coordination. Mitochondrial mutations also lead to selective damage to neurons and muscle. The particular pattern of vulnerability depends on the exact type of mitochondrial mutation and the resulting defects in the electron transport chain.

b. Genetic Susceptibility

Considerable heterogeneity has already been identified in the susceptibility of individuals to toxins. Individuals have different kinds and amounts of liver enzymes to detoxify exogenous and endogenous toxins. Just as genetic mutations can lead to disease, normal genetic variation can lead to disease susceptibility. Some of the best examples of this is susceptibility to cancer. DNA repair enzymes differ in their properties. If an individual is never under undue stress, no consequences of the genetic differences are apparent. If, however, the individuals are exposed to toxins, then those whose repair enzymes are not as active or efficient as others have a higher incidence of certain kinds of cancer such as colon cancer. Investigators are now looking furiously for such factors in neurodegenerative diseases such as Alzheimer's and Parkinson's disease. Variants for the gene for ApoE, for instance, appear to confer different degrees of susceptibility to Alzheimer's disease.[12] Whether this susceptibility arises from a differential sensitivity to an endogenous toxin is as yet unknown but it is certainly a likely possibility.

In familial amyotrophic lateral sclerosis (ALS), a genetic defect occurs in the enzyme superoxide dismutase, a key enzyme in the control of free radical formation.[13-14] Animals expressing the mutant human gene develop a degenerative disorder mimicking familial ALS. This is the first chronic neurodegenerative disorder in which a gene defect in the free radical pathway has been identified. The gene is expressed in all cells but for some as-yet unknown reason the motor neurons are particularly vulnerable to the neurodegenerative process. This single example lends the most credence to the hypothesis that free radical mechanisms may play a role in neurodegenerative diseases. It also supports the hypothesis that oxidative stress or excitotoxicity due to glutamate may also play a role in these diseases since substantial experimental data suggest these two factors are intimately connected to the free radical mechanism.

D. EXOGENOUS TOXINS

Over the last few decades several toxins have been identified that act selectively on brain and are of interest regarding the potential role of environmental agents in neurodegenerative disorders.

1. The ALS/Parkinsonism/Dementia Complex of Guam

During World War II, the Chamoro population of Guam was isolated from its normal nutritional sources, and many individuals relied heavily (moreso than usual) on flour from the cycad nut for sustinence.[15] Subsequently, relatively large numbers of individuals from this population were found to develop motor neuron disease resembling ALS often accompanied by a certain degree of parkinsonism. The incidence of this illness gradually decreased over the next 2 decades, but then the incidence of parkinsonism increased and then was often accompanied by dementia. More recently, the incidence of parkinsonism has decreased, but the incidence of dementia has remained high in persons exposed to cycad flour. The pathology of the illnesses resembles certain features of ALS, Parkinson's disease and Alzheimer's disease, but differences also exist. In the Guam dementia, for instance, amyloid plaques and neurofibrillary tangles occur, but their distribution and ultrastructural characteristics differ from that seen in Alzheimer's disease.

The cause of the neuronal degeneration was thought initially to be secondary to excessive amounts of an amino acid β-*N*-methylamino-L-alanine (BMAA) which when carboxylated acts as an NMDA agonist.[15] Subsequently, the concentrations of this amino acid in cycad flour have been found to be too low to account for the illness. Alternative theories have proposed that the culprit may be zinc from the utensils used to prepare the flour or may be cycasin itself which is known to damage DNA.[16] Regardless of which chemical substance proves to be the villain in this illness, the fact that an environmental toxin is responsible for a series of perhaps related neurodegenerative disorders is trully remarkable and is likely to yield clues about the nature of the sporadic illnesses.

2. Domoic Acid Poisoning

Domoic acid is a potent agonist for the kainate subtype of excitatory amino acid receptors. In 1990, a report of a group of people exposed to domoic acid was reported from Canada.[17] The individuals all ate mussels that had grown in algae-rich waters near Prince Edwards Island. There had been a period of drought which had raised the concentration of domoic acid in the fungi. The individuals all developed intestinal symptoms, but several also developed seizures, memory loss, and delerium. The delerium cleared, but profound recent memory loss persisted, and one individual was recently documented to have developed intractable partial complex seizures and bilateral hippocampal sclerosis.[18]

Kainate receptors are very dense in hippocampus, and when several of these individuals died, the damage in hippocampus paralleled the distribution of kainate receptors. It is as yet unclear whether individuals who were exposed to the toxin but did not develop severe symptoms acutely will eventually develop similar problems as they age.

3. Lathyrism and African Konzo

A syndrome of upper motor neuron dysfunction (spasticity — especially of the legs) of acute onset has been observed after ingestion of large amounts of *Lathyrus sativa* (a drought-resistant chickpea) or improperly prepared cassava.[19-20] In the first instance, the toxin is the amino acid β-oxalyl-amino-alanine (BOAA) which is a potent agonist at the AMPA subtype of excitatory amino acid receptors. In the second instance, the toxin appears to be cyanide. Obviously, all neurons in the brain are exposed to these toxins after ingestion, but only certain ones develop disease. It is also known that almost all neurons have AMPA receptors, and yet only certain neurons are significantly damaged by the toxin. Presumably the selective damage results from an interplay of vital metabolic pathways that differ from neuron to neuron. Definition of these differences may well provide clues to interventions that can stop or retard these types of illnesses.

II. SUMMARY

In this chapter, I have not reviewed all the details concerning a potential role for endogenous and exogenous toxins in Alzheimer's disease and related neurodegenerative disorders, but rather set forward the principles and broad outlines of data on which the hypotheses are based. As our understanding of the vast heterogeneity of brain biochemistry and pathology becomes more sophisticated and detailed, we are likely to find cascades of interdependent pathways that are crucial for neuronal survival and optimal function. Toxins and genetic defects may interfere at several points in these pathways and thus lead to clinical illness. Indeed, multiple different defects may lead to the same phenotypic disease. By the same token, there are likely to be multiple strategies for interfering therapeutically to correct defective pathways in disease. It is anticipated that such therapies will start to become available in the near future.

REFERENCES

1. Olney, J. W., Brain lesion, obesity and other disturbances in mice treated with monosodium glutamate, *Science*, 164, 719, 1969.
2. Choi, D. W., Calcium-mediated neurotoxicity: relationship to specific channel types and role in ischemic damage, *Trends Neurosci.*, 11, 465, 1988.
3. Novelli, A., Reilly, J. A., Lysko, P. G., and Henneberry, R. C., Glutamate becomes neurotoxic via the *N*-methyl-D-aspartate receptor when intracellular energy levels are reduced, *Brain Res.*, 451, 205, 1988.
4. Schwarcz, R., Whetsell, W. O., and Mangano, R. M., Quinolinic acid: an endogenous metabolite that produces axon sparing lesions in rat brain, *Science*, 219, 316, 1983.
5. Mouridian, M. M., Heyes, M. P., Pan, J.-B., Henser, I. J.-E., Markey, S. P., and Chase, T. N., No changes in central quinolinic acid levels in Alzheimer's disease, *Neurosci. Lett.*, 105, 233, 1989.
6. Heyes, M. P., Rubinow, D., Lane, C., and Markey, S. P., Cerebrospinal fluid quinolinic acid concentrations are increased in Acquired immunity deficiencey syndrome, *Ann. Neurol.*, 26, 275, 1989.
7. Greenamyre, J. T., and Young, A. B., Excitatory amino acids and Alzheimer's disease, *Neurobiol. Aging*, 10, 593, 1989.
8. Carlson, M. D., Penney, J. B., and Young, A. B., NMDA, AMPA and benzodiazepine binding site changes in Alzheimer's disease visual cortex, *Neurobiol. Aging*, 14, 343, 1993.
9. Ulas, J., Brunner, L. C., Geddes, J. W., Choe, W., and Cotman, C. W., *N*-Methyl-D-aspartate receptor complex in the hippocampus of elderly, normal individuals and those with Alzheimer's disease, *Neuroscience*, 49, 45, 1992.
10. Packer, L., Prilipko, L., and Christen, Y., Eds., *Free Radicals in the Brain*, Springer-Verlag, Berlin, 1992.
11. Beal, M. F., Does impairment of energy metabolism result in excitotoxic neuronal death in neurodegenerative disorders?, *Ann. Neurol.*, 31, 119, 1992.
12. Poirier, J., Apolipoprotein E in animal models of CNS injury and Alzheimer's disease, *Trends Neurosci.*, 17, 525, 1994.
13. Rosen, D. R., Siddique, T., Patterson, D., Figlewicz, D. A., Sapp, P., Hentati, A., Donaldson, D., Goto, J., O'Regan, J. P., Deng, D. X., Rahmani, Z., Krizus, A., McKenna-Yasek, D., Cayabyab, A., Gaston, S. M., Berger, R., Tanzi, R. E., Halperin, J. J., Herzfeldt, B., Van den Bergh, R., Hung, W. Y., Bird, T., Deng, G., Mulder, D. W., and Brown, R. H., Mutations in Cu/Zn superoxide dismutase gene are associated with familial amyotrophic lateral sclerosis, *Nature*, 362, 59, 1993.
14. Gurney, M. E., Pu, H., Chiu, A. Y., Dal Canto, M. C., Polchow, C. Y., Alexander, D. D., Caliendo, J., Henati, A., Kwon, Y. W., Deng, H. X., Chen, W., Zhai, P., Sufit, R. L., and Siddique, T., Motor neuron degeneration in mice that express a human Cu, Zn superoxide dismutase mutation, *Science*, 264, 1772, 1994.
15. Spencer, P. S., Nunn, P. B., Hugon, J., Ludolph, A. C., Ross, S. M., Roy, D. N., and Robertson, R. C., Guam amyotrophic lateral sclerosis-parkinsonism-dementia linked to a plant excitant neurotoxin, *Science*, 237, 517, 1987.
16. Kisby, G. E., Ellison, M., and Spencer, P. S., Content of the neurotoxins cycasin (methylazoxymethanol β-D-glucoside) and BMAA (β-*N*-methylamino-L-alanine) in cycad flour prepared by Guam Chamorros, *Neurology*, 42, 1336, 1992.
17. Teitelbaum, J. S., Zatorre, R. J., Carpenter, S., Gendron, D., Evans, A. C., Gjedde, A., and Cashman, N. R., Neurologic sequelae of domoic acid intoxication due to the ingestion of contaminated mussels, *N. Engl. J. Med.*, 322, 1781, 1990.
18. Cendes, F., Andermann, F., Carpenter, S., Zatorre, R. J., and Cashman, N. R., Temporal lobe epilepsy caused by domoic acid intoxication: evidence for glutamate receptor-mediated excitotoxicity in humans, *Ann. Neurol.*, 37, 123, 1995.
19. Spencer, P. S., Ludolph, A., Dwivedi, M. P., Roy, D. N., Hugon, J., and Schaumburg, H. H., Lathyrism: evidence for role of the neuroexcitatory amino acid BOAA, *Lancet*, 2, 1066, 1986.
20. Tylleskär, T., Légué, F. D., Peterson, S., Kpizingui, E., and Stecker, P., Konzo in the Central African Republic, *Neurology*, 44, 959, 1994.

Chapter **19**

TRACE ELEMENTS IN ALZHEIMER'S DISEASE

William R. Markesbery

CONTENTS

I. INTRODUCTION

The etiology (cause) and pathogenesis (cellular and molecular mechanisms occurring in the development of a disease) of Alzheimer's disease (AD) are not known. The central question in AD is what causes selective neuron death. A clear understanding of the etiologies and pathogenetic mechanisms of AD must be gained in order for treatment or prevention to be established on a rational basis. Numerous hypotheses about the etiology and pathogenesis of Alzheimer's disease have been suggested, including genetic defect, slow or unconventional virus disorder, defective membrane metabolism, endogenous toxins, amyloid precursor protein abnormality, calcium metabolism abnormality, mitochondrial defect, free radical mediated neurodegeneration, and trace element neurotoxicity. It is most likely that AD is a multifactorial disorder and that more than one of these mechanisms are present in the disorder.

Trace element neurotoxicity has been hypothesized to play a role in AD for many years. Numerous elements have been reported to be imbalanced in AD. The elements receiving the most attention in AD are aluminum (Al), mercury (Hg), zinc (Zn), and iron (Fe). Emphasis is usually placed on elevated concentrations of elements in AD, with the suggestion that they have a direct toxic effect on neurons. However, it is well known that excess concentrations of some elements are capable of producing harmful biologic effects by displacing other essential elements. Thus, an increase in one nonessential element in the brain in AD could displace an essential element important in a specific metabolic pathway leading to disruption of structure and function.

II. ALUMINUM

Aluminum is the element that has received the most emphasis in AD, but its role in the pathogenesis of this disorder has never been defined. Aluminum is one of the most common elements in our universe, making up 8.1% of the earth's crust. It is a nonessential but ubiquitous element, commonly encountered in cookware, cans, beer, cheese, tea, baking powder, antacids, analgesics, antiperspirants, and drinking water. Aluminum is absorbed through the gastrointestinal tract, lungs, nose, and skin. Aluminum was first thought to be important in AD in 1965 when it was found that intracerebral injection of Al in rabbits caused neurofibrillary tangle formation. Subsequent early studies revealed an increase in Al concentration in the brain in AD where neurofibrillary tangles were most prominent. More recently, studies of bulk brain Al concentrations in AD have shown a lack of agreement with some studies showing elevation and others no elevation. Microprobe studies at the cellular level have shown variable results as well. Several epidemiological studies have shown an increased risk of AD in regions where Al concentrations in drinking water were higher. However, these were fraught with inherent difficulties, and the results are not easy to interpret. It is possible that there are mild elevations of Al in AD and that some of these are in focal brain areas or "hot spots". The major unanswered question is whether Al deposition is an early or primary event or a late event superimposed on degenerating neurons. It is most likely that Al is not a primary etiologic agent in AD. However, Al is known to be toxic to neurons and if superimposed on degenerating neurons it could accentuate the degenerative process causing more rapid neuron death.

III. MERCURY

Another element that has been postulated to possibly be involved in AD is mercury. Mercury, an ubiquitous, nonessential element, has long been known to be toxic to the central nervous system in its inorganic (elemental or mercuric salt) or organic (methylmercury) forms. The most common source of elemental Hg is in dental amalgams. Toxicity can occur from inhalation of Hg vapors. Of inhaled Hg vapor, 80% is retained. Mercuric salts are found in medications, in catalytic agents used in plastic manufacturing, and in food. Organic Hg, primarily in the form of methylmercury, is in food, paint, fungicides, seeds, cosmetics, and medications. Exposure to methylmercury in the food chain, primarily in seafood, represents one of the major forms of exposure for humans.

The toxicity of Hg to humans has been appreciated for centuries. Poisoning from inhalation of Hg vapors is characterized by tremor, irritability, moodiness, and other personality changes. These symptoms occurred in workers in the felt hat and fur industries and were referred to as *erethism* or the "Mad Hatter syndrome".

Environmental methylmercury contamination occurred in Japan when Hg was discharged into Minamata Bay, and consumption of contaminated fish resulted in poisoning. Another major environmental intoxication occurred in Iraq when Hg-treated wheat seed, distributed for planting, was eaten by farmers, resulting in widespread poisoning. The clinical manifestations of methylmercury intoxication include sensory changes, ataxia, visual field constrictions, weakness, and inability to concentrate.

Recent instrumental neutron activation analysis studies have shown an elevation of Hg in AD in the cerebral cortex and several of the deep nuclei including the nucleus basalis of Meynert, the major cholinergic projection nucleus in the cerebral hemispheres. Selenium (Se) and zinc (Zn) play a protective role against Hg in biological tissue. One study indicated that when Hg was elevated in the brain in AD, Se and Zn were decreased, suggesting that they were utilized to detoxify Hg.

Mercury is known to be toxic to neurons. It can be toxic by causing a decrease in protein synthesis, by interfering with membrane enzyme function, by diminishing other essential elements, or by binding to tubulin and interfering with assembly of microtubules, a major cytoskeletal structure of neurons.

It has been established by several studies that defective microtubule assembly occurs in the brain in AD. Guanosine triphosphate (GTP) is an absolute requirement for tubular polymerization, but the GTP binding site on β-tubulin has been shown to be blocked or absent in homogenate of brain from most AD patients. Mercury bound to ethylenediaminetetraacetic acid blocks GTP binding to β-tubulin in homogenate of normal brain similar to that observed in AD. This suggests that Hg may play a role in altered microtubule assembly and be a possible pathogenetic factor in AD.

IV. ZINC

It has been suggested that a deficiency of zinc (Zn) may play a role in AD. However, multiple studies of bulk brain Zn have not found significant deficiencies or elevations in Alzheimer's disease. Microprobe studies have shown no significant alterations in Zn at the cellular level in AD.

More recent studies have shown that Zn ions *in vitro* can cause one form of the amyloid beta peptide to form clumps resembling the amyloid plaques found in the brain in AD. This has led to the hypothesis that altered Zn regulation could cause Zn to build up, come in contact with amyloid β-peptide, and cause it to form clumps in the brain in AD. In one report, AD patients given Zn supplements showed deterioration of cognitive function within several days.

V. IRON

Another element that could be important in the pathogenesis of AD is iron, one of the most common elements in the earth's crust and an essential element in plant and animal life. It is utilized in a broad spectrum of biochemical reactions. Normal adult humans are estimated to contain 4 to 5 grams of Fe, with the highest concentrations being in the liver and spleen. Once absorbed, Fe is bound to transferrin, which delivers it to tissue, where it is stored as ferritin. Brain cells have a high-affinity receptor for transferrin. This system is postulated to be the way that the brain accesses Fe from the general circulation to meet its high metabolic requirements.

Studies using a variety of techniques have suggested disturbed Fe metabolism in the brains of AD patients. Iron is increased in cerebral cortical grey matter, amygdala, and olfactory pathway in

AD. A microprobe study detected a significant elevation of Fe in neurofibrillary tangles in AD. Ferritin, a protein to which Fe is bound, contains more Fe in the brain of patients with AD than control subjects.

The role of Fe is of considerable interest in relationship to free radical formation. Free radicals are atoms or molecules containing an orbit with one or more unpaired electrons. Free radicals are catalyzed by free ions of transition metals such as Fe and copper. Some free radicals are capable of removing an electron from neighboring molecules to complete their orbits and in the process damage lipids, proteins, or DNA. There is a fine balance between free radical formation and antioxidant defense, and when the balance is tipped in favor of reactive oxygen species, oxidative stress results. Neurons are especially vulnerable to free radical attack. It has been postulated that free radicals may play a role in neuron death following central nervous system ischemia and trauma, and in Parkinson's disease and amyotrophic lateral sclerosis. The oxygen-rich environment of the brain plus the presence of excess Fe ions could hypothetically set the stage for increased free radical formation and subsequent neuron degeneration.

There is an increase in lipid peroxidation in the brain in AD which is most pronounced in the medial temporal lobe, where neuron degeneration is most prominent. Protein oxidation is increased in the aged brain and in AD. Glutamine synthetase, an enzyme sensitive to oxidation, is significantly reduced in the frontal lobe in AD. Mitochondrial DNA oxidation is increased in some areas of the brain in AD compared with age-matched control subjects. In addition it has been shown that aggregated amyloid beta peptide is capable of generating free radicals that can alter oxidative sensitive enzymes and possibly damage membranes. These studies indicate that the brain is under increased oxidative stress in Alzheimer's disease.

Thus, the increase in Fe in the brain in AD and the increasing body of information indicating enhanced free radical formation and oxidative stress in the brain in AD suggest that Fe could play a role in the pathogenesis of AD. Importantly these findings bring about the possibility of amalgamating the neurotoxic trace element, free radical, amyloid, and altered calcium metabolism hypotheses in the pathogenesis of AD.

ACKNOWLEDGMENT

Supported by National Institutes of Health grants P01AG05119 and P50AG05144.

REFERENCES

1. Markesbery, W. R. and Ehmann, W. D., Brain trace elements in Alzheimer's disease, in *Alzheimer Disease,* Terry, R. D. Ed., Raven Press, New York, 1994, 353.
2. Bush, A. L., Pettingell, W. H., Multhaup, G., et al., Rapid induction of Alzheimer Aβ amyloid formation by zinc, Science, 265, 1464, 1994.
3. Markesbery, W. R. and Ehmann, W. D., Aluminum and Alzheimer's Disease, *Neuroscience,* 1, 212, 1993.

TREATMENT

Chapter **20**

CLINICAL DRUG TRIALS IN ALZHEIMER'S DISEASE: METHODOLOGICAL CONSIDERATIONS

———————————— Leon J. Thal

CONTENTS

I. INTRODUCTION

Alzheimer's disease (AD) is a major public health issue largely because of the life expectancy of the U.S. population. In 1990, 12.5% of the U.S. population was over the age of 65, and by 2040 this will increase to approximately 22.5% of the U.S. population. In the elderly, acquired cognitive disorders occur in approximately 15% of the over age 65 population. Of these, two-thirds will develop dementia secondary to AD. Thus, for 1990, with a population of 232 million individuals, approximately 4.4 million were demented, and 3 million of these had AD. By the year 2040, with the expected growth in the population over the age of 65 to 22.5% of the U.S. population, the number of AD patients will increase to approximately 6 million. In 1990, estimated cost of care for this population was approximately $80 billion. If these population projections are correct and effective treatments are not found, the cost will double in the next 50 years. These demographic and economic factors, coupled with our expanding knowledge of the biology of this disease, has sparked both public and scientific interest in this disorder leading to many spectacular scientific advancements as well as the realization that an effective treatment for this disease must be developed.

II. PROBLEMS INHERENT IN THE CONDUCT OF CLINICAL DRUG TRIALS IN ALZHEIMER'S DISEASE

A. ABSENCE OF A BIOLOGICAL MARKER

At the present time, there is no biological marker for AD. A review of the available clinical pathological series reveals that the disorder can be diagnosed with approximately 85% accuracy during life using clinical criteria. This means that some individuals who have disorders other than AD will be included in AD drug trials. This relatively high degree of accurate diagnosis has come about largely because of advances in understanding the neuropsychological changes characteristic of this disorder, the use of a standardized evaluation for patients, and the development of clinical criteria for diagnosis. Currently, three sets of diagnostic criteria exist including those developed from a workshop sponsored by the National Institute of Neurologic Communicative Disorders and Stroke and the Alzheimer Disease and Related Disorders Association (NINCDS-ADRDA); from the American Psychiatric Association in their diagnostic and statistical methodology (DSM-IV); and from the World Health Organization (ICD-10). The criteria espoused by these organizations is fairly similar. Those of NINCDS-ADRDA and DSM-IV are most widely used in the U.S. In general, these criteria require the presence of dementia which is acquired and progressive in nature, and involves multiple cognitive domains in the presence of a normal level of consciousness. In addition, appropriate laboratory evaluations must be carried out to eliminate other potential causes of the dementia syndrome.

In most clinical series, diagnostic accuracy is about 85% for clinical research purposes such as clinical drug trials. Diagnostic accuracy greater than 90% can be achieved by eliminating atypical cases. However, while useful for clinical drug testing, any approach that increases specificity will also decrease sensitivity. This approach is therefore suitable for clinical drug trials, but not for the diagnosis of subjects in a community setting.

The development of a biological marker capable of distinguishing patients with AD with extremely high specificity and sensitivity would be quite useful. Given the already excellent clinical criteria for diagnosing this disorder, a useful biological marker would need to have specificity and sensitivity exceeding 95%. Such a biological marker, however, would also have uses far beyond confirming a clinical diagnosis. If the biological marker were dependent upon a unique biological characteristic of the disorder, it might be useful for diagnosing very early cases or even asymptomatic individuals who are destined to develop disease at a later date. Presymptomatic diagnosis may be possible because the pathological changes characteristic of AD are likely to be present many years before the clinical expression of the disorder. Although there are a number of candidate molecules currently being studied as potential markers for this disease, none has yet been demonstrated to be clinically useful.

B. VARIATIONS IN PRESENTATION AND COURSE

The course of AD is quite variable. This variability introduces significant variance in trials of agents designed to slow the rate of progression in AD and dictates the use of large sample sizes to detect significant differences. Although on average individuals survive for 8 to 10 years after diagnosis, some individuals decline quite precipitously and expire in as little as 3 to 4 years, while others decline quite slowly and survive for 20 to 30 years following diagnosis. At present, the factors controlling the rate of decline are poorly understood. Control of the rate of decline is almost certainly multifactorial. In some instances, genetic influences are clearly operative. Thus, age of onset and rate of progression are often similar when several individuals within the same family are afflicted by the disorder. Age of onset appears to affect rate of decline with young patients declining more rapidly than older ones. Recently, the gene dosage of the cholesterol-carrying protein apolipoprotein E_4 was demonstrated to have a major effect on age of onset of AD. Individuals carrying two alleles for apolipoprotein E_4 develop the disease approximately 10 years earlier than individuals who carry no alleles for this form of cholesterol-carrying protein. Apolipoprotein E_4 status may therefore affect the rate of decline as well as the age of onset. However, empirical data supporting the effect of apolipoprotein E_4 on rate of decline is as yet lacking.

A number of clinical variables have been examined to determine whether or not they affect rate of decline. Features such as psychotic behavior, myoclonus, and extrapyramidal features have all been found to be associated with a more rapid rate of decline. Recently, approximately 20 to 25% of AD patients have been found to have cortical Lewy bodies at autopsy, the pathological hallmark of Parkinson's disease. These individuals generally develop mild extrapyramidal features such as masked faces, slowness of movement, and increased tone, characteristic of Parkinson's disease. The rate of decline for this cohort is approximately 50% more rapid than for individuals with AD pathology but without accompanying Lewy bodies. Thus, many factors affect the rate of decline. The high degree of variability in rate of decline complicates the detection of small differences in rate of decline in clinical drug trials.

C. WHAT TO TREAT IN A SYMPTOMATIC TRIAL

In addition to memory impairment, patients with AD have a wide variety of cognitive and behavioral impairments. Other common areas affected include language, visuospatial relations, and behavioral disturbances. Therapeutic trials designed to improve symptomatology must decide which of these cognitive disorders to target since the underlying pathophysiology and biochemistry is likely to differ. Most subjects with AD present with a combination of many of these clinical features. In particular, behavioral disturbances have been recognized as occurring in one-third to one-half of all subjects. The treatment of behavioral disturbances remains an important area of unmet need in caring for patients with AD, since behavioral disturbances often precipitate institutionalization.

III. PRINCIPLES OF PHARMACOLOGICAL INTERVENTION

A. PHARMACOKINETICS

In the design of clinical drug trials, issues related to the pharmacokinetics of the compounds must be considered. Questions such as the distribution of the drug and its half-life are quite important. Dosing for AD patients should generally be via the oral route. The half-life of the drug should be sufficiently long so that excessively frequent dosing is not required. In some cases, drugs may be administered through the skin using transdermal preparations. Transdermal preparations offer the advantage of being able to deliver constant dosing over prolonged periods of time without the need for frequent administration. Dose–response curves need to be established in early clinical trials. For some classes of drugs such as cholinesterase inhibitors, inverted U-shaped dose response curves with suboptimal response at both low and very high dosing occurs. Thus, dose titration or exposure to a broad range of doses must be carried out in early trials with new drugs.

B. PATIENT SELECTION CRITERIA

Which patients enter clinical drug trials? At present, the vast majority of AD clinical trials are restricted to ambulatory outpatients with mild to moderate dementia who are free of other significant medical illnesses and who do not require use of psychoactive medications. The use of these restrictive inclusion-exclusion criteria means that at any one time only approximately 10% of the U.S. population of ambulatory AD outpatients would meet criteria for inclusion in an AD trial. While this seems like a large number, the use of these inclusion/exclusion criteria gives rise to a series of problems. First, individuals with moderately advanced or advanced dementia are rarely if ever included. Nursing home patients are virtually never included. Thus, results from patients with mild to moderate dementia may or may not be applicable to those with more severe disease. Second, subjects on concomitant psychoactive medications are excluded. This allows for a better estimate of the effect of the drug to be tested without contamination by other potentially psychoactive medications. While this approach is preferable for measuring the effect size of drug treatment, the results of such trials may or may not be generalized to other populations which are being treated with a broad range of psychoactive medications. Third, subjects with specific conditions such as severe aphasia, advanced dementia, or other unusual problems are often excluded. Individuals with advanced dementia are generally excluded because currently available assessment instruments are unable to detect change in these individuals. Thus, the usefulness of a drug in populations not included in controlled clinical trials must be adduced by observational postmarketing studies. While postmarketing observational studies may work in drugs with large effect sizes, this approach is not likely to work well in AD where treatment effect sizes will probably remain quite small for the next several decades.

C. DURATION

The duration of a trial depends largely upon the primary question to be answered and the study design. Trials designed to produce short-term improvement in cognitive functioning may be relatively brief and involve only 3 to 6 months of testing. Many current trials, however, are designed to alter the rate of decline in AD. Since the rate of decline is highly variable, improved estimates of the rate of decline can be obtained by lengthening the duration of the study. In addition, shorter studies require larger numbers of subjects, adding to the difficulty in conducting the study and to increased cost. Most trials designed to alter the rate of cognitive decline require at least 1 year of treatment in a double-blind placebo-controlled randomized condition. Some recent trials have even extended to 2 years. In a typical 1-year trial, a difference in the rate of decline of approximately 50% between the placebo and the drug treated group can be detected with a total sample size of approximately 400 subjects.

In the future, some trials will be carried out in an attempt to delay onset of disease. These trials will require the enrollment of elderly individuals who are free of dementia, but are expected to develop it in future years. The development of new cases will therefore depend on the incidence of AD in the population studied. If an agent existed that could delay the onset of clinically recognizable disease by 50%, such a trial would require approximately 4000 subjects with follow-up of 5 years to detect clinically and statistically significant differences between treatment and placebo groups for preventing the appearance of new cases of AD. Such large sample sizes are not unusual for trials of cardiovascular agents.

IV. HOW TO CHOOSE DRUGS

A. EMPIRIC

In past decades, drug treatment often proceeded on an empiric basis. Drugs available to treat one particular condition were often utilized to treat a second condition even though the underlying cause of the disorder was quite different.

B. SCIENTIFIC

In the last 20 years, the treatment of many diseases has become more scientifically based. The application of modern neurochemical techniques to the brains of patients with AD has revolutionized our approach to the therapeutics of this disorder. Drug development for AD shifted to a scientific basis after the 1976 observation that the brains of patients with AD were deficient in the enzyme responsible for the synthesis of the neurotransmitter acetylcholine. For almost the next two decades, drug treatment of this disorder focused largely on attempts to increase cholinergic neurotransmission. This strategy resulted in the development of tetrahydroaminoacridine (tacrine, Cognex) as the first FDA-approved drug for the treatment of AD. Numerous other cholinesterase inhibitors are also under development.

Other neurobiological findings have provided clues to rational drug development. The discovery that β protein, the principle component of senile plaque cores in AD, may be neurotoxic has lead to the screening of hundreds of compounds that might block the formation of β protein from its precursor protein, influence clearance of protein, interfere with the formation of amyloid fibrils, or block toxicity. When successful lead compounds have been identified, they will be tested in animal models, then eventually in humans. Similar programs are under way in an attempt to develop compounds that might alter brain levels of apolipoprotein E or interfere with mechanisms of interaction between apolipoprotein E and β protein to decrease AD pathology. Thus, our improved understanding of the biology of the disease has resulted in rational drug design.

V. TRIAL DESIGN

Over the years, the types of trial designs used to test drugs in AD patients have undergone considerable modification and change. Early trials in AD were often poorly designed. Flaws in these early trials included inadequate blinding, small sample size, and the use of multiple outcome variables. Psychometric measures that were not meaningful in the life of AD patients were often chosen as outcome measures. These outcome measures lacked "face validity". Over the past decade, increasing attention has been paid to trial design so that most current trials are well designed and include appropriate randomization, adequate blinding, a few select outcome measures, and a meaningful relationship between the outcome variable and a key feature of the disease.

In early AD trials, cross over designs were frequently used. In a cross over design, the population to be studied is divided into two groups and each group is exposed to both treatments in an opposite order. For example, if the two groups are group A and group B, group A receives a placebo followed by drug while group B receives drug followed by placebo. Often a washout period is interspersed between the two periods of treatment. While this design may seem attractive since fewer patients are needed because each patient can serve as his or her own control, it has a number of major flaws. First, a crossover trial is more useful in a stable disorder where there is no change in the baseline. This is not true of AD. When using the crossover design in AD, the patients' baseline scores may not be the same in the drug and placebo phases of the trial because the subject changes during the course of the trial. Second, a crossover trial assumes that there are no carryover effects. In AD trials, there frequently are carry-over defects. These may occur either because a drug effect carries over from one period to another or because a subject learns something permanently while under drug treatment which then fails to wash out during a subsequent crossover to placebo. The use of crossover trials in AD has almost ceased because of these many confounds.

A second design combining some features of a crossover and a parallel design has been termed an "enrichment design". This design was used in the first multicenter tacrine trial. This design is particularly useful for compounds with an inverted U-shaped dose–response curve. In an enrichment design, subjects are exposed to varying doses of an agent based on the supposition that each subject will obtain the optimal effect if the treatment dose can be individualized. At the end of the dose-ranging phase all subjects undergo a washout period during which treatment response is determined. Individuals failing to respond to any dose are dropped from the study. Individuals responding to a particular dose are subsequently rerandomized to treatment with either their optimal dose or to placebo. This allows for a second independent confirmation of the effect of the drug during treatment of the subject with the optimal dose. Since nonresponding subjects are dropped, subjects entering the double-blind, placebo-controlled, efficacy portion of the trial are considered to be an "enriched" population. While this design has many advantages, such as allowing for the determination of the optimal dose and for discarding nonresponding subjects, it has one significant disadvantage in that all subjects in the trial are exposed to drug during the dose titration phase. Thus, carry-over effects from the dose-titration phase to the double-blind efficacy phase may occur, interfering with the final interpretation of the data. In addition, since all subjects are exposed to drug during some portion of the trial, there is no true placebo group to use when comparing the frequency of adverse events.

The most widely utilized and robust clinical trial design is that of a parallel study. In this type of trial, subjects are randomized to receive either drug or placebo, then followed over time. If the randomization is carried out appropriately, there should be no bias in the allocation of subjects to treatment group. Subject characteristics should be equally represented in the two groups and any differences that emerge should be due to the application of the treatment rather than to other random factors. Parallel design studies suffer from none of the disadvantages of carryover that might occur in crossover or enrichment designs. In addition, side effects of the drug can be accurately gauged by comparing them to the frequency of the same adverse events in the matched placebo group. The only disadvantage of a parallel trial design is that it generally requires a somewhat larger sample size. If properly performed, however, results from this design are the easiest to interpret.

VI. OUTCOME MEASURES

Each trial requires a series of outcome measures that are reliable, reproducible, objective, and measure meaningful change in the disease state. For a drug to be considered effective for the treatment of AD, it must improve cognitive and overall performance or prevent decline.

A. PRIMARY OUTCOME MEASURES

For most AD trials, improvement in cognition or slowing the rate of cognitive decline is a key primary outcome measure. Clinical trials generally utilize composite cognitive measures designed to track the cognitive deficits characteristic of the disease. For pharmacological trials, the most widely used global cognitive measure is the Alzheimer Disease Assessment Scale, cognitive subsection (ADAS, COS). This instrument contains 70 points and is heavily weighted toward verbal memory, a key deficit in this disorder. It also measures orientation, praxis, and language. It was developed for psychopharmacological trials of AD and validated on an AD population. Its longitudinal characteristics have been well defined and AD patients decline by approximately 7 to 9 points per year. It requires 30 to 45 minutes to administer. Other global cognitive instruments include the Mini-Mental State Examination (MMSE) and the Blessed Information-Memory-Concentration Test (BIMC). Rates of cognitive decline are 3 to 4 points per year for these two brief

(10-minute) tests which contain 30 and 33 test points, respectively. Although briefer, these tests were not specifically designed for psychopharmacological studies of AD and they are less sensitive to change. A fourth global cognitive instrument, the Dementia Rating Scale of Mattis, contains 144 points. It requires approximately 45 minutes to administer and AD subjects decline by approximately 11 points per year. The advantage of the Mattis Dementia Rating Scale is that it was designed for the longitudinal evaluation of patients with AD and individuals who reach a floor on other composite instruments can still be rated on the Mattis.

All four of these scales perform similarly in some respects. The average rate of change for AD patients for each of these scales over 1 year is approximately equal to the standard deviation of that rate of change. All of the scales have ceiling and floor effects so that AD patients tracked longitudinally on any of these scales appear to decline more slowly at first when they are near the ceiling, more rapidly when they are on the middle portions of the scale, then more slowly at the end when a floor effect is reached. Rate of change on each scale is not linear over the entire scale range, but approaches linearity during the middle stages of dementia. The rate of decline is independent of residence, sex, and location, and appears to be a good predictor of disease progression. The rate of change is quite predictable for groups and knowledge of the rate of decline allows for the accurate estimation of sample sizes for studies designed to slow decline in AD.

Global measures are also necessary to estimate whether or not the effect size demonstrated in an AD trial is sufficient to be clinically meaningful. Adequate instrumentation for the measurement of global change in AD does not exist. Virtually all AD clinical trials currently utilize some form of a clinician's global impression of severity or change. This instrument was adopted from pharmacological trials of psychiatric conditions, then applied to the AD population, usually without validation. These instruments are useful in capturing overall improvement of domains not specifically tested on formal psychometric testing that might improve during a clinical trial. A number of semi-structured global instruments are currently in development for use in AD patients. Finally, a staging instrument, the Clinical Dementia Rating Scale, which examines performance in the areas of memory, orientation, judgment, community affairs, and home and hobbies has been used as a global instrument in many recent AD trials, testing compounds designed to alter the rate of decline in AD.

B. SECONDARY OUTCOME MEASURES

There are many other domains that one might wish to measure in subjects with AD. Among the most important are activities of daily living. Here, too, appropriately validated scales do not exist for the AD population. In general, scales developed to measure either basic activities of daily living or instrumental activities of daily living in older individuals have been applied to the AD population. The functional hallmark of a drug that successfully enhances cognition would be to improve an individual's ability to perform activities of daily living. Alternately, a drug that slows the rate of decline should preserve an individual's ability to perform these activities. In AD, higher-order instrumental activities of daily living such as handling money, paying bills, filling out insurance or social security forms, remembering telephone numbers, making business decisions, or handling legal affairs are lost early in the course of the disease. More basic activities of daily living such as dressing, feeding, ambulating, and toileting become impaired later in the course of the illness. Appropriate scales to measure both instrumental and basic activities of daily living are currently being developed and validated.

Other secondary measures that may be appropriate for AD clinical drug trials include measurement of depression, attention, caregiver burden, and quality of life.

A recent FDA symposium on the assessment of antidementia drugs concluded that a drug marketed for the treatment of dementia must demonstrate improvement on a rating scale that captures the cardinal cognitive factors of AD to ensure specificity as well as improvement on a clinical global instrument to ensure a sufficient effect size to be clinically meaningful.

VII. DATA ANALYSIS

Criteria must be established to conclude that a drug is beneficial in treating patients with AD. For short-term clinical trials designed to improve cognitive functioning improvement on a cognitive scale such as the ADAS-Cog and on a global measure such as the Clinical Global Impression of Change in a sufficient amount to be clinically meaningful should be demonstrated.

For drugs designed to slow the rate of decline, similar measures could be applied on changes in the rate of decline, or slope can be computed. For example, if on average patients decline by four points per year on the Blessed Information-Memory-Concentration Test and the application of a drug reduces the rate of decline to two points per year, then the rate of decline has decreased by approximately 50%. Most caregivers, family members, and experts in the field of AD believe that the development of a compound that could slow the rate of decline by even 25% would be clinically useful. Hopefully, such an agent would continue to be effective over many years so that the actual performance of subjects on drug would continue to diverge from that of a placebo-treated group.

A third method of analyzing data uses survival analysis. In classical survival analysis used in the testing of anticancer agents, actual survival is utilized. A drug is deemed useful if it statistically significantly prolongs survival in the drug-treated as opposed to the placebo-treated group. In AD, survival would not be a useful measure because quality of life in the late stages of the disease is extremely poor. However, there are many other events for which survival analysis could be utilized. For example, a drug that delayed institutionalization in AD patients might be both clinically useful and highly cost effective. One trial currently under way is utilizing death, institutionalization, loss of basic activities of daily living, and progression of dementia from moderate to severely demented as outcome measures that will be analyzed by survival analysis. A delay in any of these outcomes would be welcome for the patient afflicted with AD.

VIII. DRUG DEVELOPMENT AND SAMPLE SIZE CONSIDERATIONS

The process of drug development is regulated by law. A series of federal laws has been passed over the years to ensure that marketed products are both safe and effective. Although many believe that this standard has always been required, it was not until the passage of the 1962 Kefauver-Harris Amendment that a requirement for efficacy was added to the 1938 Federal Food Drug and Cosmetic Act, which only required that marketed compounds must be safe.

The testing of drugs for AD usually begins with testing in the laboratory. The drug may be screened for certain types of activity or for toxicity in cell culture models. Subsequently, the compound often undergoes laboratory assessment in models of learning and memory or in models designed to simulate a biochemical change or disorder in AD. Testing for toxicity must be carried out in two animal species prior to human clinical exposure. Initial testing in humans called phase I testing is carried out exposing a small number of subjects, usually several dozen, to the compound in order to determine bioavailability, maximum tolerated dose, and side effects. Determination of efficacy is not of primary importance in phase I testing. Phase II testing generally involves exposing several dozen to several hundred individuals in order to gain more information regarding dose requirements and also to gain an initial indication of efficacy. Phase III testing is generally carried out after the appropriate dose or doses have been determined. In Phase III testing, several hundred subjects are exposed to the drug for a final determination of efficacy. In recent years, there has been a trend to combine phases II and III into a single study phase to expedite the process. Two phase III trials are generally necessary to make certain that the results of a single trial are not due to chance.

The number of subjects needed to determine drug efficacy in phase III testing depends on the relationship between the effect size and the variation in the outcome measure. For example, the standard deviation for the rate of change of commonly used cognitive instruments such as the BMIC, MMSE,

ADAS, and Mattis Dementia Rating Scale is approximately equal to the decline over 1 year. Thus, in a 1-year study designed to slow decline in AD, a typical trial designed to reduce the rate of decline by 25 to 50% will require 300 to 500 subjects. Studies of this size are always multicenter in order to accrue the required sample size.

After a compound is approved, additional information primarily regarding side effects and interactions with other compounds may be gained during phase IV testing where the compound is administered to many thousands of individuals. Thus, the development of drugs is a lengthy and costly process. The clinical testing of a drug for AD often requires 7 to 10 years to collect sufficient evidence to prove safety and efficacy. Total cost estimates range from $150 to 300 million per compound. In the future, considerations of cost, effect size, and effect on quality of life are likely to be important considerations in AD drug trials.

ACKNOWLEDGMENT

Supported by NIA grants AGO 5131 and 10483.

REFERENCES

1. Friedman, L. M., Furberg, C. D., and DeMets, D. L., *Fundamentals of Clinical Trials*, 2nd ed., PSG Publishing, Littleton, MA, 1985.
2. *Diagnostic and Statistical Manual of Mental Disorders*, 4th ed., American Psychiatric Association, Washington, DC, 1994.
3. Corey-Bloom, J., Galasko, D., and Thal, L. J., Longitudinal changes in cognition, in *Dementia*, Burns, A., and Levy, R., Eds., Chapman & Hall, New York, 1994, 79.
4. Galasko, D., Hansen, L. A., Katzman R., et al., Clinical-neuropathological correlations in Alzheimer's disease and related dementias, *Arch. Neurol.*, 51, 888, 1994.
5. Folstein, M. F., Folstein, S. E., and McHugh, P. R., Mini-Mental State: a practical method for grading the cognitive status of patients for the clinician, *J. Psychiatr. Res.* 12, 189, 1975.
6. Green, C. R., Mohs, R. C., Schmeidler, J., et al., Functional decline in Alzheimer's disease: a longitudinal study, *JAGS*, 41, 654, 1993.
7. Mattis, S., Mental status examination for organic mental syndrome in the elderly patient, in *Geriatric Psychiatry: A Handbook for Psychiatrists and Primary Care Physicians*, Bellak, L., and Karasu, T.E., Eds., Grune & Stratton, New York, 1976, 77.
8. Rosen, W. G., Mohs, R. C., and Davis, K. L., A new rating scale for Alzheimer's disease, *Am. J. Psychiatry,* 141, 1356, 1984.
9. Blessed, G., Tomlinson, B.E., and Roth, M., The association between quantitative measures of dementia and of senile change in the cerebral grey matter of elderly subjects, *Br. J. Psychiatry,* 114, 797, 1968.
10. Hansen, L., Salmon, D., Galasko, D., et al., The Lewy body variant of Alzheimer's disease: a clinical and pathological entity, *Neurology,* 40, 1, 1990.
11. Ernst, R. L. and Hay, J. W., The US economic and social costs of Alzheimer's disease revisited, *Am. J. Public Health,* 84, 1261, 1994.
12. Meeting Report: Antidementia Drug Assessment Symposium, Ad Hoc FDA Dementia Assessment Task Force, *Neurobiol. Aging,* 12, 379, 1991.
13. Corder, E. H., Saunder, A. M., and Strittmatter, W. J., Gene dose of apolipoprotein E type 4 allele and the risk of Alzheimer's disease in late onset families, *Science,* 261, 921, 1993.
14. McKhann, G., Drachman, D., Folstein, M., et al., Clinical diagnosis of Alzheimer's disease: report of the NINCDS-ADRDA Work Group under the auspices of Department of Health and Human Services Task Force on Alzheimer's Disease, *Neurology,* 34, 939, 1984.

Chapter 21

PHARMACOLOGICAL APPROACHES TO BEHAVIORAL SYMPTOMS IN ALZHEIMER'S DISEASE

Douglas Galasko

CONTENTS

I. THE CLINICAL APPROACH TO BEHAVIORAL SYMPTOMS

A. BEHAVIORAL SYMPTOMS ARE AN INTEGRAL PART OF ALZHEIMER'S DISEASE

In addition to cognitive symptoms such as memory loss and language impairment, patients with Alzheimer's disease (AD) often develop behavioral symptoms. While cognitive symptoms are required for the diagnosis of AD and are relentlessly progressive, behavioral symptoms are not inevitable, usually fluctuate in severity, and may be intermittent or transient. Because behavioral symptoms are difficult to define uniformly, estimates of their frequency in patients with AD vary. About 50 to 75% of patients with AD will have significant disruptive behavior at some stage of the illness. The repertoire of behavioral symptoms depends on the degree of severity of AD. For example, early in the course of dementia, depression and anxiety are the most common behavioral symptoms. As AD progresses to an intermediate stage, additional symptoms such as delusions, hallucinations, and insomnia may emerge. In more severely demented patients, agitation is likely to be the most prominent abnormal behavior, manifesting as insomnia, nocturnal confusion or "sundowning", restlessness, verbal outbursts, or physical behaviors such as pacing and wandering. It is not always easy to classify these symptoms since patients may show a mixture of several types of behavioral symptoms. Together with incontinence, agitation and related abnormal behaviors are among the most common factors that make patients with AD difficult to manage at home and likely to be moved to a long-term care facility. Successful management of agitation may stall or avert the need for institutional placement of patients.

Although behavioral symptoms vary in appearance and severity among patients with AD, they should be regarded as an integral part of the disease. The pathology of AD affects areas of the brain and neurotransmitter circuits which are likely to predispose patients to behavioral symptoms. For example, depression may be related to degeneration of neurons that use catecholamines as neurotransmitters, while hallucinations may reflect degeneration of neurons in the temporal lobe. In addition, the cortical atrophy responsible for the dementia of AD impairs patients' ability to monitor and interpret their surroundings and behavior. A patient's specific symptoms probably arise from the interaction between AD, premorbid personality, environmental stress, and interpersonal relationships. All of these elements need to be considered when formulating a treatment plan. Not all behavioral symptoms need to be treated. Intervention is usually required when the symptoms cause discomfort to patients, make patients dangerous to themselves or to others, provoke caregiver distress, or increase the level of care that patients require.

1. Clinical Evaluation Should Precede Medical Therapy

Before initiating treatment, the physician must determine whether physical illness, medications, or environmental or interpersonal factors are contributing to the behavioral symptoms. The list of potential underlying conditions is large and requires thorough evaluation. For example, medical conditions such as infections, electrolyte imbalance, stroke, heart attack, and chronic pain may be associated with symptoms of depression, insomnia, or agitation. Impaired vision or hearing may worsen behavioral symptoms. Medications that act on the brain may provoke behavioral symptoms or delirium. A wide range of prescription drugs falls into this category, including theophylline, beta-stimulants, antihypertensive agents such as beta-blockers, and clonidine, digitalis, narcotic analgesics, and corticosteroids. In addition, drugs that act on the central nervous system and are used to treat behavioral symptoms may themselves have behavioral side effects. For example, neuroleptics, tricyclic antidepressants, and benzodiazepines may produce delirium and sometimes may paradoxically increase agitation. It is often worthwhile to decrease or withdraw unnecessary medications before prescribing new ones for symptom control. Changes in a patient's environment may contribute to behavioral symptoms; a move to unfamiliar surroundings or changes in daily routines may lead to anxiety and insomnia. By searching for remediable precipitating factors, the clinician may reduce the need for medications to control behavioral symptoms.

Nonpharmacological approaches are an important adjunct to medical therapy, as discussed in Chapter 23. Caregivers are active partners in developing a treatment plan and should receive counseling and education to enhance their understanding of the behavioral symptoms. They need to realize that the behaviors are related to the neurodegenerative process of AD, that symptoms such as delusions and agitation do not result from the caregiver-patient interaction and therefore should not cause guilt, and that medications may or may not succeed in bringing the symptoms under control. When caregivers overreact to relatively minor behavioral symptoms, counseling may be the major — and only — therapeutic intervention.

2. General Principles of Medication Use in the Elderly

Elderly patients are more sensitive than younger adults to medication effects and side effects. The combination of aging and AD produces marked deficits of brain neurotransmitter systems, particularly acetylcholine, dopamine, norepinephrine, and serotonin. Medications that act on the brain may further block these neurotransmitter circuits, which may result in side effects. Almost every pharmacokinetic process changes with aging, from gastrointestinal absorption of drugs and their binding to plasma proteins, tissues, and receptors to metabolism and excretion. This often results in prolonged half-life, increased accumulation and storage of the drug in various tissues, increased blood levels of the drug, and unwanted side effects. These factors influence the choice of specific drugs.

Interactions between medications may potentiate efficacy, toxicity, or side effects by a variety of mechanisms, including changes in absorption, transport and metabolism, and drug interactions at the level of receptors. Elderly patients often take a large number of medications, which increases the risk of interactions. Special care should be taken when prescribing two or more psychotropic drugs, particularly agents with sedative, hypotensive, or anticholinergic properties. A basic tenet is to use the lowest effective dose of medication for behavioral symptoms. This usually means initiating treatment with a very low dose and increasing the medication gradually. The effective dose in elderly demented patients is often lower than that standardly recommended for younger adults.

Most psychotropic medications act on a broad range of neurotransmitter systems, which may produce side effects such as sedation, poor balance and gait, confusion, orthostatic hypotension, urinary retention, and weight loss. Neuroleptics can also cause extrapyramidal side effects that resemble Parkinson's disease, and tardive dyskinesia characterized by involuntary movements of the tongue, mouth, and face. After initiating treatment for behavioral symptoms, the clinician should therefore monitor blood pressure (both lying and standing) and weight, check the patient's general alertness and cognition, assess gait and balance, and in the case of neuroleptics, look for extrapyramidal findings. If an adequate trial of one medication does not result in symptomatic improvement, a different agent should be tried. After symptom control is achieved, the clinician should reassess the patient at intervals and consider tapering and withdrawing the drug if possible. Because of cognitive impairment, patients with AD may have difficulty complying with medications. To counter this, strategies include simplifying dosing schedules, using day-by-day pill dispensers, and enlisting caregivers to supervise medications. Injectable forms of neuroleptics and sedative medications are used as a last resort, because they have long half-lives and produce drug levels that are difficult to control.

In patients with AD, behavioral symptoms may overlap; for example, agitation may coexist with insomnia. It is important to decide which behaviors require management, as this allows therapy to be aimed at a defined target. Guidelines for tailoring specific medications to behavioral symptoms in patients with AD are tentative at best (Table 1). Most research studies in this area are difficult to interpret because of varying definitions of symptoms, crude measurement of symptom severity, side effects and outcomes, and small numbers of patients. Moreover, few studies have met the "gold standard" of being double-blind and placebo-controlled. Many of the recommendations that follow describe medications that have been incompletely evaluated for the control of behavioral symptoms in patients with AD or are extrapolated from studies of treatment of behavioral symptoms in cognitively normal elderly patients.

TABLE 1   Medications for Behavioral Symptom Control in Alzheimer's Disease

Symptom	Class of medication
Depression	Cyclic antidepressants
	SSRI agents
	MAO inhibitors
Psychosis	Neuroleptics
	Atypical neuroleptics
Insomnia	Benzodiazepines
	Sedatives
	Sedating antidepressants
Anxiety	Benzodiazepines
Agitation	Neuroleptics
	Atypical neuroleptics
	Sedating antidepressants

II. TREATMENT OF SPECIFIC BEHAVIORAL SYMPTOMS

A. DEPRESSION

Although over 50% of patients with AD develop apathy and loss of interest, clinicians are uncertain about whether to interpret these as mild forms of depression or as symptoms intrinsic to AD. Sustained major depression is uncommon and affects about 15 to 20% of patients with AD, usually early in the course of illness. Depression may be underrecognized in patients with more severe dementia because they have difficulty expressing their symptoms. Many studies have shown that drug treatment of depression in nondemented people over the age of 60 is efficacious and safe, with response rates of 60 to 70%, regardless of which agent is used. Treatment studies of depressed patients with AD are scant and generally have not followed a double-blind, placebo-controlled design.

Cyclic antidepressants have been a mainstay in the treatment of depression. They have a wide range of potential side effects in the elderly. Antihistamine actions may cause sedation, although this sometimes is beneficial for patients with depression and insomnia. Antiadrenergic effects may lead to orthostasis; anticholinergic actions may result in confusion, urinary retention, constipation, or tachycardia. Tricyclic agents slow cardiac conduction and should be avoided if the EKG shows bundle branch block because of the risk of causing high-grade heart block. For these reasons, when treating elderly patients, clinicians prefer to prescribe nortriptyline or desipramine, which are secondary amines with less-pronounced side effects than tertiary amines such as imipramine or amitriptyline.

Monoamine oxidase inhibitors (MAO-Is) are efficacious in depressed elderly patients, despite concerns about their potentially serious side effects of increasing blood pressure. Dietary restrictions accompanying the use of MAO-Is prohibit foods with a high content of tyramine (including cheese, chocolate, coffee, and alcohol) and may be difficult to enforce in demented patients. MAO-Is therefore remain second-order choices for treating depression in patients with AD.

A recent theme in antidepressant drug development is to augment serotonin neurotransmission, thought to be impaired in depression. Selective serotonin reuptake inhibitors (SSRIs) have recently achieved success in clinical trials of young depressed patients and are currently widely used in clinical practice. The first of these agents, fluoxetine, has efficacy comparable to that of tricyclics in elderly depressed patients, but fewer cardiovascular and minimal anticholinergic side effects. Other medications in the SSRI class are sertraline and paroxetine. The newest selective antidepressant is velnafaxine, which inhibits reuptake of serotonin and norepinephrine. These agents have not been formally studied in AD, and although free of the adverse effects typical of tricyclic antidepressants, they can produce a different profile of side effects that includes insomnia, tremor, and loss of appetite. They are also more expensive than other antidepressant medications.

There is little evidence that cognition improves in patients with AD as a result of treating depression. The choice of medication usually is guided by side effect profiles and considerations of cost. In patients with AD whose depression is refractory to medications, electroconvulsive therapy (ECT) may be used.

B. PSYCHOTIC SYMPTOMS

Delusions and hallucinations occur most often in patients with AD who have mild to moderately severe dementia. These symptoms, although dramatic, do not always disrupt the patient or the caregiver and should not automatically be treated with medications. For example, visual hallucinations or delusions that people are hiding the patient's belongings are unlikely to need medication. On the other hand, delusions that people are trying to harm the patient or that the patient's spouse has been replaced by an impostor are more likely to need pharmacological suppression. Neuroleptic medications are usually the first choice for controlling psychotic symptoms. In an attempt to avoid the side effects of neuroleptics on the motor system, namely Parkinsonism and tardive dyskinesia, novel antipsychotics have recently been developed. These include clozapine and risperadone. Aspects of treatment with these agents are discussed under agitation.

C. INSOMNIA

Sleep research has demonstrated that the structure of sleep breaks down in association with aging and especially affects patients with AD. Although many ingenious interventions have been developed to entrain patients to more regular sleep-wake cycles, including bright light therapy and careful scheduling of daytime activity, at times medications are needed. The earliest sedative drugs included long-acting benzodiazepines and barbiturates. Although effective for short-term use, they produced drowsiness that carried over into daytime, and impaired gait and balance, predisposing patients to falls. These long-acting agents are therefore contraindicated in AD. Of the older sedatives, chloral hydrate remains in current use, usually on an intermittent dosing schedule. Newer approaches to pharmacological management include using short-acting benzodiazepines, such as lorazepam or temazepam. These medications have not been rigorously studied for treating insomnia in patients with AD, although several short-term studies have reported on their use to control agitation. All benzodiazepines can produce confusion and cognitive worsening in patients with AD, and low doses should be used whenever possible. When benzodiazepines are used chronically, tolerance frequently develops, with declining effects of a previously stable dose. To counteract the development of tolerance, an important recommendation is to use benzodiazepines discontinuously; for example, temazepam should be given no more than 4 to 5 days per week. Another popular medication for treating insomnia is trazodone, a cyclic antidepressant with sedating properties.

D. ANXIETY

Anxiety is relatively uncommon in patients with AD. Several classes of medications may be used, most of which can produce tolerance with long-term use. Among the benzodiazepines, the factor of shorter half-life favors agents such as lorazepam and oxazepam over diazepam. Several newer agents have been developed. Buspirone, an azapirone derivative, is an effective anxiolytic which may carry less risk of tolerance than benzodiazepines. Alprazolam has an excellent safety profile in young patients and may also be useful in treating anxiety in patients with AD.

E. AGITATION

Neuroleptics are widely used in managing agitation. These agents may produce serious side effects, including Parkinsonism, tardive dyskinesia, confusion, and falls. They have been overused for chemical restraint, especially in institutions, and have been linked to serious consequences of falls such as hip fractures. Patients with AD who have Parkinsonism may be especially sensitive to neuroleptics and may develop severe rigidity and bradykinesia after treatment.

A recent meta-analysis of double-blind, placebo-controlled studies of neuroleptics in agitated demented patients showed that these medications, used in relatively low doses, had a significant, though small, symptomatic effect. Overall, 41% of patients improved with placebo, compared with 59% on neuroleptics; in other terms, 18 of 100 dementia patients with behavioral symptoms clearly responded to neuroleptics beyond chance. Comparative analyses did not suggest that any specific neuroleptic had relatively greater overall efficacy than any other. Many clinicians prefer to prescribe high-potency agents such as haloperidol or fluphenazine because they are less likely to produce sedation and anticholinergic activity than low potency agents such as thioridazine; as a trade-off, high potency agents are more likely to produce parkinsonism. Neuroleptics in dementia are a double-edged sword, but the evidence favors their careful use.

Atypical neuroleptics were recently introduced into clinical practice to treat psychosis. These agents bind poorly to the D2 type of dopamine receptor in the brain and therefore are far less likely to produce extrapyramidal side effects. Clozapine, the first of these, can cause bone marrow depression. Extensive blood monitoring is required, which dampens enthusiasm for using clozapine in elderly demented patients. Risperadone was recently released in the U.S. for the treatment of psychotic symptoms. In clinical trials in schizophrenic patients, this medication showed efficacy in controlling psychosis with very few side effects when used at low doses. Although this drug shows promise, it has not been tested for psychosis or agitation in patients with AD. Since risperadone retains modest D2-binding activity, its side effect profile in elderly patients could pose problems.

Trazodone, as discussed earlier, has antidepressant and sleep-promoting actions. It has been shown to improve agitation as well as mood in several studies which included elderly patients with dementia. Even though high doses, ranging from 150 to 500 mg/day, were often used, the safety profile of trazodone was fairly good. The sedating action of trazodone may be advantageous in patients who show nocturnal agitation or sundowning.

Chloral hydrate, sedative-hypnotics, and benzodiazepines can be helpful in controlling agitation in patients with AD. Because their calming effect is achieved by sedation, these medications may be best suited for use as adjuncts to neuroleptics or trazodone or for short-term control of particularly severe episodes of agitation.

III. FUTURE DIRECTIONS

Research in psychopharmacology is maturing to an extent that receptor- and neurotransmitter-specific medications are becoming available for clinical application. As a result, recommendations for treating behavioral symptoms are likely to change rapidly in the next few years. The discovery of SSRI agents for treating depression and atypical neuroleptics for psychosis heralds an exciting future. However, enthusiasm for bringing new and supposedly improved drugs from bench to bedside must be tempered by insisting that the efficacy of these drugs is documented by systematic testing in appropriate groups of patients, using formal clinical trials with double-blind, placebo-controlled design, to determine their merits and potential side effects.

REFERENCES

1. Salzman, C., Neuropsychopharmacology, in *The Clinical Neurology of Aging*, Katzman, R. and Rowe, J., Eds., F.A. Davis, Philadelphia, 1992, 59.
2. Cohen-Mansfield, J. and Billig, N., Agitated behavior in the elderly: a conceptual review, *J. Am. Geriat. Soc.*, 34, 711, 1986.
3. Salzman, C., Treatment of agitation in the elderly, in *Psychopharmacology: A Generation of Progress*, Meltzer, H.Y., Ed., New York, Raven Press, 1987, 1167.
4. Wragg, R.E., and Jeste, D.V., Overview of depression and psychosis in Alzheimer's disease, *Am. J. Psychiat.*, 146, 577, 1989.

5. Schneider, L.S., Pollock, V.E., and Lyness, S.A., A metaanalysis of controlled trials of neuroleptic treatment in dementia, *J. Am. Geriat. Soc.*, 38, 553, 1990.

6. Prinz, P.N., Vitiello, M.V., Raskind, M.A., and Thorpy, M.J., Geriatrics: sleep disorders and aging, *N. Engl. J. Med.*, 323, 520, 1991.

7. Song, F., Freemantle, N., Sheldon, T.A., House, A., Watson, P., Long, A., and Mason, J., Selective serotonin reuptake inhibitors: meta-analysis of efficacy and acceptability, *Br. Med. J.*, 306, 683, 1993.

Chapter 22

TREATMENT OF ALZHEIMER'S DISEASE

Lina Shihabuddin
Kenneth L. Davis

CONTENTS

I. INTRODUCTION

There are currently two main approaches to the treatment of Alzheimer's disease. The first, presumably a palliative one, is neurotransmitter replacement, most commonly based on the cholinergic deficits demonstrated in this disease. The second is a neuroprotective approach, aimed at protecting neurons from further degeneration and thus stopping cognitive deterioration.

Several studies have documented the role of cholinergic system in Alzheimer's disease, as well as in memory and learning. It is known that (1) centrally active anticholinergic agents produce attention and memory deficits (Dundee and Pandit 1972, Drachman and Leavitt 1974), (2) the cholinergic system modulates memory and learning (Deutsch 1971), and (3) lesions in the central cholinergic system cause memory and learning impairment which are relieved with cholinergic agonists, acetylcholinesterase inhibitors, and acetylcholine releasing agents (Haroutunian et al., 1990; Bartus et al., 1987; Collerton, 1986; Olton and Wenk, 1987). Moreover, post-mortem studies of Alzheimer's disease patients demonstrated that cholinergic abnormalities correlate with the degree of cognitive impairment (Davies and Maloney, 1976; Perry et al., 1977, 1978). The findings of central cholinergic depletion in Alzheimer's disease, together with the role of the cholinergic system in memory and learning, lead to the cholinergic enhancement treatment approach. The replacement strategies have yielded some promising findings, yet the results have not demonstrated robustness and universality (Eagger et al., 1992; Chatellier et al., 1990; Farlow et al., 1992; Davis et al., 1992). The variable results seen with cholinergic replacement may be in part due to other neurotransmitters involved in the disease process. This hypothesis lead to combination therapies aiming at several neurotransmitter deficiencies.

The alternative to this palliative approach is the neuroprotective strategy which interferes with the degenerative process and aims at modifying the course of the disease by altering the fundamental pathophysiological processes. There is evidence of involvement of the immune system in Alzheimer's disease (Aisen et al., 1994). Several markers of inflammation have been demonstrated in the brains of Alzheimer's disease patients on histochemical studies (Aisen et al., 1994). Moreover, there is a decreased incidence of Alzheimer's disease in patients on chronic anti-inflammatory medications. These hypotheses lead to trials of anti-inflammatory drugs in the treatment of Alzheimer's disease. Another rationale for the neuroprotective approach is the fact that Alzheimer's disease is characterized by senile plaques and neurofibrillary tangles. It has been proposed that amyloid beta protein (AB), which is the principle constituent of senile plaques, causes cell death and neurofibrillary tangles (Hardy and Higgins, 1992; Wisniewski et al., 1990). AB is derived from processing of the transmembrane protein amyloid precursor protein (Goldgaber et al., 1987). The presence of AB in Alzheimer's disease may result from several causes. Amyloid precursor protein (APP) can undergo secretory processing that occurs within the domain of AB, thereby precluding amyloidogenesis (Suzuki et al., 1992). In contrast, lysosomal processing of amyloid precursor protein can produce amyloidogenic fragments (Estus et al., 1992; Golde et al., 1992; Haass et al., 1992). Increased synthesis of APP in certain cell types would in turn overwhelm the capacity of the cell to degrade its substrate through regular pathways. A disrupted balance between protease and protease inhibitors in the brain could lead to abnormal degradation of APP and increased production of AB (Robakis et al., 1991). Two forms of APP contain a Kunitz-type protease inhibitors (KPI) insert that may provide protease inhibitor activity to APP. Protease inhibitors have been shown to modulate cell growth and might be involved in the neuronal sprouting activity associated with plaques (Monard, 1987; Probst et al., 1983). The presence of ACT in plaques further supports a role of plasma proteinase inhibitors in amyloidogenesis. Thus, agents that interfere with AB production or deposition could alter the course of Alzheimer's disease.

In this chapter the agents used in replacement therapy are discussed followed by the combination therapy and the therapies aimed at modifying the course of the disease.

II. B-NEUROTRANSMITTER REPLACEMENT

A. CHOLINERGIC AGONISTS:

Alzheimer's disease patients consistently show cholinergic abnormalities correlating with cognitive impairment (Davies and Maloney, 1976; Perry et al., 1977, 1978). Both muscarinic and nicotinic receptors have been implicated in cognition in Alzheimer's disease. Five muscarinic receptors subtypes, known as M1 to M5, have been demonstrated and localized in the CNS (Fukada et al., 1989; Bonner et al., 1987; Bonner, 1989; Ashkenazi et al., 1989; Birdsall et al., 1989; Yasuda et al., 1993). Studies with pharmacological agonists have identified four classes of muscarinic receptors that are known as M1, M2, M3, M4 (Waelbroeck et al., 1990). The subtypes identified by antisera (M1 to M5) show substantial overlap with the receptors identified pharmacologically (M1 to M4) (Yasuda et al., 1993). The postsynaptic M1 receptors, the main subtype found in the cerebral cortex, have been implicated in memory processes (Nordberg et al., 1992; Potter et al., 1987). Activation of the M1, M3, and M5 receptors causes cellular excitation, whereas activation of the M2 and M4 subtypes produces inhibitory effects (Bonner, 1989). The excitatory role of the M1 and M3 receptors combined with their location in the cortex and hippocampus make these sites potential targets for pharmacological treatment of the cognitive deficits in Alzheimer's disease.

There are at least three different subtypes of nicotinic receptors in the human frontal cortex (Sugaya et al., 1990). The nicotinic receptors can be divided into three types called super-high, high, and low affinity (Nordberg et al., 1992). The high-affinity nicotinic sites in the brain of Alzheimer's disease patients are reportedly decreased (Sugaya et al., 1990; Nordberg et al., 1992). In animal studies, the nicotinic antagonist produces a dose-dependent impairment of memory comparable to those observed with scopolamine (Elrod and Buccafusco, 1991). The nicotinic and muscarinic systems appear to jointly modulate performance in learning and memory (Riekkinen et al., 1990). Animal data suggest that presynaptic nicotinic receptors mediate a positive feedback mechanism that modulates cholinergic activity (Elrod and Buccasfusco, 1991).

1. Bethanacol

Bethanacol is a synthetic β-methyl analog of acetylcholine. It is a relatively short-acting cholinergic agonist with muscarinic selectivity. Bethanacol has poor blood-brain barrier permeability; thus, it needs to be administered by intracerebral ventricular route. This route of administration carries some risks, including those related to anesthesia, pneumocephalus, seizures, and chronic subdural hematomas. Studies on small samples of patients showed modest improvement of cognition with Bethanacol (Read et al., 1990; Harbaugh et al., 1987).

2. Arecoline

Arecoline is a natural alkaloid with both muscarinic and nicotinic agonist properties. Arecoline administration to normal volunteers improves learning (Sitaram et al., 1978). Modest improvement in verbal and spatial memory has been observed after continuous intravenous infusion of arecoline for 5 days in patients with Alzheimer's disease (Raffaele et al., 1991).

3. RS-86

RS-86 (2-ethyl-8-methyl-2,8-diazospiro-4,5-decan-1,3-dionhydrobromide) is a long-acting cholinergic agonist with good blood-brain barrier permeability. RS-86 is selective for muscarinic receptors. Oral administration of RS-86 has no effect (Bruno et al., 1985, Mouradian et al. 1988, Hollander et al. 1987) or minimal effect (Wettstein and Spiegal, 1984) on cognitive function in patients with Alzheimer's disease.

4. Oxotremorine

Oxotremorine is a synthetic nonselective muscarinic agonist with a half-life of several hours. Oral administration of oxotremorine to Alzheimer's disease patients did not improve cognitive function and was associated with significant side effects including depression and anxiety (Davis et al., 1987).

5. Nicotine

Although muscarinic receptors play a significant role in memory, there is evidence to suggest involvement of nicotinic receptors as well in Alzheimer's disease. The nicotinic and muscarinic systems jointly modulate learning and memory (Elrod and Buccafusco, 1991). The infusion of 0.5 µg/kg of nicotine per hour produced significant effects on mood in Alzheimer's disease patients. The same dose rarely had such effects in normal non-age-matched control subjects (Sunderland et al., 1988). Intravenous nicotine administration to Alzheimer's disease patients has been shown to improve performance in recall (Newhouse et al., 1988). The toxic effects of nicotine manifested by anxiety and depressive symptoms limit the clinical utility of this drug.

6. Other Agonists

F102B [*cis*-2-methylspiro-(1,3-oxathiolane-5,3')quinuclidine] is a structurally rigid analog of acetylcholine. It is a selective M1 agonist and crosses the blood-brain barrier. F102B reverses the cognitive impairment observed in hypocholinergic animals (Fisher et al., 1991). It has not yet been tested in Alzheimer's disease.

Xanomeline, an arecoline derivative, is a muscarinic agonist with selective affinity for central M1 receptors. It is orally bioavailable with a high degree of individual variability after first pass. In a study of approximately 300 patients with Alzheimer's disease, xanomeline was shown to be safe and efficacious. In this study clinical efficacy was dose dependent. Baseline to end-point improvement in cognition with xanomeline 75 mg tid was superior to placebo on neuropsychological testing, CIBIC, and CGI (Tollefson et al., personal communications).

BIBN 99 is a lipophilic compound which readily crosses the blood-brain barrier. It is a muscarinic receptor blocker with higher affinity to M2 than M1. It is speculated that such properties will be warranted in treatment of Alzheimer's disease.

Other drugs which are partial M1 agonists and partial M2 antagonists which might alleviate central cholinergic deficits in Alzheimer's disease with less peripheral side effects are under development. Since the deficits in Alzheimer's disease involve both the muscarinic and the nicotinic system, agents that stimulate the nicotinic receptors as well are worth consideration.

B. CHOLINESTERASE INHIBITORS

1. Tetrahydroaminoacridine (THA)

1,2,3,4-Tetrahydro-9-acridinamine (THA), known as tacrine, is a synthetic aminoacradine. Tacrine is the first drug approved by the FDA (1993) for the treatment of cognitive impairment in Alzheimer's disease. The commercially available drug Cognex is tacrine monohydrochloride monohydrate. This is a reversible noncompetitive ACHE inhibitor with an elimination half-life of 2 to 4 hours; it is rapidly absorbed when administered orally. The mechanism by which THA increases brain ACH levels is not clear. Various mechanisms including its blocking effect on slow K+ channels and its M1 cholinergic effects have been implicated. It has also been suggested that THA may lead to increased ACH synthesis (Peterson, 1990). THA has been shown to bind to muscarinic and nicotinic receptor sites. The affinity for muscarinic receptors is about 100 times higher than for nicotinic receptors. The clinical relevance of the direct effects of THA at the cholinergic receptor site depends on the actual concentration of THA in human brain tissue *in vivo*. Recent findings of high concentration of THA in the brain strengthens the possibility that THA's effects may be mediated by its activity at cholinergic receptor sites (for review see Adem, 1992; Freeman and Dawson, 1991). The enzymatic activity of monoamine oxidases (MAO) type A and B have been shown to be reduced by THA. MAO-A seems to be inhibited to a larger degree than MAO-B. At therapeutic concentrations THA is believed to produce a significant decrease in MAO activity leading to an enhanced monoaminergic activity. Knowing that some cognitive deficits in Alzheimer's disease are believed to be due to a monoaminergic deficit, this enhancement might also contribute to the therapeutic effect of THA in Alzheimer's disease. In addition, THA has been shown to induce monoamine release and inhibit monoamine uptake leading to an increase in several monoamine neurotransmitters including dopamine, serotonin, and norepinephrine (Drukarch et al., 1987, 1988).

Eight large placebo-controlled studies have assessed the efficacy of tacrine in large samples of AD patients (see Table 1). A 6-week parallel trial using an enriched-population design (Davis et al., 1992) found that patients treated with THA showed significantly less decline in cognitive function than the placebo-treated group as assessed by the Alzheimer's Disease Assessment Scale cognitive subscale. A 12-week parallel group design demonstrated a significant dose-related cognitive improvement with THA (Farlow et al., 1992). Similar results were reported in a study of 30-weeks' duration (Knapp et al., 1994). Two recently published studies, one with a crossover design and the other with a parallel design, failed to find statistically significant differences between THA and placebo (Wilcock et al., 1994; Maltby et al., 1994). THA in combination with lecithin resulted in significant improvement in Mini-Mental Status scores in two studies (Gauthier et al., 1990; Eagger et al., 1992) and in minimal to no cognitive improvement in two others (Chatellier et al., 1990; Maltby et al., 1994). From the above studies, it is suggested that lecithin is not essential and probably does not contribute to the therapeutic effect of THA. Moreover, these studies suggest that THA in a dose of 80 to 160 mg for at least 2 weeks produces a significant improvement in cognitive performance tests as well as in global clinical measures.

Side effects of THA include nausea, abdominal distress, tachycardia, and liver toxicity. The elevation in liver transaminases is dose-dependent and is reversible with stopping the drug.

2. Physostigmine

Physostigmine is a natural alkaloid that is absorbed in the gastrointestinal tract, subcutaneous tissue, and mucous membrane. It readily crosses the blood-brain barrier and reaches maximal levels in short time; it is hydrolyzed and inactivated within 2 hours. Most studies using parenteral administration of physostigmine have documented transient cognitive improvement in at least a subgroup of patients with AD (Mohs and Davis, 1987). Oral administration of the drug has shown to have some efficacy as well (Mohs et al., 1985). It has been speculated that long-term treatment with physostigmine, or any cholimemetic, may delay deterioration in Alzheimer's disease: four out of five patients who received the drug over a 3-year period did not significantly deteriorate in their performances on the Buschke selective reminding task (Beller, 1988). Two out of six patients treated with oral physostigmine for 29 months also did not show deterioration, whereas all six drug free subjects did (Jenike, 1990). However, these observations are little more than intriguing anecdotes. Oral physostigmine administration is associated with problems. For example, the blood, and therefore CNS, levels achieved with a given dose are quite variable and necessitate individual titration of medication. Blood levels required to achieve CNS concentrations necessary for cognitive enhancement may be associated with significant adverse effects. Physostigmine short half-life is also a problem further intensifying fluctuations in drug levels and necessitating the frequent administration.

3. Galanthamine

Galanthamine is a tertiary amine of the phenthrene group which is a competitive cholinesterase inhibitor with no butrylcholinesterase activity. It has a half-life of 7 hours which is longer than that of THA and physostigmine (Thomsen et al., 1990). Studies show that it has good bioavailability after oral administration (Mihailova et al., 1989). Galanthamine 30 mg PO per day in divided doses over 2 months administered to nine AD patients was well tolerated and appeared to be beneficial (Rainer et al., 1989). In an open trial of 30 mg Galanthamine in 18 AD patients treated for 2 months showed no significant changes on neuropsychological tests; however, after being on the drug for 1 year, six patients showed a positive change in competency of everyday routine and in emotional situations (Dal-Bianco et al., 1991). Preliminary reports from a recent double-blind trial with over

TABLE 1

Study	Sample size	Scales	Tacrine before, mean(SD)	Tacrine after, mean(SD)	Change	Placebo before, mean(SD)	Placebo after, mean(SD)	Change
Davis et al.	215, 80 mg/d for 6 wks	ADAS, c	30.7(19.0)	31.1(20.6)	0.5*	29.2(17.6)	32.2(17.6)	3.0
		CGIC	NA	3.9	NA	NA	4.0	NA
		ADAS, to	35.5(23.5)	36.2(23.5)	0.7*	33.9	37.7(20.6)	3.8
		PDS	46.8	46.7	-0.1*	(20.6) 46.6	44.1	-2.5
		IADL	17.5	17.5	0.0*	17.6	18.1	0.5
		PSMS	8.5(4.41)	8.8(4.4)	0.3	8.3(3.0)	8.2(3.0)	-0.1
		MMSE	16.1(8.82)	16.0(8.8)	-0.1*	16.3(7.3)	15.3(7.3)	-0.9
Farlow et al.	98, 20 mg/d for 12 wks	ADAS, nc	6.3(5.0)	5.4(5.0)	-0.9	6.1(6.0)	5.5(4.5)	-0.6
		ADAS, to	32.5(13.8)	31.4(14.8)	-1.1	34.2(15.7)	34.2(16.5)	0.1
		MMSE	19.0(6.0)	19.0(6.0)	0.0	17.9(5.2)	17.9(6.7)	-0.1
		CGIC	NA	3.9	NA	NA	4.2(1.1)	NA
		PDS	51.9(18.8)	50.5(19.8)	-1.4	46.6(17.2)	42.9(20.2)	-3.7
Farlow et al.	82, 40 mg/d for 12 wks	ADAS, nc	6.0(4.5)	5.3(6.3)	-0.7*	6.1(6.0)	5.5(4.5)	-0.6
		ADAS, to	33.3(14.4)	31.6(16.2)	-1.7*	34.2(15.7)	34.2(16.5)	0.1
		MMSE	18.3(4.5)	18.8(5.4)	-0.5	17.9(5.2)	17.9(6.7)	-0.1
		CGIC	NA	3.7(1.1)	NA*	NA	4.2(1.1)	NA
		PDS	51.4(19.8)	50.9(20.7)	-0.5	46.6(17.2)	42.9(20.2)	-3.7
Farlow et al.	37, 80 mg/d for 12 wks	ADAS, nc	5.0(4.3)	4.9(4.9)	-0.1*	6.1(6.0)	5.5(4.5)	-0.6
		ADAS, to	32.5(16.5)	28.8(17.1)	-3.7*	34.2(15.7)	34.2(16.5)	0.1
		MMSE	19.0(4.9)	19.8(5.5)	0.8	17.9(5.2)	17.9(6.7)	-0.1
		CGIC	NA	3.5	NA*	NA	4.2(1.1)	NA
		PDS	53.4(17.7)	49.2(20.1)	-4.1	46.6(17.2)	42.9(20.2)	-3.7
Gauthier et al.	52, up to 100 mg/d for 8 wks	MMSE	17.3(5.8)	16.9(6.8)	0.94	NA	NA	NA
		3MMSE	55.1(18.3)	49.3(23.1)	5.82*	NA	NA	NA
		HDS	149.6(23.1)	135.1(33.8)	14.52*	NA	NA	NA
		RDRS–II	26.7(6.7)	30.1(7.7)	-3.33*	NA	NA	NA
		BSAD, sy	5.9(6.9)	7.52(6.65)	-1.56*	NA	NA	NA
		BSAD, gl	1.2(1.2)	1.30(1.11)	-0.13	NA	NA	NA
Chatellier et al.	49, mean 114 mg for 4 mo	MMSE	15.0(6.2)	17.2(6.2)	-2.2	13.7(5.8)	14.9(6.4)	-1.2
		SGS	23.4(13.6)	21.7(13.8)	1.7	33.9(19.8)	30.2(15.7)	3.7

Study	Dose	Scale						
Knapp et al.	263, 80 mg/d for 30 wks	CIBI	NA	NA	-0.3*			
		ADAS, co	30.6(14.1)	NA	-2.3*			
		FCCA	NA	NA	-0.3*			
		GDS	NA	NA	0.05			
		CGIC	NA	NA	6.6			
		PDS	NA	NA	3.1*			
		ADAS, nc	NA	NA	-0.1			
		ADAS, to	16.8(4.6)	NA	-2.4			
		MMSE			1.3			
Knapp et al.	263, 120 mg/d for 30 wks	CIBI	NA	NA	-0.3			
		ADAS, co	30.6(14.1)	NA	-1.8			
		FCCA	NA	NA	-0.4*			
		GDS	NA	NA	-0.1			
		CGIC	NA	NA	3.5			
		PDS	NA	NA	4.5*			
		ADAS, nc	NA	NA	0.9			
		ADAS, to	16.8(4.6)	NA	-0.4			
		MMSE			0.6			
Knapp et al.	263, 160 mg/d for 30 wks	CIBI	NA	NA	-0.5*			
		ADAS, co	30.6(14.1)	NA	-5.3*			
		FCCA	NA	NA	-0.6*			
		GDS	NA	NA	-0.2*			
		CGIC	NA	NA	9.4			
		PDS	NA	NA	4.6*			
		ADAS, nc	NA	NA	-0.8			
		ADAS, to	16.8(4.6)	NA	-6.4*			
		MMSE			2.5*			
Eagger et al.	73 up to 125 mg/d for 13 wks	MMSE	15.93(6.8)	17.7(8.00)	-1.77	18.5(6.3)	17.4(6.0)	1.05
		AMTS	5.58(3.1)	6.88(3.44)	-1.3	5.7(2.6)	6.5(2.7)	-0.8
		ADL	34.50(5.8)	33.83(6.63)	0.6	35.0(7.7)	34.4(8.1)	0.63

Note: ADAS,c = Alzheimer's disease assessment scale, cognitive; ADAS, nc = Alzheimer's disease assessment scale, noncognitive; ADAS, to = Alzheimer's disease assessment scale, total; CGIC = clinical global impression of change; IADL = instrumental activities of daily living; PDS = progressive deteriorating scale; PSMS = physical self maintainance scale; MMSE = mini mental status exam; 3MMSE = modified mini mental status exam; HDS = hierarchic dementia scale; RDRS-II = rapid disability rating scale II; BSAD, sy = behavioral scale for Alzheimer's disease, symptoms; BSAD, gl = behavioral scale for Alzheimer's disease, global impression; SGS = Stockton geriatric score; GDS = global deterioration scale; CIBI = clinical interview based impression; AMTS = abbreviated mental test score; ADL = activities of daily living.

100 patients indicate that galathamine 30 to 50 mg PO per day for up to 13 weeks showed significant improvement in cognitive performance assessed by cADAS, MMSE, CGI, and SKT. Unlike tacrine galanthamine was without hepatotoxicity (Kewitz et al., 1994).

4. E2020

E2020 1-bezyl-4-(5,6-dimethoxy1-indanon)-2-yl)-methylpiperidine hydrochrolide is another ACHE inhibitor. The drug has a half-life of 50 hours and is substantially bound to plasma proteins. In a 14-week randomized double-blind study of 160 patients, E2020 was well tolerated with no significant effects on physical or laboratory results. In that study, E2020 5 mg daily produced significant improvement in cognition and quality of life as measured by ADAS-cog, MMSE, and QOL while CGIC revealed a 50% reduction in patients showing clinical decline. Trends for improvement were also present on the Clinical Dementia Rating and Activities of Daily Living scales. Some dose related improvement, without statistical significance, was observed in the 1 and 3 mg groups (Rogers et al., 1994).

C. CHOLINERGIC RELEASING AGENTS
1. DuP 996

Linopiridine [DuP996; 3,3-bis(4-pyrindinlmethyl)-1-phenylindolin-2-one] enhances potassium-stimulated release of acetylcholine, dopamine, and serotonin without effecting basal neurotransmitter release (Nicholson et al., 1990). DuP 996 has been shown to protect against hypoxia-induced passive avoidance deficits in rodents (Cook et al., 1990). The drug also seems to enhance ACH synthesis to replenish neurotransmitter storage (Vickroy, 1993). Autoradiographic studies demonstrating linopirdine binding sites in the cortex and hippocampus support the potential usefulness of this agent for the treatment of cognitive deficits in Alzheimer's disease (DeSouza et al., 1992). In humans, administration of DuP 996 induces EEG changes consistent vigilance-improving properties (Saletu et al., 1989). Unpublished clinical results have been mixed with only sporadic statistically significant differences of active drug over placebo (DuPont Merck Pharmaceutical Co., data on file).

2. ENA 713

The SANDOZ compound ENA 713, a centrally selective acetylcholine inhibitor, has been studied in two international multicenter studies in Europe, one involving 402 patients recruited at more than 50 centers in 11 European countries, the other one involving 114 patients from 11 centers in 5 countries. Experience up to this time shows the compound to have the expected effects of a centrally active acetylcholine inhibitor: good tolerability up to a single dose of 3 mg in young and elderly subjects, CNS-related effects starting at a single dose of 1.0 mg, adverse events such as nausea and vomiting at a single dose of 4 mg and higher. Long-lasting inhibition of cholinesterase is observed in volunteers and patients. The compound is biologically well tolerated, after due titration, up to 12 mg per day in patients with Alzheimer's disease. No hepatotoxicity is observed. Pharmacokinetics parameters show marked individual variability. Plasma levels of the compound and its main metabolite do not appear to be related to its tolerability. There is evidence of a statistically significant effect of ENA 713 on some of the core cognitive and behavioral symptoms in a certain percentage of Alzheimer's patients (Spiegel et al., 1994).

D. COMBINED TREATMENT APPROACH

There is ample evidence demonstrating that multiple neurotransmitter systems are involved in Alzheimer's disease; thus a combined treatment strategy is likely to be more efficacious than cholinergic monotherapy. Animal research shows that noradrenergic brain lesions negate cholino-mimetic enhancement of memory in hypocholinergic animals (Haroutunian et al., 1985). Admin-istration of alpha adrenergic agonist clonidine in turn restores the efficacy of cholinomimetic treatment in animals with a large noradrenergic and modest cholinergic lesions (Haroutunian et al.,

1990). The alpha adrenergic antagonist idazoxan, which enhances locus cereleus firing and nore-pinephrine turnover, has been shown to improve memory in rodents (Sara et al., 1989). Moreover, post-mortem studies showed major neurotransmitter losses of the noradrenergic systems in Alzheimer's disease patients. All these findings support the use of a combination of cholinergic and noradrenergic agents to treat AD.

A pilot study with clonidine and physostigmine treatment in nine patients showed the safety and feasibility of combining these agents in AD (Davidson et al., 1989). In another study the combination of physostigmine and yohimbine, an alpha 2 antagonist, was well tolerated in AD patients (Bierer et al., 1993). Studies evaluating the efficacy of this treatment have primarily used cholinesterase inhibitors and monoamine oxidase inhibitor L-deprenyl. Several double-blind placebo-controlled studies done on small patient samples showed that treatment with 10 mg/day of L-deprenyl improves performance on attention, memory, and learning tasks (Angoli et al., 1990; Mangoni et al., 1991; Piccinin et al., 1990; Tariot et al., 1987a, 1987b; Marin et al., 1993). Higher doses were associated with more side effects and were not as efficacious (Tariot et al., 1987a). The beneficial effects of L-deprenyl do not appear to be related to its antidepressant effects since the MAO-A inhibitor tranylcypromine did not improve cognitive performance in AD patients (Tariot et al., 1988b).

The possible additive effects of L-deprenyl and cholinesterase inhibitors is suggested by the double-blind placebo-controlled 4-week crossover study which demonstrated that augmentation of either THA or physostigmine with L-deprenyl significantly improved performance on the cognitive subscales of the ADAS (Schneider et al., 1993). L-Deprenyl improved cognitive performance in physostigmine nonresponders in a double-blind study of 17 AD patients, suggesting monoaminergic therapy may be appropriate for a subgroup of patients (Marin et al., 1993). In another double-blind placebo-controlled study of 16 AD patients, no significant improvement with the combination of deprenyl and physostigmine was found (Sunderland et al., 1992). However, plasma levels of physostigmine were below therapeutic levels in many patients.

1. ESTROGEN

Studies have suggested that estrogen may have an effect on cognition and mood in women. *In vivo* studies showed estrogen effects on several neurotransmitters including serotonin and acetylcholine (Luine et al., 1975; 1980). Cognitive improvement has been reported in Alzheimer's disease female patients with estrogen replacement therapy (Fillit et al., 1986; Honjo et al., 1989). In a 30-week randomized clinical trial of tacrine, patients who received estrogen replacement therapy had a 50% greater response to tacrine than the patients who did not (Schneider et al., 1994).

III. NEUROPROTECTIVE AGENTS

A. ANTIOXIDANTS

Increased free radical production in AD and normal aging has been demonstrated (Palmer and DeKosky, 1993). Increased superoxide dismutase-derived hydrogen peroxide fluxes, metal ions, and damaged mitochondria can contribute to cell damage mediated by free radicals (Melhorn and Cole, 1984). Free radical production in AD might also be caused by amyloid beta protein, glutamate, increased levels of monoamine oxidase, or another toxic event (Behl et al., 1992). These findings support the usage of antioxidants in treating AD.

L-Deprenyl posseses antioxidant properties through its inhibition of monoamine oxidase B. It is believed to have neuroprotective effect by acting as a scavenger of free radicals (Knoll, 1992).

Vitamin E and idebenone are also potential antioxidants for treatment of Alzheimer's disease since they prevent cell death caused by glutamate and amyloid beta protein (Behl et al., 1992; Oka et al., 1993). Alpha tocopherol, a biologically active constituent of vitamin E, interferes with the effects of lipid peroxidation by trapping free radicals (Wilson, 1983). Both L-deprenyl and vitamin

E have been studied in Parkinson's disease. A multicenter double-blind placebo-controlled trial has demonstrated that deprenyl given at 10 mg/day delays the onset of disability associated with early Parkinson's disease (The Parkinson Study Group, 1983). This effect could be attributed to the acute effect of monoamine oxidase inhibition leading to increased dopamine particularly in the patients who were receiving L-dopa. A multicenter double-blind placebo-controlled study is being completed to investigate the ability of L-deprenyl and vitamin E, administered alone or in combination, to slow the progression of Alzheimer's disease.

B. GLUTAMATERGIC AGENTS

Glutamate is the major excitatory neurotransmitter in the brain (Fonnum, 1984). The postsynaptic effects of glutamate are mediated via several receptor subtypes that can be classified according to their prototypic agonists, i.e., *N*-methyl-D-aspartate (NMDA), quisqualate (QUIS) and kainate (KAIN) (Foster and Fagg, 1987). Studies of brains of AD patients have shown extensive loss of NMDA sites (Greenamyre et al., 1987). The glutamenergic system has been implicated in memory and learning. For example, spatial learning is disrupted by the NMDA receptor blocker aminophosphonopentanioc acid (Collingridge and Bliss, 1987; Morris et al., 1986). Antagonists of QUIS and KAIN receptors interfere with passive avoidance training in rodents (Danysz et al., 1988).

Glutamate is also neurotoxic and has been speculated to be involved in the pathogenesis of several CNS degenerative diseases. This neurotoxic effect can occur both through NMDA and non-NMDA receptors (Rothman and Olney, 1987; Sheardon et al., 1990). Altering glutamenergic activity is a potential approach to the therapeutics of Alzheimer's disease. However, given that glutamate can enhance learning as well as produce neurotoxicity, any attempts at using it in treatment needs to consider this completely. Antagonism of the glycine site of the NMDA receptor could decrease glutamate neurotoxicity. 1-Hydroxy-3-amino 2-pyrolidine (HA-966) and I-aminocyclobutane (ACBC) inhibit NMDA binding and block NMDA responses (Hood et al., 1989; Watson et al., 1989). The glycine antagonist kynurenic acid (KYNA) and 7-chloro-kynurenic acid (7-cl-KYNA) do not interfere with passive avoidance in mice. Thus, the antagonism of glycine site may interfere with glutamate toxicity without causing cognitive impairment (Chiamulera et al., 1991). Non-NMDA receptors antagonists might provide a potential therapeutic strategy as well. Several of these antagonists have been shown to protect against ischemia (Sheardon et al., 1990). Clinical trials are needed to determine whether these agents can influence the course of AD.

C. ANTI-INFLAMMATORY AGENTS

There is evidence from histological studies that the immune system plays a role in AD. Increased numbers of reactive glia and microglia as well as activated T lymphocytes have been observed in post-mortem brain tissue (Haga et al., 1989; Rogers et al., 1988). Complement proteins including the membrane attack proteins C5-C9 have also been identified in senile plaques, tangles, and dystrophic neurites (Eikelenboom et al., 1989; McGeer et al., 1992). It seems that the process involves the complement cascade through the activation of c1q by AB (Eikelenboom et al., 1989; Rogers et al., 1992; Rogers et al., 1992). Elevated concentrations of tumor necrosis factor, Interleukin 1(Il-1) and interleukin 6 (Il-6) have also been demonstrated (Fillit et al., 1991; Bauer et al., 1991). Since interleukins can enhance APP production, their presence in the AD brain may be important (Alstiel and Sperber, 1991). Acute phase reactants are also elevated in AD, and alpha 2 macroglobulin and alpha 1 antichymotrypsin (ACT) have been demonstrated in amyloid deposits in AD (Abraham et al., 1988; Rozemuller et al., 1990; Bauer et al., 1991).

A retrospective survey of the prevalence of AD in rheumatoid arthritis clinic patients who had received antiinflamatory therapy found the prevalence to be significantly lower than that of the general population over the age of 64 (McGeer et al., 1992). Furthermore, elderly leprosy patients who had received treatment with dapsone, an anti-inflammatory agent, had a significantly lower rate of dementia than that of drug-free patients (McGeer et al., 1992). These are intriguing but very preliminary observations.

A 6-month double-blind study with the nonsteroidal anti-inflammatory agent indomethacin demonstrated that AD patients who received active drug had significantly less decline than did patients who received placebo (Rogers et al., 1993). However, in that study, 20% of the indomethacin-treated patients developed severe gastrointestinal side effects which warranted their removal from the study. Moreover, they used idiosyncratic outcome measures, a combination of videotaped evaluation and mental status examination, which makes it difficult to evaluate the real value of that study. In a co-twin control study among 50 elderly twin pairs, the onset of AD was inversely associated with prior use of anti-inflammatory agents including steroids, aspirin, or nonsteroidal anti-inflammatory drugs taken for arthritis or related conditions (Breitner et al., 1994). Since steroids are used in treating several inflammatory diseases, it could be a logical choice in AD. The systemic toxicity of steroids limit their use at high doses for a long time. Low-dose steroid therapy may be the safest strategy; 10 mg/day of prednisone is a well-tolerated and effective dose in rheumatoid arthritis. Initial pilot studies of prednisone in AD suggest that to suppress acute phase proteins an initial dose of 20 mg is needed followed by a 10-mg maintenance dose. A multicenter double-blind placebo-controlled trial of prednisone in AD patients is currently under way. In this study 150 patients will be enrolled at 20 sites in the U.S., prednisone will be administered at an initial daily dose of 20 mg for 1 month followed by a taper to a maintenance dose of 10 mg which is continued for 1 year (Aisen et al., in preparation).

Colchicine is used in treating familial Mediterranean fever and renal amyloidosis. Both these illnesses involve chronic inflammation, elevated acute phase reactants, and amyloid deposition. These similarities to AD pathology suggest that colchicine may be worth testing in AD.

Hydroxychloroquine is an antimalarial agent which is proven to be a safe and effective drug for the treatment of rheumatoid arthritis and lupus erythematosus. This agent suppresses cytokine and acute phase reactant levels in these illnesses (Salmeron and Lipsky, 1983). Hydroxychloroquine is a lysomotropic agent that interferes with lysosomal enzymatic activity by increasing the pH in these organelles (Deduve et al., 1974) and by stabilizing lysosomal membranes (Matsuzawa and Hostetler, 1980). Since AB production may involve lysosomal enzymes hydroxycholoquine may have unexpected utility in AD.

D. ANTI-AMYLOID AGENTS

AD is characterized by neurofibrillary tangles and extracellular deposits of amyloid beta protein (AB). AB, which constitutes the plaques, has been implicated in cell death (Hardy and Higgins, 1992; Wisniewski et al., 1991). AB is derived from processing of the transmembrane amyloid precursor protein (APP)(Goldgaber et al., 1987; Kang et al., 1987; Robakis et al., 1987). Lysosomal processing of APP may produce amyloidogenic fragments (Estus et al., 1992; Golde et al., 1992; Haass et al., 1992). Thus, agents interfering with AB production and/or toxicity could have a beneficial effect in altering the course of AD. The effects of colchicine and hydroxychloroquine on lysosomal processing suggest that these agents are candidates for clinical trials in AD. Cholinergic agonists were shown to alter the processing of the amyloid precursor protein by increasing the secretory breakdown pathway of the protein (Buxbaum et al., 1992). Thus, manipulation of the cholinergic activity may have its beneficial effect in AD not only through augmentation of cholinergic neurotransmission but also through interfering with amyloid deposition.

E. CHELATING AGENTS

Several findings suggest an association between aluminum and neurodegenerative diseases including AD (Martyn et al., 1989). Aluminum administration has been shown to be neurotoxic to the cholinergic system (Clayton et al., 1992). These data suggest that aluminum is associated with AD; although probably a secondary effect, it has nevertheless stimulated using a chelating agent in the treatment of AD.

Desferrioxamine mesylate is a chelating agent with a particular affinity for aluminum; it is used in iron and aluminum overdoses (Chang et al., 1983; Propper et al., 1977). In a 2-year double-blind controlled trial on 48 AD patients, intramuscular desferrixamine was compared to placebo or no treatment (Crapper et al.; 1991). There was a significant reduction in the rate of cognitive decline in daily living skills in the patients who received desferrioxamine when compared to the placebo group. The therapeutic effects observed with this compound may not be due to its chelating action since it has been shown to inhibit free radical formation and inflammation as well (Crapper et al., 1991). The study was not blinded because of the need for intramuscular injections of the active medications which was not approved for the placebo group. Consequently "blinded" videotapes of patient interviews served as the basis for evaluation.

F. CALCIUM CHANNEL BLOCKERS

Excessive calcium influx has been suggested as the final common pathway of neuronal death after a variety of insults, including hypoglycemia and hypoxia (Schanne et al., 1979; Mattson et al. 1991; Cheng and Mattson 1992). Thus, calcium channel blockers are a therapeutic option for AD. In a double-blind placebo-controlled multicenter trial of 227 AD patients, there was a prophylactic benefit over the 12-week duration of the trial of 30 mg tid nimodipine (Tollefson, 1990). Higher doses of nimodipine were not as efficacious.

G. NERVE GROWTH FACTOR

Several neurotrophic factors which are proteins capable of altering neuronal survival, innervation, and function have been identified (Vantini, 1992). The cell loss in AD and other neurodegenerative illnesses suggests a role for neurotrophic factors in their pathophysiology and treatment. NGF is one of these neurotrophins and has been most studied in relation to AD. NGF is primarily located in the hippocampus, cortex, and basal forebrain and it acts selectively on cholinergic neurons (Vantini, 1992). The basal forebrain cholinergic neurons have the NGF receptor and express increased choline acetyltransferase activity in response to NGF (Hefti et al., 1986, Mobley et al. 1986). NGF administration has been demonstrated to attenuate degenerative changes in cholinergic cells caused by transactions of the septohippocampal pathway (Koliastsos et al., 1991). NGF treatment also elevates choline acetyltransferase activity, acetylcholine synthesis, and release following partial lesions of the fimbria (Lapchak and Hefti, 1991). Some, but not all post-mortem studies have shown a decrease in NGF mRNA or MGF-like protein in AD (Phillips et al., 1991; Goedert et al., 1989; Allen et al., 1991). However, NGF-like activity has recently been shown to be significantly elevated in AD brains, suggesting a possible compensatory increase in response to degenerative changes in the basal forebrain cholinergic system (Crutcher et al., 1993).

Nerve growth factor (NGF) is a 118 amino acid polypeptide with no blood-brain barrier penetrance necessitating intracerebroventricular administration. Basic studies support the use of NGF in the treatment of AD. ICV administration of NGF has been shown to reverse lesions-induced deficits of cortical acetylcholine and cholineacetyltransferase (Lapchak and Hefti, 1991), to promote survival of cholinergic neurons after fimbrial transection in rats, and to reverse behavioral deterioration in these rats (Koliatsos et al., 1991). Recently NGF has been produced by recombinant techniques (Bruce and Heinrich, 1989) and is now available for trials in AD. In addition genetically modified, NGF-secreting fibroblasts grafts have been shown to prevent degeneration of cholinergic neurons after surgical lesions of the fimbria-fornix in rats (Rosenberg et al., 1988). This opens the possibility of infusing or grafting a genetically engineered designer cell which would secret *in situ* the factor or neurotransmitter required (for review see Olson and Hoffer, 1993). Lately, NGF conjugated to an antibody to the transferrin receptor was shown to cross the blood-brain barrier with peripheral injection. In this study NGF increase the survival of cholinergic and noncholinergic neurons (Friden et al., 1993). A case report of a patient treated with NGF for 1 month was associated with improvement in verbal episodic memory, increased nicotine binding in frontal and temporal cortices and increased cerebral blood flow (Olson et al., 1992). In a Swedish study, NGF was administered to two patients by an infusion pump connected to the right lateral ventricle via a subcutaneous catheter. The patients were treated for 3 months (total amount of NGF, prepared from male mouse salivary glands, was 6.6 mg). Tests of verbal episodic memory were improved, whereas no global cognitive improvement was observed. Serious side effects of weight loss, pain, and confusion were an important problem. A significant increase in "C-nicotine receptor binding" as well as increased blood flow as measured by PET was observed in some cortical areas as well as progressive decrease of slow-wave EEG activity (Winblad et al., 1994). Other substances with neutrophic activity such as epidermal growth factors, brain-derived neutrophic factor, gangliosides, and the B1-28 peptide of the B-amyloid protein (Whitson et al., 1989) might also have a therapeutic potential. A trial with intrathecal ganglioside GM1 has been initiated. The first patient in that study has had intraventricular treatment for 18 continuous months (Gottfries, 1994).

REFERENCES

Adem, A, Putative mechanisms of action of tacrine in Alzheimer's disease, *Acta Neurol. Scand. Suppl.*, 139, 69, 1992.

Abraham, C. R., Selkoe, D. J., and Potter, H, Immunohistochemical identification of the serine protease inhibitor alpha-1-antichymotrypsin in the brain amyloid deposits of Alzheimer's disease, *Cell*, 52, 487, 1988.

Allen, S. J., MacGowen, S. H., Treanor, J. J. S, et al., Normal B-NGF content in Alzheimer's disease cerebral cortex and hippocampus, *Neurosci. Lett.*, 131, 135, 1991.

Altstiel, L. and Sperber, K., Cytokines in Alzheimer's disease, *Prog. Neurol. Psychopharmacol. Biol. Psychiat.*, 15, 481, 1991.

Aisen, P. S. and Davis, K. L., Inflammatory mechanisms in Alzheimer's disease. Implications for therapy, *Am. J. Psychiatry*, 151, 1105, 1994.

Aisen, P. S., Anti-inflammatory therapy for Alzheimer's disease, in preparation.

Agnoli, A., Martucci, N., Fabbrini, G., et al., Monoamine oxidase and dementia: treatment with an inhibitor of MAO-B activity, *Dementia*, 109, 1990.

Ashkenazi, A, Peralta, E. G., Winslow, J. W., et al., Functional diversity of muscarinic receptor subtypes in cellular signal transduction and growth, *Trends Pharmacol. Sci. Suppl.*, 16, 1989.

Bartus, R. T., Dean, R. L., Pontecorvo, M. J., et al., The cholinergic hypothesis: a historical overview, current perspective and future directions, *Ann. N.Y. Acad. Sci.*, 444, 332, 1985.

Bartus, R. T., Dean, R. L., and Flicker, C., Cholinergic psychopharmacology: an integration of human and animal research on memory, in *Psychopharmacology: The Third Generation of Progress*, Meltzer, H. Y., Ed., Raven Press, New York, 1987, 219.

Bauer, J., Strauss, S., Schreiter-Gasser, U., et al., Interleukin-6 and alpha-2-macroglobulin indicate an acute phase response in Alzheimer's disease cortices, *FEBS Lett.*, 285, 111, 1991.

Behl, C., Davis, J., Cole, G. M., et al., Vitamin E protects nerve cells from amyloid B protein toxicity, *Biochem. Biophys. Res. Commun.*, 186, 944, 1992.

Beller, S. A., Overall, J. E., Rhoades, H. M., et al., Long term outpatient treatment of senile dementia with oral physostigmine, *J. Clin. Psychiat.*, 49, 400, 1988.

Birdsall, N. and Committee, Nomenclature for muscarinic receptor subtypes recommended by symposium, *Trends Pharmacol. Sci. Suppl.*, VII, 1989

Bonner, T. I., New subtypes of muscarinic acetylcholine receptors, *Trends Pharmacol. Sci. Suppl.*, 11, 1989.

Bonner, T. I., Buckley, A., Young, A. C., et al., Identification of a family of muscarinic acetylcholine receptor genes, *Science*, 237, 527, 1987.

Bruno, G., Mohr, E., Gillepsie, M., et al., RS-86 therapy of Alzheimer's disease, *Arch. Neurol.*, 43, 659, 1985.

Buccafusco, J. J. and Jackson, W., Beneficial effects of nicotine administered prior to a delayed matching-to-sample task in young and aged monkeys, *Neurobiol. Aging*, 12, 233, 1991.

Buckley, N. J., Bonner, T. I., and Brann, M. R., Localization of a family of muscarinic receptor mRNAs in rat brain, *J. Neurosci.*, 4646, 1988.

Bierer, L. M., Aisen, P. S., Davidson, M., et al., A pilot study of oral physostigmine plus yohimbine in patients with Alzheimer's disease, *Alz. Dis. Assoc. Dis.*, 7, 98, 1993.

Breitner, J. C., Gau, B. A., Welsh, K. A., et al., Inverse association of anti-inflammatory treatments and Alzheimer's disease: Initial results of a co-twin control study, *Neurology*, 44, 227, 1994.

Bruce, G. and Heinrich G, Production and characterization of biologically active recombinant human nerve growth factor, *Neurobiol. Aging*, 10, 89, 1989.

Bruno, G., Mohr, E., Gillespie, M., et al., RS-86 therapy of Alzheimer's disease, *Arch. Neurol.*, 43, 659, 1985.

Buxbaum, J. D., Oishi, M., Chen, H. I., Pinkas-Karamarski, R., Jaffe, E. A., Gandy, S. E., and Greengard, P., Cholinergic agonist and interleukin 1 regulate processing and secretion of the Alzheimer's B/A4 amyloid protein precursor, *Proc. Natl. Acad. Sci. U.S.A.*, 89, 10075, 1992.

Chang, T. M. S. and Barre, P., Effect of desferrioxamine on removal of aluminum and iron by coated charcoal haemoperfusion and hemodialysis, *Lancet*, 1051, 1983.

Chatellier, G. and Lacomblez, L., Tacrine (tetrahydroaminoacridine; THA) and lecithin in senile dementia of the Alzheimer's type: a multi-center trial, *Br. Med. J.*, 495, 1990.

Chatellier, G. and Lacomblez, L., on behalf of groupe Francais d'Etude de la Tetrahydroaminoacridine, Tacrine (tetrahydroaminoacridine,THA) and lecithin in senile dementia of Alzheimer's type: a multi-center trial, *Br. Med. J.*, 495, 1990.

Cheng, B. and Mattson, M. P., Glucose deprivation elicits neurofibrillary tangle-like antigenic changes in hippocampal neurons: prevention by NGF and bFGF, *Exp. Neurol.*, 117, 114, 1992.

Chiamulera, C., Costa, S., and Reggiani, A., Effect of NMDA and strychnine-insensitive glycine site antagonist on NMDA-mediated convulsions and learning, *Psychopharmacology*, 102, 551, 1991.

Christie, J. E., Shering, A., and Ferguson, J., et al., Physostigmine and arecoline: effects of intravenous infusions in Alzheimer's presenile dementia, *Br. J. Psychiat.*, 138, 46, 1981.

Collerton, D., Cholinergic function and intellectual decline in Alzheimer's disease, *Neuroscience*, 19, 1, 1986.

Collingridge, G. L. and Bliss, T. V. P, NMDA receptors-their role in long-term potentiation, *Trends Neurosci.*, 10, 288, 1987.

Cutler, N. R., Murphy, M. F., and Nash, R. J., et al., Clinical safety, tolerance and plasma levels of the oral anticholinesterase 1,2,3,4-tetrahydro-9-aminoacradin-l-olmaleate (HP 029) in Alzheimer's disease: preliminary findings, *J. Clin. Pharmacol.*, 556, 1990.

Clayton, R. M., Sedowofia, S. K. A, Rankin, J. M., and Manning, A., A long term effect of aluminum in the fetal mouse brain, *Life Sci.*, 51, 1921, 1992.

Cook, L., Nicholson, V. J., and Steinfels, G. F., et al., Cognitive enhancement by acetylcholine release Du996, *Drug. Rev. Res.*, 19, 301, 1990.

Crapper, D. R., Dalton, A. J., Kruck, T. P. A., et al., Intramuscular desferroxamine in patients with Alzheimer's disease, *Lancet*, 337(8753), 1304, 1991.

Crutcher, K. A., Scott, S. A., Liang, S., et al., Detection of NGF-like activity in human brain tissue:increase levels in Alzheimer's disease, *J. Neurosci.*, 13, 2549, 1993.

Dal-Bianco, P., Maly, J., Wober, C., et al., Galanthamine treatment in Alzheimer's disease, *J. Neurol. Transm.*, 33(Suppl.), 59, 1991.

Danysz, W., Wroblewski, J. T., and Costa, E., Learning impairment in rats by N-methyl-D-aspartate receptor antagonist, *Neuropharmacology*, 27, 653, 1988.

Davis, K. L., Hollander, E., Davidson, M., et al., Induction of depression with oxotremorine in patients with ALzheimer's disease. *Am. J. Psychiat.*, 144(4), 468, 1987.

Davis, K. L., Thal, L. J., Gamzu, et al., Tacrine in patients with Alzheimer's disease: a double blind placebo controlled multicenter study, *N. Engl. J. Med.*, 1374, 1992.

Davies, P. and Maloney, A. J., Selective loss of central cholinergic neurons in Alzheimer's disease, *Lancet*, 2, 1403, 1976.

Davidson, M., Bierer, L. M., Kaminsky, R., et al., Combined administration of physostigmine and clonidine to patients with dementia of the Alzheimer's type: a pilot safety study, *Alzheimer's Dis. and Assoc. Dis.*, 1, 1, 1989.

Deduve, C., Debarsy, T., Pode, B., et al., Lysomotropic agents, *Biochem. Pharmacol.*, 23, 2495, 1974.

DeSouza, E. B., Rule, B. L., Tam, S. W., 3H Linopiridine (DuP996) labels a novel binding site in rat brain involved in the enhancement of stimulus-induced neurotransmitter release: autoradiographic localization studies, *Brain Res.*, 582, 335, 1992.

Drukarch, B., Kits, S., Van Der Meer, E. G., et al., 9-amino-1,2,3,4-tetrahydroacridine (THA), an alleged drug for the treatment of Alzheimer's disease, inhibits acetylcholinesterase activity and slow woutwars K$^+$ current, *Eur. J. Pharmacol.*, 141, 153, 1987.

Durkarch, B., Leysen, J. E., and Stoof, J. C., Further analysis of the neuropharmacological profile of 9-amino-1,2,3,4-tetrahydroacridine (THA), an alleged drug for the treatment of Alzheimer's disease, *Life Sci.*, 42, 1011, 1988.

Dundee, J. W. and Pandit, S. K., Anterograde amnesic effects of pethidine, hyoscine, and diazepam in adults, *Br. J. Pharmacol.*, 44, 140, 1972.

Deutsch, J. A., The cholinergic synapse and the site of memory, *Science*, 174, 788, 1971.

Drachman, D. A. and Leavitt J., Human memory and the cholinergic system, *Arch. Neurol.*, 30, 113, 1974.

Eagger, S., Morant, N., Levy, R., and Sahakian, B., Tacrine in Alzheimer's disease time course of changes in cognitive function and practice effects, *Br. J. Psychiat.*, 160, 36, 1992.

Eikelenboom, P., Hack, C. E., Rozemuller, J. M., et al., Complement activation in amyloid plaques in Alzheimer's dementia, *Virch. Arch. B*, 56, 259, 1989.

Elrod, K. and Buccafuso, J. J., Correlation of the amnestic effects of nicotinic antagonists with inhibition of regional brain acetylcholine synthesis in rats, *J. Pharmacol. Exp. Ther.*, 403, 1991.

Estus, S., Golde, T., Kunishita, T., et al., Potentially amyloidogenic, carboxyl-terminal derivatives of the amyloid protein precursor, *Science*, 255, 726, 1992.

Farlow, M., Gracon, S. I., Hershey, L. A., Lewis, K. W., Sadowsky, C. H., and Dolan-Ureno, J, A controlled trial of tacrine in Alzheimer's disease, *JAMA*, 2523, 1992.

Fonnum, F., Glutamate: a Neurotransmitter in mammalian brain, *J. Neurochem.*, 42, 1, 1984.

Foster, A. C. and Fagg, G. E., Taking apart the NMDA receptor, *Nature*, 329, 395, 1987.

Fillit, H., Ding, W., Buee, L., et al., Elevated circulating tumor necrosis factor levels in Alzheimer's disease, *Neurosci. Lett.*, 129, 318, 1991.

Fillit, H., Weiner, H., Cholst, I., et al., Observation in a preliminary open trial of estradiol therapy for senile dementia-Alzheimer's type, *Psychoneuroendocrinology,* 11(3), 337, 1986.

Fisher, A., Brandeis, R., Karton, I., et al., (±)-*cis*-2-Methyl-spiro(1,3-oxathiolane 5,3')quinuclide, an M1 selective cholinergic agonist, attenuates cognitive dysfunction in an animal model of Alzheimer's disease, *J. Pharmcol. Exp. Ther.,* 392, 1991.

Freeman, S. E. and Dawson, R. M., Tacrine: a pharmachological review, *Prog. Neurobiol.,* 36, 257, 1991.

Friden, P. M., Walus, L. R., Watson, P., et al., Blood-brain barrier penetration and *in vivo* activity of an NGF conjugate, *Science,* 259, 373, 1993.

Fukada, K., Kubo, T., Maeda, A., et al., Selective effector coupling of muscarinic acetylcholine receptor subtypes, *Trends Pharmacol. Sci. Suppl.,* 4, 1989.

Gauthier, S., Bouchard, R., Lamontagne, A., et al., Tetrahydroaminoacridine-Lecithin combination treatment in patients with intermediate stage Alzheimer's disease, *N. Engl. J. Med.,* 1272, 1990.

Goedert, M., Fine, A., Dawbarn, D., et al., Nerve growth factor receptor MRNA distribution in human brain: Normal levels in the basal forebrain in Alzheimer's disease, *Mol. Brain Res.,* 5, 1, 1989.

Goldgaber, D., Harris, H., Hla, T., et al., Interleukin-1 regulates synthesis of amyloid beta protein precursor mRNA in human endothelial cells, *Proc. Natl. Acad. Sci. U.S.A.,* 86, 7606, 1989.

Golde, T. E., Estus, S., Younkin, L. H., Selkoe, D. J., and Younkin, S. G., Processing of the amyloid precursor for potentially amyloidogenic derivatives, *Science,* 155, 728, 1992.

Gottfries, C. G., Serotonergic approach and intrathecal treatment with gangliosides for Alzheimer's type dementia, *Neuro-psychopharmacology,* 10(35), S176, 1994.

Greenamyre, J. T., D'Amato, C. J., and Shoulson, I, Alterations in L-glutamate binding in Alzheimer's and Huntington's diseases, *Science,* 227, 1496, 1985.

Greenamyre, J. T. and Young, A. B., Excitatory amino acids and Alzheimer's disease, *Neurobiol. Aging,* 10, 593, 1989.

Hardy, J. A. and Higgins, G. A., Alzheimer's disease: the amyloid cascade hypothesis, *Science,* 10, 256 (5054), 1992.

Harbaugh, R. E., Roberts, D. W., Cooms, D. W., et al., Preliminary report: intracranial cholinergic drug infusion in patients with Alzheimer's disease, *Neurosurgery,* 15, 514, 1984.

Hefti, F., Hartikka, J., Salvatierra, A., Localization of nerve growth factor receptors in cholinergic neurons of the human basal forebrain, *Neurosci. Lett.,* 69, 37, 1986.

Hefti, F., and Schneider, L. S., Nerve growth factor and Alzheimer's disease, *Clin. Neuropharmacol.,* 14(Suppl. 1), 62, 1991.

Haratounian, V., Kanof, P. D., and Davis, K. L., Pharmacological alleviation of cholinergic lesion induced memory deficits in rats, *Life Sci.,* 37, 945, 1985.

Haroutanian, V., Santucci, A. C., and Davis, K. L., Progress in Brain Research Implication of multiple transmitter system lesions for cholinomimetic therapy in Alzheimer's disease, Aquilonius, S. M. and Gillberg, P. G., Eds., *Elsevier Science,* 1990, 333.

Haass, C., Koo, E. H., Mellon, A., Hung, A. Y., and Selkoe, D. J., Targeting of cell-surface B-amyloid precursor protein to lysosomes: alternative processing into amyloid-bearing fragments, *Nature,* 357, 500, 1992.

Haga, S., Akai, K., and Ishii, T., Demonstration of microglia cells in and around senile (neurotic) plaques in the Alzheimer's brain: an immunohistochemical study using a novel monoclonal antibody, *Acta Neuropathol.,* 77, 569, 1989.

Hollander, E., Davidson, M., Mohs, R. C., et al., RS 86 in the treatment of Alzheimer's disease: cognitive and biological effects, *Biol. Psychiat.,* 22, 1067, 1987.

Hood, W. F., Sun, E. T., Compton, R. P., et al., 1-aminocyclo-butane 1-carboxylase (ACBC): a specific antagonist of the *N*-methyl-D-aspartate receptor coupled glycine receptor, *Eur. J. Pharmacol.,* 161, 281, 1989.

Honjo, H., Ogino, Y., Naitoh, K., et al., *In vivo* effects by estrone sulfate on the central nervous system-senile dementia (Alzheimer's Type), *J. Steroid Biochem.,* 34, 521, 1989.

Knapp, M. J., Knopman, D. S., and Solomon, P. R., et al., A 30 weeks randomized controlled trial of high dose tacrine in patients with Alzheimer's disease, *JAMA,* 271, 985, 1994.

Knoll, J., The pharmacological profile of L-deprenyl (Selegiline) and its relevance for humans: a personal review, *Pharmacol. Toxicol.,* 70, 317, 1992.

Koliastsos, V. E., Clatterbuck, R. E., Haring, J. W., et al., Human nerve growth factor prevents degeneration of basal forebrain cholinergic neurons in primates, *Ann. Neurol.,* 30, 831, 1991.

Kewitz, H., Berzewski, H., Rainer, M., et al., Galanthamine, a selective nontoxic acetylcholinesterase inhibitor is significantly superior over placebo in the treatment of senile dementia Alzheimer's type, *Neuropsychopharmacology,* 10, 58, 1994.

Jenike, M. A. and Alberts, M. S., and Baer, L., Oral physostigmine as treatment for Alzheimer's disease: A long term outpatient trial, *Alz. Dis. Assoc. Dis.,* 1990.

Lapchak, P. A. and Hefti, F., Effect of recombinant human nerve growth on presynaptic cholinergic function in rat hippocampal slices following partial septohippocampal lesions: measures of [H]acetylcholine release and choline acetyltransferase activity, *Neuroscience,* 42, 639, 1991.

Leber, P., Guidelines for the clinical evaluation of antidementia drugs, first draft, U.S. Food and Drug Administration, Rockville, MD, 1990.

Leslie, S. W., Chandler, L. J., Barr, E. M., et al., Reduced calcium uptake by rat brain mitochondria and synaptosomes in response to aging, *Brain Res.,* 329, 177, 1985.

Luine, V. N., Khylchevskaya, R. I., and McEwen, B. S., Effect of gonadal steroids on activities of monoamine oxidase and choline acetylase in rat brain, *Brain Res.*, 86, 293, 1975.

Luine, V. N., Park, D., Joh, T., et al., Immunochemical demonstration of increased choline acetyltransferase concentration in rat preoptic area after estradiol administration, *Brain Res.*, 191, 273, 1980.

Maltby, N., Broe, A. G., Creasey, H., et al., Efficacy of tacrine and lecithin in mild to moderate Alzheimer's disease: double blind trial, *Br. Med. J.*, 308, 879, 1994.

Mangoni, A., Grassi, M. P., Frattola, L., et al., Effects of a MAO-B inhibitor in the treatment of Alzheimer's disease, *Eur. Neurol.*, 100, 1991.

Marin, D. B., Bierer, L. M., Ryan, T. M., Markofsky, R. E., Schmeidler, J, Mohs, R. C., and Davis, K. L., Combination L-deprenyl and physostigmine for the treatment of Alzheimer's disease. Presented at Biological Psychiatry Meeting, San Francisco, 1993.

Martyn, C. N., Barker, D. J. P., Osmond, C., Harris, E. C., Edwardson, J. A., and Lacey, R. F., Geographical relation between Alzheimer's disease and drinking water, *Lancet*, 59, 1989.

Mattson, M. P. B, Rychlik, B., and Engle, M. G., Effects of elevated intracellular calcium levels on the cytoskeleton and tau in cultural human cortical neurons, *Mol. Chem. Neuropathol.*, 15, 117, 1991.

Matsuzawa, Y. and Hostetler, K. Y., Inhibition of lysosomal phospholipase A and phospholipase C by chloroquine and 4-4 bis(diethylaminoethoxya, B-diethyldiphenylethane), *J. Biol. Chem.*, 255, 5190, 1980.

Melhorn, R. J. and Cole, G., Adv free radical biology and medicine 1, 165, 1985.

McGeer, P. L., Akiyama, H., Itagaki, S., and McGeer, E. G., Activation of the classical complement pathway in the brain of Alzheimer's patients, *Neurosci. Lett.*, 107, 341, 1989.

McGeer, P. L. and McGeer, E. G., Complement proteins and complement inhibitors in Alzheimer's disease, *Res. Immunol.*, 143, 621, 1992.

McGeer, P. L., McGeer, E. G., Rogers, J., et al., Does anti-inflammatory treatment protect against Alzheimer's disease?, in *Alzheimer's Disease: New Treatment Strategies*, Khachaturian Z. S., Blass J. P., Eds., Marcel Dekker, New York, 1992, 165.

Mihailova, D., Yamboliev, I., Zhivkova, Z., Tencheva, J., and Jovovich, V., Pharmacokinetics of Galanthamine hydrobromide after single subcutaneous and oral dosage in humans, *Pharmacology*, 39, 50, 1989.

Mobley, W. C., Rutkowski, J. L., Tennenkoon, G. I., et al., Nerve growth factor increases cholinergic acetyltransferase activity in developing basal forebrain neurons, *Mol. Brain Res.*, 1, 53, 1986.

Mohs, R. C., Davis, B. M., John, C. A., et al., Oral physostigmine treatment of patients with Alzheimer's disease, *Am. J. Psychiat.*, 142, 28, 1985.

Monard, D., Role of protease inhibition in cellular migration and neuritic growth, *Biochem. Pharmacol.*, 36, 1389, 1987.

Morris, R. G. M, Anderson, E., Lynch, G. S., et al., Selective impairment of learning and blockade of long-term potentiation by an *N*-methyl-D-aspartate receptor antagonist, AP5, *Nature*, 319, 774, 1986.

Mouradian, M. M., Mohr, E., Williams, A. J., et al., No response to high dose muscarinic agonist therapy in Alzheimer's disease, *Neurology*, 38, 606, 1988.

Murphy, M. F., Hardiman, S. T., Nash, R. J., et al., Evaluation of HP 029 (Velnacrine Maleate) in Alzheimer's disease, *Ann. N.Y. Acad. Sci.*, 253, 1991.

Newhouse, P. A., Sunderland, T., Triot, P. N., et al., Intravenous nicotine in Alzheimer's disease: a pilot study, *Psychopharmacology*, 95, 171, 1988.

Nicholson, V. J., Tam, S. W., Myers, M. J., et al., Du996 (3,3-bis(4-pyrindinylmethyl)-1-phenylindolin-2-one) enhances the stimulus-induced release of acetylcholine from rat brain *in vitro* and *in vivo*, *Drug Rev. Res.*, 19, 285, 1990.

Nordberg, A., Alafuzoff, I., Winblad, B., Nicotinic and muscarinic subtypes in the human brain: changes with aging and dementia, *J. Neurosci. Res.*, 103, 1992.

Oka, A., Belliveau, M. F., Rosenberg, P. A., et al., Vulnerability of oligodendroglia to glutamate. Pharmacology, mechanisms and prevention, *J. Neurosci.*, 13, 1441, 1993.

Olton, D. S., Wenk, G. L., Dementia: Animal models of the cognitive impairments produced by degeneration of the basal forebrain cholinergic system, in *Psychopharmacology: The Third Generation of Progress*, Meltzer H. Y., Ed., Raven Press, New York, 1987, 941.

Olson, L. and Hoffer, B. J., The potential use of neurotrophic factors in the treatment of Alzheimer's disease, in Alzheimer's Disease, New Treatment Strategies, Khachaturian, Z. S. and Blass, J. P., Eds., Marcel Dekker, New York, 1993, 125.

Olson, L., Nordberg, A., Von Holst, H., et al., Nerve growth factor affects C-nicotine binding, blood flow, EEG, and verbal episodic memory in an Alzheimer's patient, *J. Neurol. Transm.*, 4, 79, 1992.

The Parkinson Study Group, Effect of deprenyl on the progression of disability in early Parkinson's disease, *N. Engl. J. Med.*, 321, 1464, 1989.

Palmer, A. M. and DeKosky, S. T., Monoamine Neurons in aging and Alzheimer's disease, *J. Neural. Trans. Gen. Sect.*, 91(2–3), 135, 1993.

Perry, E. K., Perry, R. H., Blessed, G., et al., Necropsy evidence of central cholinergic deficits in senile dementia, *Lancet*, 1, 189, 1977.

Perry, E. K., Tomlinson, B. E., Blessed, G., et al., Correlation of cholinergic abnormalities with senile plaques and mental test scores in senile dementia, *Br. Med. J.*, 2, 1457, 1978.

Peterson, C., Tetrahydroaminoacridine increases acetylcholine synthesis and glucose oxidation by mouse brain slices *in vitro*, *Neurosci. Lett.*, 31, 115(2–3), 274, 1990.

Piccinin, F. L., Finali, G., and Piccirilli, M., Neuropsychological effects of l-deprenyl in Alzheimer's type dementia, *Clin. Neuropharmacol.*, 147, 1990.

Phillips, H. S., Hains, J. M., Armanini, M., et al., BDNF MRNA is decreased in the hippocampus of individuals with Alzheimer's disease, *Neuron*, 7, 695, 1991.

Pomara, N., Mendels, J., Lewitt, P. A., et al., Multicenter trial of milacemide in the treatment of Alzheimer's disease, *Biol. Psychiat.*, 29(Suppl.), 718, 1991.

Potter, L. T., Muscarinic receptors in the cortex and hippocampus in relation to the treatment of Alzheimer's disease, in *International Symposium on Muscarinic Cholinergic Mechanisms*, Cohen, S. and Sokolovsky, M., Eds., Freud Publishing, London, 1987, 294.

Probst, A., Basler, V., Bron, B., et al., Neurotic plaques in senile dementia of Alzheimer's type: a golgi analysis in the hippocampal region, *Brain Res.*, 268, 249, 1983.

Propper, R., Cooper, B., Rufo, B., et al., Continuous subcutaneous administration of desferoxamine in patients with iron overload, *N. Engl. J. Med.*, 297, 418, 1977.

Raffaele, K. C., Berardi, A., Morris, P., et al., Effects of acute infusion of the muscarinic cholinergic agonist on verbal and visuo-spatial function in dementia of the Alzheimer's type, *Prog. Neuro-Psychopharmacol. Biol. Psychiat.*, 15, 643, 1991.

Read, S. L., Frazee, J., Shapiro, J., et al., Intracerebroventricular bethanechol for Alzheimer's disease. Variable dose-related responses, *Arch. Neurol.*, 1025, 1990.

Robakis, N. K., Anderson, J. P., Lawrence, M. R., et al., Expression of the Alzheimer amyloid precursor in the brain tissue and effects of NGF and EGF on its metabolism, *Clin. Neuropharmacol.*, 14(Suppl.), 15, 1991.

Rogers, J., Luber-Narod, J., Styren, S. D., et al., Expression of immune system associated antigen by cells of the human central nervous system. Relationship to the pathology of Alzheimer's disease, *Neurobiol. Aging*, 9, 330, 1988.

Rogers, J., Schultz, J., Brachova, L., et al., Complement activation and B-amyloid-mediated neurotoxicity in Alzheimer's disease, *Res. Immunol.*, 143, 624, 1992.

Rogers, J., Cooper, N. R., Webster, S., et al., Complement activation by B-amyloid in Alzheimer's disease, *Proc. Natl. Acad. Sci. U.S.A.*, 89, 10016, 1992.

Rogers, J., Kirby, L. C., Hempelman S. R., et al., Clinical trial of indomethacin in Alzheimer's disease, *Neurology*, 43, 1609, 1993.

Rogers, S. and Friedboff, L., E2020 improves cognition and quality of life in patients with mild to moderate Alzheimer's disease: results of a phase-II trial, *Neurology*, 44(Suppl. 2), 156S, 1994.

Rosenberg, M. B., Freidman, T., Robertson, R. O., et al., Grafting genetically modified cells to the damaged brain: restorative effects of NGF expression, *Science*, 242, 1575, 1988.

Rothman, S. M. and Olney, J. W., Excitoxicity and the NMDA receptor, *Trends Neurosci.*, 7, 299, 1987.

Rozemuller, J. M., Stam, F. C., and Eikelekboom, P., Acute phase proteins are present in amorphous in the cerebral but not in the cerebellar cortex of patients with Alzheimer's disease, *Neurosci. Lett.*, 109, 75, 1990.

Saletu, B., Darragh, A., Salmon, P., et al., EEG brain mapping in evaluating the time course of the central action of Du996: a new acetylcholine release drug, *Br. J. Pharmacol.*, 28, 1, 1989.

Salmeron, G. and Lipsky, E., Immunosuppressive potential of antimalarials, *Am. Med.*, 75(1A), 19, 1983.

Sara, S. J. and Debaugesw, B., Idazoxam, an alpha 2 agonist, facilitates memory retrieval in the rat, *Behav. Neurol. Biol.*, 51, 401, 1989.

Schanne, F. A. X., Kane, A. B., and Young, E. E., et al., Calcium dependence of toxic cell death: a final common pathway, *Science*, 206, 700, 1979.

Schneider, L., Small, G., Farlow, M., et al., Does estrogen augment psychopharmachologic response in elderly patients?, *Neurology*, in press.

Sheardon, M. J., Nielsoen, E. O., Hansen, A. J., et al., 2,3-Dihydroxy-6-nitro-7-sulfamoyl-benzo (F) quinoxaline: a neuroprotectant for cerebral ischemia, *Science*, 247, 571, 1990.

Sitaram, N., Weingartner, H., and Gillin, J. C., Human serial learning: enhancement with arecoline and impairment with scopolamine correlated with performance on placebo, *Science*, 201, 274, 1978.

Spiegel, R., Enz, A., Meier, D., and Emre, M., The cholinergic approach in ATD: focus on international multicenter drug studies, *Neuropsychopharmacology*, 10(3S), S176, 1994.

Sunderland, T., Tariot, P. N., and Newhouse, P. A., Differential responsivity of mood, behavior and cognition to cholinergic agents in elderly neuropsychiatric populations, *Brain Res.*, 472, 371, 1988.

Sunderland, T., Molchan, S., and Lawlor, B., et al., A strategy of "combination chemotherapy" in Alzheimer's disease: rationale and preliminary results with physostigmine plus deprenyl, *Int. Psychogeriatr.*, Suppl. 2, 291, 1992.

Suzuki, T., Nairn, A. C., Gandy, S. E., and Greengard, P., Phosphorylation of Alzheimer amyloid precursor protein by protein kinase C, *Neuroscience*, 48, 755, 1992.

Sugaya, K., Giacobini, E., and Chiappinelli, V. A., Nicotinic acetylcholine receptor subtypes in human frontal cortex: changes in Alzheimer's disease, *J. Neurosci. Res.*, 349, 1990.

Tariot, P. N., Cohen, R. M., Sunderland, T., et al., L-Deprenyl in Alzheimer's disease, *Arch. Gen. Psychiat.*, 44, 427, 1987.

Tariot, P. N., Sunderland, T., Weingartner, H., et al., Cognitive effects of L-deprenyl in Alzheimer's disease, *Psychopharmacology*, 91, 489, 1987.

Tariot, P. N., Sunderland, T., Cohen, R. M., et al., Tranylpromine compared with L-deprenyl in Alzheimer's disease, *J. Clin. Psychopharmacol.*, 8, 23, 1988.

Thomsen, T., Bickel, U., Fischer, J. P., et al., Galanthamine hydrobromide in a long term treatment of Alzheimer's disease, *Dementia*, 1, 46, 1990.

Tollefson, G. D., Short-term effects of the calcium channel blocker nimodipine (Bay-e-9736) in the management of primary degenerative dementia, *Biol. Psychiat.*, 27, 1133, 1990.

Vantini, G., The pharmacological potential of neurotrophins: A perspective, *Psychoneuroendocrinology*, 17, 401, 1991.

Vickroy, T. W., Presynaptic cholinergic actions by the putative cognitive enhancing agent DuP996, *J. Pharmacol. Exp. Ther.*, 264, 910, 1993.

Waelbroeck, M., Taslenoy, M., Camus, J., et al., Binding of selective antagonists to four muscarinic receptors (M1 to M4) in rat brain, *Mol. Pharmacol.*, 38, 267, 1990.

Watson, G. B., Bolanowski, M. A., Baganoff, M. P., et al., Glycine antagonist action of 1-aminocyclobutane1-1-carboxylate (ACBC) in *Xenopus oocytes* injected with rat brain mRNA, *Eur. J. Pharmacol.*, 167, 291, 1989.

Wettstein, A. and Spiegal, R., Clinical studies with the cholinergic drug RS-86 in Alzheimer's disease (AD) and senile dementia of the Alzheimer type (SDAT), *Psychopharmacology*, 84, 572, 1984

Whitson, J. S., Selkoe, D. J., and Cotman, C. W., Amyloid B protein enhances survival of hippocampal neurons *in vitro*, *Science*, 243, 1488, 1989.

Winblad, B., Seiger, A., Nordberg, A., et al., NGF in the treatment of Alzheimer's disease, *Am. Coll. Neuropsychopharmacol.*, 54, 1994.

Wilcock, G. K., Surnom, D. J., Scott, M., et al., An evaluation of the efficacy and safety of tetrahydroaminoacridine (THA) without lecithin in the treatment of Alzheimer's disease, *Age Ageing*, 22, 316, 1993.

Wilson, R. L., Free radical protection: why vitamin E, not vitamin C, B-carotene or gluthathione?, in *Biology of Vitamin E*, Pitman Ed., Ciba Foundation Symposium 101, London, 1983, 19.

Wisniewski, H, Wegiel, J., Strojny, P., et al., Ultrastructural morphology and immunohistochemistry of beta amyloid classical, primitive and diffuse plaques, in *Frontiers of Alzheimer's Research*, Ishii, T., Ed., Elsevier, Amsterdam, 1991, 99.

Yasuda, R. R., Ciesla, W., Flores, L. R., et al., Development of antisera selective for M4 and M5 muscarinic cholinergic receptors: distribution of M4 and M5 receptors in rat brain, *Mol. Pharmacol.*, 43, 149, 1993.

Chapter **23**

PSYCHOSOCIAL INTERVENTIONS

Mary S. Mittelman
Steven H. Ferris

CONTENTS

I. INTRODUCTION

Alzheimer's disease (AD) has devastating effects on both the patients who suffer from the disease and on the families who care for them. The promising current research to discover and evaluate pharmacological treatments for the cognitive and behavioral symptoms of AD are described elsewhere in this book. It is clear that great strides are being made in the direction of understanding the basic pathophysiology of AD and in translating these results into potential therapeutic strategies. However, currently available pharmacologic treatments produce only modest improvements in symptoms. The possibility of halting the progression of the disease or achieving the ultimate goal of preventing onset of symptoms remains far in the future. In the meantime, the financial and emotional cost of AD to patients and families as well as to the federal health care budget continues to grow as the population continues to age. It is essential that innovative interventions be developed to mitigate the *impact* of the disease on patients, families, and society as a whole. The focus of these interventions should be to avoid excess disability of patients and improve the ability of families to care for them without deleterious consequences to themselves. Successful efforts will have a marked effect on the social and economic impact of AD on families and on the health care system.

II. INTERVENTIONS FOR PATIENTS

A. RATIONALE FOR NONPHARMACOLOGIC INTERVENTIONS

AD patients commonly manifest a variety of behavioral ("noncognitive") symptoms, particularly during the middle stages of illness. The nature of these symptoms and the psychotropic medications currently available for their management have been described in a previous chapter of this book. However, these medications generally are not fully effective and frequently have undesirable side effects as well. Paradoxically, these side effects can even include an increase in the cognitive and behavioral symptoms of dementia. Many of the behavioral symptoms associated with AD, including depression, agitation, wandering, and incontinence, potentially can be managed or minimized using nonpharmacologic treatment methods. Some of these symptoms may not be direct consequences of the impact of AD on the neurologic system, but rather result from the frustration of the impaired individual who can no longer function competently in his environment. Therefore, it is essential to develop nonpharmacologic interventions to be used either alone or in conjunction with pharmacologic interventions. Nonpharmacologic interventions have the potential advantages of optimizing the use of the remaining intact areas of functioning of the patient while avoiding the undesirable side effects of medications and of involving family caregivers and paid caregivers with the patients in constructive and gratifying ways. However, although the behavioral concomitants of AD have been well documented, very few systematic, controlled trials of nonpharmacologic interventions to control these symptoms have been reported in the literature.

B. INTERVENTIONS FOR EARLY STAGE PATIENTS

In the early stages of AD the primary symptom of the disease is memory loss. Awareness of deterioration may lead to depression, anger, and grief. At this time, patients have to cope not only with symptoms of disease, but also with loss of jobs and changing relationships with family members. Loving relatives may deny that the patients are ill or try to shield the patients from awareness of their illness. They frequently avoid discussing the patient's illness. Thus, the patient at this stage may feel that he or she has lost any meaningful role in society and has become isolated from former work-related relationships and from family members as well.

1. Alleviating Depression

Depression is a frequent symptom of the early stages of AD. At this point in the disease, patients are generally aware that they are not able to function normally. Many caregivers in support groups have suggested that patients in the early stages of dementia would also benefit from support groups. These caregivers say that they feel inadequate to the task of broaching the subject of the illness, having difficulty adjusting to the diagnosis themselves, although they sense that the patients want to talk about it. Caregivers also express the belief that patient support groups would assist them in their own caregiving responsibilities and would alleviate their sense of guilt and helplessness. The results of several recent pilot studies suggest that participation in *patient* support groups can alleviate patient depression associated with the early stages of the disease.

There have been several clinical reports of cognitive therapy strategies for alleviating depression in AD patients with mild impairment. Patients were seen individually by therapists in structured sessions in which they were encouraged to identify positive experiences and pleasant activities. Depression rating scales employed before and after treatment suggest a decline in symptoms of depression.

Education and training of caregivers may alter their responses to the patients and diminish the symptoms of depression in both patients and caregivers. In one treatment/control study, training the caregivers to provide cognitive stimulation to AD patients prevented the development of symptoms of depression in patients as well as in caregivers. Another study of behavioral management strategies for caregivers of patients at this stage of the illness also showed a reduction in patient depression.

2. Sheltered Workshops

Many people in the early stages of AD are forced, because of functional limitations, to quit their jobs. They are not incapacitated enough for day care centers and may remain at home when they would prefer to work. Sheltered workshops, which enable patients to do productive work, have been shown to be effective for both the mentally ill and the mentally retarded. A pilot study of a sheltered workshop for AD patients improved the morale of patients and family members. Although they are expensive to run, requiring a low patient to staff ratio to operate successfully, sheltered workshops may provide a sense of usefulness for patients and make the transition to day care easier to accept.

C. INTERVENTIONS FOR MIDDLE STAGE PATIENTS

Behavioral problems such as agitation, wandering, and violence are particularly prevalent in the middle stages of AD. By this point in the disease, patients are no longer as aware that they are ill, but may be much more frustrated by their inability to communicate their needs. They can no longer comprehend complicated environments. To some extent, the behavioral symptoms of AD can be managed by proper education of caregivers. At this stage, family members and paid caregivers must be trained to simplify the environments of patients and to interpret nonverbal cues.

1. Behavioral Management

There have been clinical reports of interventions to provide patients in the middle stages of AD with pleasant events and activities in which they were still able to participate. Day care centers which include physical activities, art, and music therapy and a club-like environment report positive reactions from both patients and families. Additional intervention strategies involve training family members or paid caregivers in the use of "operant" learning techniques to reduce or eliminate agitation, aggressivity, and other disruptive behaviors. Current research is evaluating the potential effectiveness of these behavioral management techniques.

2. Environmental Restructuring

As AD progresses, patients become easily confused and disoriented if they are presented with complicated external stimuli. Innovative efforts at simplifying the environment have been implemented in congregate care facilities, such as pictures of toilets on the doors of bathrooms, and pictures of the contents of dresser drawers on the outside. Case reports suggest that these visual cues help avoid agitation in patients.

D. INTERVENTIONS FOR LATE STAGE PATIENTS

1. Nonpharmacological Management of Incontinence

Urinary incontinence is one of the most psychologically distressing and socially disruptive problems faced by elderly persons. This loss of function is an inevitable consequence in patients who survive to the most severe stages of AD. The incontinence of an elderly family member has adverse effects on the family caregiver, including burden and stress, health deterioration, economic worries, and the potential for abuse or neglect of the patient. Thus, it is not surprising that incontinence has frequently been cited as a predictor of institutionalization of AD patients. Nevertheless, it is generally agreed that incontinence can often be cured, usually improved, and always managed. Research in nursing homes suggests that behavioral management interventions can be effective. For example, when paid caregivers were trained to develop individualized schedules for toileting patients based on diaries of observations of the patients' mean times to voiding, there was a significant reduction in incontinent episodes. Education was an important component of this intervention and produced a significant increase in knowledge about urinary incontinence among nursing home staff. The use of color and form to identify the bathroom, use of appropriate containment garments or devices, substitution of Velcro fasteners for buttons and zippers, controlling fluid intake, and learning to recognize nonverbal cues have also reduced the problem of incontinence among nursing home patients in demonstration projects. These interventions can be adapted to fit the needs of family caregivers and have the potential to prolong the caregiver's ability to care for the dementia patient in the community.

2. Preventing Contractures

Contractures (which can be defined as a permanent limitation of passive range of motion) can be caused or exacerbated by immobilization of the limbs. It is generally assumed that patients in the last stages of AD can no longer walk, sit unsupported, or feed themselves. However, it is possible that in addition to the role of neurological impairment in causing contractures, these disabilities are at least partly due to the fact that their joints have become contracted and muscles weakened due to inactivity. Thus, hypertonus (increased muscle tone) of the skeletal muscles in combination with inactivity is the presumed cause of contractures in these patients. Patients with head or spinal cord injuries develop hypertonus through a neurologic mechanism which is similar to the mechanism causing hypertonus in AD patients. Studies of these patients have demonstrated that contractures can be prevented by regular range of motion exercises. This suggests that regular active or passive exercise of the limbs also may prevent contractures among AD patients and enable them to continue with some physical activities, such as walking, into later stages of dementia than now appears feasible. By so doing, this intervention might alter the downward spiral of functioning, in which lack of motion causes contractures which in turn make motion painful and leads to more contractures. Case histories of AD patients who have had optimum care have shown remarkable levels of physical functioning in the late stages of the disease. Although such care may be too expensive for the majority of patients, the principles underlying the care, avoiding inactivity to avoid excess disability, could have major cost-saving effects if applied widely.

III. EFFECTS OF ALZHEIMER'S DISEASE ON FAMILY CAREGIVERS

Alzheimer's disease has many deleterious effects on the family members of patients. As the patients deteriorate, they become less and less aware of their disabilities. Families continue to suffer the effects of the illness and are forced to become increasingly more responsible for the health, welfare, and ultimately for the most fundamental activities of daily living of their Alzheimer's relatives. As a result, caring for a family member with AD has severe adverse effects on the mental health of caregivers. As many as 80% of caregivers of dementia patients have been reported to be suffering from chronic fatigue, depression, or anger. Depression has been the most frequently reported outcome of caregiving, to which spouse-caregivers appear to be particularly vulnerable.

In addition, some investigators have also reported that caregiving has a negative impact on the physical health of family caregivers.

Spouse caregivers are particularly affected by the decline of the patient because they have the closest bond to the patient and almost always live with the patient. Spouse caregivers suffer unusually high levels of certain chronic diseases such as diabetes, arthritis, ulcers, and anemia. There is some evidence that the physical health of male spouses of AD patients is particularly affected. For example, they are more likely to suffer such ill effects as high blood pressure.

Families generally prefer to avoid institutionalization of AD patients and spouses are also less likely than other relatives to institutionalize AD patients. However, when caregivers keep patients at home they require considerable support and assistance if their own welfare is to be maintained.

IV. INTERVENTIONS FOR FAMILY CAREGIVERS

A. RATIONALE FOR PROVIDING SUPPORT FOR CAREGIVERS

Caregivers are affected not only by the inevitable cognitive and functional deterioration of the patient caused by the illness, but also by lack of family support, family conflict, problems with roles other than the caregiving role, isolation, and constriction of social activities. Interventions can alter the secondary effects of the illness on caregivers by improving support and reducing family conflict, decreasing isolation, and directly providing assistance in the form of problem-focused strategies and empathetic understanding. There is convincing evidence in a large number of epidemiologic studies as well as from immune and neuroendocrine studies for a relationship between both physical and mental health and quality of social support.

Social support is a potential target for interventions to improve physical and mental health. Social support has been operationally defined as including tangible assistance (such as physical or financial support), emotional support, information and advice, providing someone to confide in, and socializing. Evidence suggests that the *quality* of the relationships among family members — the emotional closeness of the members of the social network, whether contacts are helpful or upsetting and the reciprocity of each relationship — are more important than the quantity of support.

B. TYPES OF INTERVENTIONS THAT HAVE BEEN INVESTIGATED

1. Support Groups

The most commonly investigated intervention to improve the well-being of caregivers has been support groups. The rationale for this intervention is that support groups provide a trusting, nonjudgmental atmosphere, an extended social network, a mutual support system, and a forum for information exchange. Thus, caregiver support groups can simultaneously decrease social isolation and teach practical solutions to common problems.

Research reports suggest that support groups are effective in increasing knowledge about dementia among participants. In some studies, there has been evidence that support groups delay institutionalization of patients and reduce burden, depression, and anxiety among caregivers who had previous high levels of stress. These results suggest that support groups can ameliorate the burden of caregiving, although they are inconsistent in their estimates of the size or the precise manifestation of the effects. However, other studies contradict these findings, showing no effectiveness of support groups when unaccompanied by other supportive treatments. Thus, there is no consistent objective evidence for efficacy, although the subjective perceptions of the helpfulness of support groups reported by participants are generally positive.

2. Individualized Services

Other interventions for family caregivers have also been tested with mixed results. Family conflict and a lack of sharing of responsibilities, major problems for caregivers, may be best treated by individualized interventions that also involve other members of the family. A study in England evaluated a program that provided individually tailored services including family counseling to elderly subjects with dementia. There were no differences between treatment and control groups in the number of admissions to nursing homes within a year of entry into the study among elderly subjects who lived with caregivers.

3. Stress Management, Education, and Respite

Stress management in either individual and family settings or in support groups appears to have no effect on measured burden. Education in small groups appears to improve sense of mastery, knowledge, and control among caregivers. However, neither education, discussion, role play in groups, nor home visits by nurses combined with home respite have demonstrated significant effects on depression in caregivers. Studies suggest that formal and informal respite services may make it possible to postpone nursing home placement of demented patients, but have not demonstrated any effect on objective measures of caregiver well-being.

C. PROBLEMS WITH INTERVENTION STUDIES FOR FAMILY CAREGIVERS

Studies designed to test the effects of interventions to improve the well-being of caregivers have yielded inconsistent results. Many intervention studies have included caregivers of all frail elderly rather than restricting themselves to those suffering from AD. Although caregivers of all disabled elderly have many problems in common, caregivers of AD patients may also experience aspects of burden unique to the characteristics of the disease. For example, AD lasts for many years and insidiously affects the patient's mind while the patient's physical functioning is spared for much of the disease's duration. In addition, the effects of caregiving depend on the relationship of the caregiver to the patient and whether the caregiver is living with the patient or not. These factors have not been taken into consideration in most intervention studies.

An AD patient can require many years of caregiving. This suggests that, in order to be effective, a treatment strategy and its evaluation must continue over a period of years. Nevertheless, most interventions to date have been conducted for only a few weeks or months. In addition, the effects of nonpharmacologic interventions may not be immediately felt, and yet studies have generally measured effectiveness for only a short period of time.

There have been many reports of interventions that seemed promising, but the evaluations were often done with neither objective measures nor control groups. Frequently the only evidence of positive outcomes are such subjective measures as caregiver satisfaction with the intervention. Study samples frequently are small, so that, although the interventions may in fact be effective, there are not enough data to show statistically significant results. This problem is compounded by the fact that, in many studies, sample size is considerably reduced by attrition before outcomes can be measured. In addition, participants in these studies are generally self-selected. Those most in need of intervention, in whom the most improvement might be shown, frequently do not participate in studies either because they are unable to leave home or because they are unaware of the potential benefits of treatment. Those least in need of intervention, because they have considerable tangible and emotional resources, are probably the most likely to use available services and therefore participate in research studies. Thus, lack of demonstrated treatment efficacy may be due to poor choice of subjects rather than poor choice of intervention.

D. THE NYU SPOUSE CAREGIVER INTERVENTION STUDY

Our own clinical experience, corroborated by the outcomes of other studies, suggested that a treatment strategy to improve the well-being of caregivers should be based on four principles: (1) each family has unique problems; (2) most caregivers would benefit from more understanding and support from their families; (3) all caregivers run the risk of isolation; and (4) it is necessary to continue to provide support for caregivers throughout the duration of the disease.

The NYU-Aging and Dementia Research Center has been conducting a study to evaluate the potential benefits of a multifaceted, structured treatment program for spouse-caregivers of AD patients since 1987. The goal of the intervention is to enable spouse caregivers to postpone or avoid nursing home placement of patients while minimizing the negative consequences of caregiving to themselves. An important component of the intervention is the involvement of other family members in addition to the spouse.

Study subjects were randomly assigned to a treatment or a control group. The treatment consists of three components: (1) *individual and family counseling* sessions tailored to each caregiver's specific situation; (2) participation in weekly *support groups* after the series of counseling sessions has concluded; (3) *continuous availability of counselors* to caregivers and families to help them deal with crises and with the changing nature of the patient's symptoms over the course of the disease. Counselors also provide *resource information and referrals* for auxiliary help, financial planning, and management of patient behavior problems. Each caregiver in the treatment group receives *all* the interventions, and each is provided with support for an unlimited period of time. Control caregivers receive resource information and help only upon request and receive no formal treatment.

At baseline and at each subsequent assessment, a battery of structured questionnaires is administered. Included are questions about the demographic characteristics of the caregiver and the patient, the responsibilities of the caregiver, the frequency of unpaid help from family and friends, other resources used for help or advice, and what caregivers do to alleviate the stress of caring for the patient. The evaluation also includes assessments of the caregiver's physical and mental health, the extent of caregiver burden, caregiver management of problem behavior, the size of the caregiver's social network and the satisfaction it provides, family cohesion and adaptability, and the safety of the home. In addition, at each assessment period the patient's level of functioning and physical health is reevaluated.

Caregivers in the treatment group have been able to postpone placement of patients in nursing homes considerably longer than control caregivers. The effect of the intervention on nursing home placements was particularly striking in the first 12 months after baseline when fewer than half as many treatment patients were placed in nursing homes as control patients. Over the eight years since the study began, the median time from entry into the study to nursing home placement was 329 days longer in the treatment group than in the control group. It was estimated that the intervention reduced the risk of placement at any given point in time by about one third. The intervention was particularly effective in preventing nursing home placement during the early to middle stages of dementia when it is generally least appropriate. The intervention also alleviated some of the deleterious effects of caregiving on caregiver depression. Although the effect was not immediate in most cases, the impact of the intervention on depression increased with each follow-up in the 1st year after subjects entered the study. Changes in depression were small for most caregivers, but the majority of caregivers who became substantially more depressed were in the control group, while the majority of caregivers who became substantially less depressed were in the treatment group.

The question remains as to what aspects of the intervention lead to the effectiveness of the treatment. Many researchers have theorized that social support mediates the stress of caring for an AD patient. We examined the effect of the intervention on the social system to help explain the effects of the treatment on depression in caregivers. The results showed that caregivers in the treatment group experienced increased family cohesion and were markedly more satisfied with their social networks.

Caregivers frequently include the family counselors in their lists of members of their social networks with whom they feel close. This suggests that the intervention, by directly providing caregivers with social support in their relationship with the family counselors, increases their satisfaction with their social networks. The difference between the treatment and control groups does not diminish with time nor does the availability of family counselors or the support groups. These results provide evidence to substantiate the theory that social support mediates between the primary stress of caregiving and outcomes such as caregiver mental health.

V. INTERVENTIONS FOR PAID CAREGIVERS

When an AD patient becomes severely impaired, some or all of the caregiving tasks are frequently performed by paid caregivers, either at home or in institutional settings such as nursing homes or day care facilities. Much of the hands-on care is performed by nurses aides, who are generally not highly educated. Their knowledge of dementia and training in caring for patients is limited. It should be possible, however, to optimize patient functioning through appropriate education and training of paid caregivers.

A. BEHAVIOR MANAGEMENT

Behavior management interventions have been used to treat a wide variety of problems in institutions, including activities of self-care, incontinence, walking, and improving participation in social activities. There has been little rigorous research documenting the results of these interventions in institutions. However, the clinical experience of health care professionals suggests that behavioral and environmental modifications can be employed effectively in modifying symptoms of dementia. For example, simplification of the environment has been reported to reduce agitation among residents of nursing homes. Physical cues have been used to direct behavior. There have been many encouraging reports of case histories in which the remaining strengths of dementia patients were identified and activities designed to capitalize on these strengths.

Occasionally, natural experiments provide evidence for changes in patient care. In recent years there has been a widespread implementation of laws that require nursing homes to stop using restraints unless they are demonstrably unavoidable. Reports from some nursing homes of the outcome of removal of restraints indicated a dramatic reduction both in the number of falls and in incontinence. A report from another nursing home concluded that, although the incidence of minor falls increased, the number of serious falls did not.

B. STAFF TRAINING

Several researchers have reported that changing the behavior of staff and families can result in improvement in the ability of patients to conduct activities of daily living and in decreased agitation. However, these studies reported no improvement in staff satisfaction as a result of these interventions. Special training and incentives for aides who provide most of the daily care is an essential element in interventions designed for institutional settings.

C. INCONTINENCE MANAGEMENT TRAINING

The cost to society of urinary incontinence has been estimated as more than $10 billion annually. This loss of function is an inevitable consequence in patients who survive to the most severe stages of AD. Studies in nursing homes have demonstrated that behavioral interventions to reduce urinary incontinence have generally had positive results. One effective intervention to reduce incontinent episodes relied on using a diary of observed voiding to develop individual pattern voiding schedules so that patients were toileted within 30 minutes of their recorded mean time. Education was an important component of this intervention and produced a significant increase in knowledge about urinary incontinence among nursing home staff. Unfortunately, the positive effects of training were generally diminished after the staff training period. These studies suggest that training nurses aides is of limited value unless they are also provided with motivation to perform these time-consuming interventions. Current nursing home management structure encourages the performance by staff of custodial, rather than therapeutic, services.

D. SPECIAL CARE UNITS

In recent years, many nursing homes have created special care units (SCUs) for dementia patients. Currently, research in these units suffers from problems of small sample size and difficulties with measurement and implementation of interventions. The SCUs have the potential to be research laboratories for innovative interventions. An NIA initiative has encouraged a collaborative multisite study of SCUs throughout the country. In addition, a group of researchers in SCUs, currently with more than 100 members, has been formed to identify and develop promising interventions, discuss measurement and assessment issues, make research and policy recommendations, and disseminate information.

VI. SUMMARY AND CONCLUSIONS

Despite the great potential of nonpharmacologic interventions for AD patients and their care-givers, research into their efficacy has been hampered by difficulties in identifying appropriate outcomes and difficulties in measuring these outcomes. In addition, while it is routine to conduct well-designed, double-blind treatment-control studies of pharmacologic interventions, it is extremely difficult to design double-blind studies of psychosocial interventions. Nevertheless, progress has been made recently in overcoming these obstacles, and creative new research strategies are currently being developed.

At best, these interventions can prevent excess disability and slow or temporarily impede the inevitable downward course of functioning resulting from the progressive loss of cognitive capacity in AD patients. Families can be provided with emotional and tangible support and taught how best to care for their demented relatives to maximize their functioning within the confines of the effects of the disease. Paid caregivers can be taught the same patient management techniques as family caregivers. Paid caregivers need to be given incentives to provide more than merely custodial care. They generally do not have the same emotional incentives to preserve the well-being of patients as family members. On the other hand, since paid caregivers spend only a limited amount of time with patients, it may be possible for them to implement interventions which family caregivers may be too burdened or exhausted to carry out effectively.

Applying the rigorous criteria of scientific research, few psychosocial interventions have proven effectiveness. However, clinical evidence suggests that they can be effective both alone and as adjuncts to pharmacologic interventions. Results of the NYU Spouse Caregiver Intervention Study provide evidence that, with large samples of subjects evaluated over a sufficiently long period of time, it is possible to demonstrate the efficacy of a nonpharmacologic intervention. Such interventions have great potential for alleviating the social and economic impact of AD.

ACKNOWLEDGMENT

We gratefully acknowledge the assistance of Lisa McElroy, Ph.D., in the preparation of this manuscript.

REFERENCES

Colling, J., Ouslander, J., Hadley, B. J., Eisch, J., and Campbell, E., The effects of patterned urge-response toileting (PURT) on urinary incontinence among nursing home residents, *J. Am. Geriat. Soc.*, 40, 135, 1992.

Cotrell, V. and Schulz, R., The perspective of the patient with Alzheimer's disease: a neglected dimension of dementia research, *Gerontologist*, 33(2), 205, 1993.

Haley, W. E., Brown, S. L., and Levine, E. G., Experimental evaluation of the effectiveness of group intervention for dementia caregivers, *Gerontologist*, 27, 376, 1987.

Lawton, M. P., Brody, E. M., and Saperstein, A. R., A controlled study of respite service for caregivers of Alzheimer's patients, *Gerontologist*, 29, 8, 1989.

Mittelman, M., Ferris, S., Steinberg, G., Shulman, E., Mackell, J., Ambinder, A., and Cohen, J., An intervention that delays institutionalization of Alzheimer's disease patients: treatment of spouse-caregivers, *Gerontologist*, 33, 730, 1993.

Mittelman, M. S., Ferris, S. H., Shulman, E., Steinberg, G., Ambinder, A., Mackell, J. A., and Cohen, J., Comprehensive support for families of AD patients: Effects on spouse-caregiver depression, *The Gerontologist,* 35, 792–802, 1995.

Teri, L. and Gallagher-Thompson, D., Cognitive-behavioral interventions for treatment of depression in Alzheimer's patients, *Gerontologist,* 31(3), 413, 1991.

Zarit, S. H., Anthony, C. R. and Boutselis, M., Interventions with care givers of dementia patients: comparison of two approaches, *Psychol. Aging,* 2(3), 225, 1987.

CARE AND MANAGEMENT

Chapter 24

INAPPROPRIATE BEHAVIOR

Jiska Cohen-Mansfield

CONTENTS

0-8493-8997-6/97/$0.00+$.50

I. DESCRIPTION OF INAPPROPRIATE BEHAVIOR

Inappropriate behaviors are those behaviors which are considered by caregivers and other observers to be socially inappropriate or bizarre, and not a direct symptom of dementia (such as a memory problem), or a result of an obvious need (e.g., wetting oneself on the way to the bathroom). Such behaviors include screaming, constant complaining, pacing back and forth, or aggressive behaviors. At times these behaviors have also been named disruptive behaviors or agitated behaviors.

Although caregivers frequently agree that a patient is agitated or behaving inappropriately, the determination of specific inappropriate behaviors is not always simple. Caregivers may disagree as to whether there is an obvious need which explains the behavior. The behavior may be subtle, such as repetitious mannerism, and as such not disruptive to others, and therefore possibly not detected by others. Such unobtrusive behaviors may still be important as they may provide clues to the patient's emotional state. Behaviors may be shaped by past habits or by cultural norms which caregivers are not always aware of.

Because of the difficulties inherent in determining the occurrence of inappropriate behavior, many research projects need to define those *a priori*, i.e., to develop a list of behaviors which are frequently inappropriate and which would be included in the study. These behaviors are rated on the basis of observations or caregivers' reports. The specific causes for the behavior, such as needs, neurologic damage attributable to dementia, and environmental features, are then investigated within the study rather than determined for each occurrence of the behavior.

Behavior problems have been classified into types or categories in several ways, based on their content (e.g, aggressive behavior, verbal behavior), their object (e.g., directed toward self, toward others, toward objects), the type of inappropriateness involved (e.g., a behavior which does not fit social standards for the situation, a behavior which would normally be appropriate but performed at an inappropriate frequency), or their assumed reason (e.g., attention seeking, due to deafness, medication induced, etc.). Based on a few research projects with nursing home residents and participants of adult day care centers, we found two dimensions to be most useful in classifying inappropriate behaviors: (1) aggressive vs. nonaggressive and (2) verbal vs. physical, so that we currently examine four types of behavior problems: physical-aggressive, verbal-aggressive, physical-nonaggressive, and verbal-nonaggressive.[1]

Inappropriate behaviors are, by definition, not completely understood by caregivers and observers. The main challenge posed by these inappropriate behaviors is to understand the cause, or multiple causes, for these behaviors. Causes may be physiological, psychological-motivational, and environmental, and it is probably the interaction of specific disease states, specific unmet needs, certain past habits, some retained abilities, and certain environmental conditions which produce the behaviors we observe. Only understanding these combinations can help us determine what the behaviors mean. Understanding their meaning is a necessary condition for clarifying the appropriate methods for handling the behavior, such as whether they should be accommodated, ameliorated, or restricted.

Whereas the need to understand the complex causes of inappropriate behaviors may seem obvious, the route to achieving this understanding is only beginning to be clarified. Understanding the motives of the noncommunicative patient who suffers from dementia is difficult detective work. Even seemingly easier tasks, such as understanding physiological status and accompanying sensations, such as pain, can be close to impossible when the person cannot communicate. All these have resulted in a correlational approach to the study of reasons for inappropriate behaviors and only partial answers concerning their causes.

II. CORRELATES OF INAPPROPRIATE BEHAVIORS

Because of the difficulties inherent in understanding the factors which cause inappropriate behaviors in persons suffering from dementia, we chose to examine personal and environmental correlates of these behaviors. These are interpreted so as to shed light on the causes of inappropriate behaviors.

Different types of behavior problems have been associated with different characteristics of older persons and different environmental characteristics. Therefore, the correlates of inappropriate behaviors are described separately for the different types described above.

A. AGGRESSIVE BEHAVIORS

Aggressive behaviors were found to correlate with *cognitive impairment*.[2-9] Aggression was associated with more severe temporal lobe atrophy in a study of Alzheimer's disease.[10] Reisberg et al.,[11] in a study of patients from mixed settings, concluded that activity disturbances and aggression were seen most often in persons with moderately severe to severe levels of cognitive impairment, with secondary peaks in persons with very severe cognitive impairment. Our results[12] differed somewhat from Reisberg's, with ours indicating that aggressive behaviors peaked with very severe levels of cognitive impairment.

Other characteristics of persons manifesting aggression were *impairment in the ability to perform activities of daily living*;[2,5] *male gender*;[2,6,13,14] and *poor quality of social interactions*.[2,3] Several studies found a relationship between aggression and the *premorbid personality* of the elderly person.[3,6,15]

Environmental correlates have also been examined for aggressive behaviors. Aggressive behaviors have been observed more frequently during times of *intimate care*, such as while being helped in performing activities of daily living.[6,15-16] These findings may suggest that aggressive behaviors may occur in response to the frustration at being helped with such elementary activities, or may be a response to touch for which the older person was not prepared or invasion of personal space. Indeed, Marx et al.[17] found an increase in nursing home residents' aggressiveness when they were touched.

In a study on aggression in community-dwelling elderly, Ryden[6] found that aggression was associated with a *noisy atmosphere*. In our observational study of nursing home residents,[18] aggressive behaviors tended to occur when there were *other persons present*; at *night when it was cold*; in environments where the resident was in close contact with another person, such as the bath; or when in touching contact with another person.

When examining specifically what triggered an aggressive event, several studies found that the majority of aggressive events could not be attributed to any clear trigger.[19,20] In contrast, Meyer et al.[21] in a study of geropsychiatric hospital patients, found that the most common antecedent to aggressive behavior was being asked to do something.

Aggressive behaviors in nursing homes tend to be directed toward staff members rather than at other persons in the environment.[8, 19-22] In contrast, residents were reported to be a more frequent target than staff in a study of incident reports in a skilled nursing facility.[23]

The most common reaction to aggressive behaviors is inaction or retreat,[3,15,19] suggesting that these behaviors are not regularly reinforced by attention, although retreat may be reinforcing to the older person when he/she is not willing to participate in an activity of daily living.

The personal and environmental correlates of aggression can be interpreted to suggest the following causes of aggressive behaviors:

1. The neurological damage associated with severe dementia may cause aggression directly, or facilitate disinhibition, especially among persons with a premorbid tendency toward antisocial or aggressive behaviors.
2. Aggression is the older person's response to a perception of danger or discomfort, such as invasion of personal space, invasion of privacy, or an uncomfortable environment. It may be an effort to dismiss the danger-causing stimuli, or an attempt to communicate about the danger, which is frustrated by inability to communicate verbally.

Although the above generalizations may apply for many aggressive behaviors, every specific instance needs to be investigated individually, with an effort to comprehend the behavior for the specific individual in a given situation. The research findings can only be used as guidelines for initial hypotheses explaining any individual's behavior. The actual understanding for the individual person needs to take into account his/her history, current problems and needs, and the environment's ability to fulfil these needs.

B. PACING AND WANDERING

Pacing and wandering were also associated with *cognitive impairment*.[10,24-29] Burns et al.,[10] in a study of Alzheimer's disease, found that wandering was linked with increased size of the sylvian fissure. Persons who wander were more likely than others to experience delusions.[30] In the nursing home, we found that persons who wandered were in *better health* than those who did not wander, i.e., they had fewer medical diagnoses, and better appetites than others. A *premorbid propensity for physical activities* was reported by Monsour and Robb,[31] who found that prior to the onset of incapacitating illness, wanderers (as compared to nonwanderers) were more active in their leisure activities than persons who did not wander; however, our research failed to replicate these findings.

In terms of environmental correlates of pacing and wandering, we[25] found that pacing/wandering occurred more frequently when there was adequate lighting and low noise levels; wandering tended to occur in corridors where there was sufficient space to ambulate.

These findings suggest that wandering and pacing behaviors are quite different from aggressive behaviors in their meaning. Within the restrictions of old age and dementia, these behaviors were correlated with relatively good health and were not associated with environmental discomfort. Furthermore, these behaviors may provide some adaptive benefit in that they provide exercise and stimulation to persons who have difficulty obtaining these otherwise, because of their difficulty communicating with the environment. Given these benefits and given that these behaviors do not have as clear a negative impact as aggressive behaviors, they may need to be considered beneficial. In this case the behaviors need to be accommodated so that they can be performed safely rather than corrected by treatment.

As was the case with aggressive behaviors, any individual person needs to be analyzed for his/her unique reasons for the wandering or pacing behavior. Clinically, one sees persons who are obviously searching for their home, or their family, and for whom the behavior is clearly associated with anguish, which requires treatment. There are other individual reasons, such as medication effects, dissatisfaction with the environment, etc., which need to be assessed and addressed.

C. VERBALLY DISRUPTIVE BEHAVIORS

Although verbally disruptive behaviors have also been associated with cognitive impairment,[12,32,33] our findings indicate a difference between aggressive verbally disruptive behaviors, such as screaming and cursing, which are related to cognitive impairment and nonaggressive verbally disruptive behaviors, such as repetitive verbalizations or milder vocalizations, where the relationship with cognitive impairment was not as clear. In the nursing home, verbally disruptive behaviors were associated with *functional impairment*,[12,32,33] and with *sleep disturbances*.[32,33] Verbally disruptive behaviors were associated with *female* gender[12,34] and with *health and affective problems*, as manifested in a larger number of physical diagnoses, more pain, and depressed affect in comparison to other nursing home residents.[34]

Environmental correlates of verbally disruptive behaviors, which included screaming, and other verbally inappropriate behaviors were being alone in the room, in the evening or at night, and being physically restrained. These behaviors were also frequent during activities of daily living, mainly toileting and bathing.[33] Most of the verbal agitation (92%) went unnoticed, without any reaction by anyone. The interpretation of verbally inappropriate behaviors is very different from that of pacing and wandering. Verbally inappropriate behaviors are related to poor health, affective problems, discomfort, and discontent, and therefore seem to indicate underlying needs which should be addressed in treatment.

III. TREATMENT FOR INAPPROPRIATE BEHAVIORS

The summary of correlates of inappropriate behaviors demonstrates that it is possible to identify likely causes of the behaviors, even when the person suffering from dementia is unable to communicate these causes. The process described, of examining medical, psychosocial, personal-historical, and environmental variables in trying to understand these behaviors, is indeed similar to the process which needs to take place in determining an intervention for any specific individual manifesting these behaviors. The reported research findings can serve as guidelines, to short-circuit the long process of finding the cause of behavior for any specific person. Therefore, in the case of verbally disruptive behavior, for example, hitherto undetected pain or other physical discomfort should be investigated first; other avenues for investigation should be fears, loneliness, and depression. Conversely, for the wanderer, the possibility that this is an adaptation of past coping skills should be investigated.

Once plausible causes are determined, treatment follows directly. Obviously, if the cause is physical in nature, a medical response, which may at least ease the pain and discomfort, is sought. When the issue is loneliness, fears, and depression, methods for soothing those persons are needed, some of which may utilize past social support, findings about past ways of relaxing, employing music therapy, activity therapy, and other modes of therapy. If, on the other hand, the behavior does not seem to indicate discomfort, the function of therapy may be reversed: rather than change the older person, therapy may be employed with the environment, physical and human, to accommodate the behavior or to channel it into routes which serve the adaptational function for the older person, without interfering with the routines of others, and without placing them in danger.

A. REPORTED INTERVENTIONS IN THE LITERATURE

In the literature, reports of interventions for behavioral problems are generally case reports or program descriptions. Controlled clinical trials are sorely lacking. Therefore, the reports from the literature should be viewed as eliciting suggestions and hypotheses, rather than as findings which can guide practice.

Generally, the interventions described in the literature can be described in five categories: behavioral interventions, environmental design, supportive interventions, educational interventions, and pharmacologic interventions.

1. Behavioral Interventions

Several studies use reinforcement to strengthen desirable behaviors. For *aggressive behaviors,* there are reports of use of a *token economy program* to reduce self-injurious behaviors among elderly long-term mental hospital patients;[35] *social reinforcement of appropriate behaviors* by staff members was also used to decrease aggressive behaviors.[36]

For *wandering* differential reinforcement of other behavior was used by Fatis et al. (as described in Hussian[37]) in a case study of an institutionalized 76-year-old female suffering from Alzheimer's disease.

Reports concerning behavioral interventions for *verbally disruptive behaviors* include *contingent positive reinforcement* for quiet time (usually social reinforcement), modified *time out, ignoring the behavior,* and *examining antecedents* to the behavior.[38-41] Other forms of behavioral treatments used were *social skills training program,* which used instructions, modeling, role playing, and feedback;[42] and *relaxation with guided imagery.*[43]

2. Environmental Design

For *wandering and pacing* a number of environmental modifications have been tried, with the goal of eliminating exit behavior and therefore keeping the older person in a safe, enclosed area. In institutions, *locked or semilocked doors* are used to assure that the elderly person ambulates freely only within the safe confines of the unit or the facility, and does not endanger him/herself outside.[44-49] Semi-locked doors include mechanisms which can only be operated by a cognitively intact person, so that the unit becomes a locked one for persons with cognitive impairment, but open for cognitively intact persons. The person who wanders usually cannot open these doors, but may get very upset trying to open them. Another environmental intervention is the use of *visual cues* on doors or floor which deter the wandering person from exiting that door. A two-dimensional grid pattern on the floor in front of doors was used by Hussian and Brown,[50] although their success was not replicated by Chafetz.[51] Other grids were used by Namazi et al.,[52] who found that a patterned cloth over the middle portion of the door, hiding the doorknob, eliminated attempts to exit. Other visual cues to decrease trespassing into other residents' rooms include large signs or pictures marking residents rooms.[53] Another method for stopping exit behavior is the use of *alarm systems*, which are activated when the older person exits through the door or is within a certain distance from the door. The system therefore alerts a caregiver, who needs to attend to the person.[55,55] Finally, rather than preventing exit behavior, *identity bracelets* assist in identifying the lost wanderer who wears them.[44,56]

Another type of environmental manipulation reported in the literature is the use of physical restraints which physically prevent the person from wandering. Because of a combination of ethical issues about limiting the autonomy of a person by restraining him/her and because of research on the ill effects of physical restraints, such as serious injuries,[57] increased agitation,[58] urinary retention, muscle atrophy, and osteoporosis,[59] there is a consensus that these are not appropriate for the management of wandering. This is also reflected in the Omnibus Budget Reconciliation Act (1987),[60] which mandated that physical restraints not be used to treat wandering and pacing in nursing home residents.

3. Supportive Interventions

Supportive interventions can also be viewed as environmental design, but, rather than concentrating on the physical environment, they also include the human environment. For *wandering and pacing*, it has been suggested that accompanying the wanderer to assure his/her safety is sometimes the appropriate intervention, when the older person has an agenda of walking outside, which should be allowed.[61] Comfort and talk with a caregiver were also identified as interventions for persons who wander or pace.[62-66]

For *verbally disruptive* behaviors, *environmental enrichment* has been described, including increasing sensory stimulation, with the use of music and touch.[43,67]

Most of the behavioral interventions (described in Section 1 above) utilize social reinforcement and other aspects which could be construed as supportive intervention. Based on the available research it is unclear whether the effective component of these treatments was the appropriate contingencies (i.e., the timing of the reinforcement to match appropriate behavior) or the provision of more supportive environments.

4. Educational Interventions

Most interventions, if found effective, require education of caregivers in their administration. This is particularly important in behavioral and supportive interventions, but is also true for the others: if an alarm system is used to safeguard persons who wander, the caregiver needs to know what to do when the alarm is activated; even the administration of pharmacologic agents is not trivial when a person is manifesting severe behavioral problems. In view of the centrality of this issue, the scarcity of research in this area is noteworthy.

For *aggressive behaviors*, several educational programs for caregivers have been described: Mentes and Ferrario[68] developed an education program for nursing aides focusing on the identification of risk factors and prevention of aggressive episodes. Ryden and Feldt[69] described a care program aimed at increasing the residents' feelings of safety and physical comfort, enabling them to experience a sense of control, thus providing optimal levels of stress, and providing them with pleasurable experiences.

5. Pharmacological Interventions

Many types of drugs have been used to manage behavioral problems, although their efficacy is not yet established.[70-72]

For *aggressive behaviors*, the following agents have been used: anxiolytic drugs for a short-term treatment;[73,74] antidepressants;[75] antipsychotic drugs, which are the most commonly used for the management of aggression;[76-78] an anticonvulsant drug (Carbamazepine[79]); beta-blockers;[78,80,81] and estrogen.[82] Obviously, adverse effects are a major concern in many of these treatments and affect the choice of treatment, its regimen, and its monitoring.

For *verbally disruptive behaviors*, the use of a combination of trazodone and tryptophan has been described.[83,84]

Another medical, though not pharmacologic, treatment reported for verbally disruptive behavior is the use of *electroconvulsive therapy*.[85]

B. CHALLENGES IN THE DEVELOPMENT OF TREATMENT PROGRAMS

The most difficult challenge in treatment of behavioral problem is the need for human and humane resources. The identification of the needs of the older person who suffers from dementia is time consuming. Moreover, many of the treatments seem to require care: the person who screams alone at night in his room and seems to be fearful and depressed requires soothing and companionship. The aggressive person who seems to feel threatened when approached for help with activities of daily living may need to be approached in a different, possibly slower, or more delicate, way. The challenge is twofold: to find ways to locate and afford the personnel who can provide this type of care and to find interventions in which these needs will be met with a minimum of staff members, possibly using videotapes, volunteers, better matching of roommates, or other methods. As a society we have yet to start addressing these challenges.

On an even more basic level, interventions for behavior problems need to be systematized and to be studied systematically. This study is difficult and expensive, because of the inherent problems in studying this population and because of the great variability among older persons and their caregivers. However, the state of knowledge is such that such studies can, and should be done, in order to guide caregivers in treating behavior problems.

Finally, we need to know how to train, treat, and support caregivers. It is evident that simple in-service training sessions are insufficient for assisting caregivers in addressing as complex and difficult a problem as inappropriate behaviors. Ongoing support systems for staff members and families need to be developed and tried.

Inappropriate behaviors are prevalent among persons suffering from dementia. The main types of such behaviors: physically aggressive behaviors, verbally aggressive behaviors, physically non-aggressive behaviors, and verbally nonaggressive behaviors, seem to stem from differing etiologies, and therefore require different treatments. Whereas physically nonaggressive behaviors frequently need to be accommodated, verbal behaviors frequently indicate unmet physical or psychological needs which should be identified and provided for. Addressing inappropriate behaviors adequately will require the devotion of considerable clinical and research resources.

REFERENCES

1. Cohen-Mansfield, J., Werner, P., Watson, V., and Pasis, S. Agitation in participants of adult day care centers: experiences of relatives and staff, *Int. Psychogeriat.*, 7(3), 447, 1995.
2. Marx, M. S., Cohen-Mansfield, J., and Werner, P. A profile of the aggressive nursing home resident, *Behav., Health Aging*, 1(1), 65, 1990.
3. Hamel, M., Gold, D. P., Andres, D., Reis, M., Dastoor, D., Grauer, H., and Bergman, H., Predictors and consequences of aggressive behavior by community-based dementia patients, *Gerontologist*, 30(2), 206, 1990.
4. Winger, J., Schirm, V., and Steward, D., Aggressive behavior in long-term care, *J. Psychosoc. Nursing*, 25(4), 28, 1987.

5. Meddaugh, D. I. Aggressive and nonaggressive nursing home patients, *Gerontologist*, 27 (special issue), 127A, 1987.

6. Ryden, M. B., Aggressive behavior in persons with dementia living in the community, *Alzheimer Dis. Assoc. Disord. Intl. J.*, 2(4), 342, 1988.

7. Swearer, J. M., Drachman, D. A., O'Donnell, B. F., and Mitchell, A. L., Troublesome and disruptive behaviors in dementia: Relationships to diagnosis and disease severity, *J. Am. Geriat. Soc.*, 36(9), 784, 1988.

8. Patel, V. and Hope, R. A., Aggressive behavior in elderly psychiatric inpatients, *Acta Psychiatr. Scand.*, 85(2), 131, 1992.

9. Fleishman, R., Rosin, A., Tomer, A., and Schwartz, R. Cognitive impairment and quality of care in long-term care institutions, *Compreh. Gerontol.*, 1, 18, 1987.

10. Burns, A., Jacoby, R., and Levy, R. Psychiatric phenomena in Alzheimer's Disease. IV. Disorders of behavior. *Br. J. Psychiat.*, 157, 86, 1990.

11. Reisberg, B., Franssen, E., Sclan, S. G., Kluger, A., and Ferris, S. H., Stage specific incidence of potentially remediable behavioral symptoms in aging and Alzheimer's disease: a study of 120 patients using the BEHAVE-AD, *Bull. Clin. Neurosci.*, 54, 95, 1989.

12. Cohen-Mansfield, J., Culpepper, W. J., and Werner, P., The relationship beween cognitive functioning and agitation in senior day care participants, *Int. J. Geriat. Psychiat.*, 10, 585, 1995.

13. Jackson, M. E., Drugovich, M. L., Fretwell, M. D., Spector, W. D., Sternberg, J. S., and Rosenstein, R. B., Prevalence and correlates of disruptive behavior in the nursing home, *J. Aging Health*, 1(3), 349, 1989.

14. Ryden, M. and Bossenmaier, M., Aggressive behavior in cognitively impaired nursing home residents, *Gerontologist*, 28(special issue), 179A, 1988.

15. Ware, C. J. G., Fairburn, C. G., and Hope, R. A., A community-based study of aggressive behavior in dementia, *Int. J. Geriat. Psychiat.*, 5, 337, 1990.

16. Nilsson, K., Palmstierna, T., and Wistedt, B., Aggressive behavior in hospitalized psychogeriatric patients, *Acta Psychiat. Scand.*, 78, 172, 1988.

17. Marx, M. S., Werner, P., and Cohen-Mansfield, J., Agitation and touch in the nursing home, *Psychol. Rep.*, 64, 1019, 1989.

18. Cohen-Mansfield, J., and Werner, P., Environmental influences on agitation: An integrative summary of an observational study, *Am. J. Alzheimer's Care Relat. Disord. Res.*, 10(1), 32, 1995.

19. Cohen-Mansfield, J., Werner, P., and Marx, M. S., The social environment of the agitated nursing home resident, *Int. J. Geriat. Psychiat.*, 7, 789, 1992.

20. Colenda, C. C. and Hamer, R. M., Antecedents and interventions for aggressive behavior of patients at a geropsychiatric state hospital, *Hosp. Commun. Psychiat.*, 42(3), 287, 1991.

21. Meyer, J., Schalock, R., and Genaidy, H., Aggression in psychiatric hospitalized geriatric patients, *Int. J. Geriat. Psychiat.*, 6, 589, 1991.

22. Bridges-Parlet, S., Knopman, D., and Thompson, T., A descriptive study of physically aggressive behavior in dementia by direct observation, *J. Am. Geriat. Soc.*, 42, 192, 1994.

23. Malone, M. L., Thompson, L., and Goodwin, J. S., Aggressive behaviors among institutionalized elderly, *J. Am. Geriat. Soc.*, 41, 853, 1993.

24. Burns, A., Jacoby, R., and Levy, R., Behavioral abnormalities and psychiatric symptoms in Alzheimer's disease: preliminary findings, *Int. Psychogeriat.*, 2(1), 25, 1990.

25. Cohen-Mansfield, J., Werner, P., Marx, M. S., and Freedman, L., Two studies of pacing in the nursing home, *J. Gerontol. Med. Sci.*, 46(3), M77, 1991.

26. Cooper, J. K., Mungas, D., and Weiler, P. G. Relation of cognitive status and abnormal behaviors in Alzheimer's disease, *J. Am. Gerontol. Soc.*, 38(8), 867, 1990.

27. Dawson, P. and Reid, D. W., Behavioral dimensions of patients at risk of wandering, *Gerontologist*, 27(1), 104, 1987.

28. Snyder, L. H., Rupprecht, P., Pyrek, J., Brekhus, S., and Moss, T., Wandering, *Gerontologist*, 18(3), 272, 1978.

29. Teri, L., Larson, E. B., and Reifler, B. V., Behavioral disturbance in dementia of the Alzheimer's type, *J. Am. Geriat. Soc.*, 36(1), 1, 1988.

30. Lachs, M. S., Becker, M., Siegal, A. P., Miller. R. P., and Tinetti, M. E., Delusions and behavioral disturbances in cognitively impaired elderly persons, *J. Am. Geriat. Soc.*, 40, 768, 1992.

31. Monsour, N. and Robb, S. S., Wandering behavior in old age: a psychosocial study, *Social Work*, 27(5), 411, 1982.

32. Cariaga, J., Burgio, L., Flynn, W., and Martin, D., A controlled study of disruptive vocalizations among geriatric residents in nursing homes, *J. Am. Geriat. Soc.*, 39, 501, 1991.

33. Cohen-Mansfield, J., Werner, P., and Marx, M. S., Screaming in nursing home residents, *J. Am. Geriat. Soc.*, 38, 785, 1990.

34. Cohen-Mansfield, J., Marx, M. S., and Werner, P., Agitation in elderly persons: an integrative report of findings in a nursing home, *Int. Psychogeriat.*, 4(2), 221, 1992.

35. Mishara, B. L. and Kastenbaum, R., Self-injurious behavior and environmental change in the institutionalized elderly, *Int. J. Aging Hum. Dev.*, 4, 133, 1973.

36. Rosberger, Z. and MacLean, J. Behavioral assessment and treatment of "organic" behaviors in an institutionalized geriatric patient, *Int. J. Behav. Geriat.*, 1(4), 33, 1983.

37. Hussian, R., Wandering disorientation, in *Handbook of Clinical Gerontology*, Carlson, L. L., Edelstein, B. A., Eds., Elmsford, NY, Pergamon Press, 1987.

38. Baltes, M. M. and Lascomb, S. L., Creating a healthy institutional environment for the elderly via behavior management: the nurse as a change agent, *Int. J. Nursing Studies*, 12, 5, 1975.

39. Christie, M. and Ferguson, G., Can't anyone stop that screaming?, *Can. Nurse*, 30, 1988.

40. Davis, A., Behavioural techniques for elderly patients. II, *Nursing Times*, 43, 26, 1983.

41. Wanlass, W. and Culver, S., Behavior modification in a demented nursing home patient, *J. Am. Geriat. Soc.*, 38(8), A18, 1990.

42. Vaccaro, F. J., Application of social skills training in a group of institutionalized aggressive elderly subjects, *Psychol. Aging*, 5(3), 369, 1990.

43. Zachow, K. M., Helen, can you hear me?, *J. Gerontol. Nursing*, 10(8), 18, 1984.

44. Butler, J. P. and Barnett, C. A., Window of wandering, *Geriat. Nursing*, 12(5), 226, 1991.

45. Coons, D. H., Wandering, *Am. J. Alzheimer's Care Relat. Disord. Res.*, 3(1), 31, 1988.

46. Cornbleth, T., Effects of a protected hospital ward area on wandering and nonwandering geriatric patients, *J. Gerontol.*, 32(5), 573, 1977.

47. Grossberg, G. T., Hassan, R., Szwabo, P. A., Morley, J. E., Nakra, B. R. S., Bretscher, C. W., Zimmy, G. H., and Solomon, K., Psychiatric problems in the nursing home, *J. Am. Geriat. Soc.*, 38(8), 907, 1990.

48. Knopman, D. S. and Saywer-DeMaris, S., Practical approach to managing behavioral problems in dementia patients, *Geriatrics*, 45(4), 27, 1990.

49. Rabins, P. V., Wandering, Paper presented at the Alzheimer's Association Annual Scientific Meeting, Chicago, 1991.

50. Hussian, R. A. and Brown, D. C., Use of two-demential grid patterns to limit hazardous ambulation in demented patients, *J. Gerontol.*, 42(5), 558, 1987.

51. Chafetz, P. K., Two-dementional grid is ineffective against demented patients' exiting through glass doors, *Psychol. Aging*, 5(1), 146, 1990.

52. Namazi, K. H., Rosner, T. T., and Calkins, M. P., Visual barriers to prevent patients from exiting through an emergency door, *Gerontologist*, 29(5), 699, 1989.

53. Bertram, M., The use of landmarks, *J. Gerontol. Nursing*, 15(2), 6, 1989.

54. Blackburn, P., Freedom to wander, *Nursing Times*, 84(49), 54, 1988.

55. Negley, E. N., Molla, P. M., and Obenchain, J., No exit: the effects of an electronic security system on confused patients, *J. Gerontol. Nursing*, 16(8), 21, 1990.

56. Gaffney, J., Toward a less restrictive environment, *Geriat. Nursing*, 7(2), 94, 1986.

57. King, T. and Mallet, L., Brachial plexus palsy with the use of haloperidol and a geriatric chair. DICP, *Ann. Pharmacother.*, 25, 1072, 1991.

58. Werner, P., Cohen-Mansfield, J., Braun, J., and Marx, M. S., Physical restraints and agitation in nursing home residents, *J. Am. Geriat. Soc.*, 37(12), 1122, 1989.

59. Rosen, H. D. and Giacomo, J. N., The role of physical restraint in the treatment of psychiatric illness, *J. Clin. Psychiat.*, 39, 228, 1978.

60. Omnibus Budget Reconciliation Act (OBRA), P. L. 100-203, Subtitle C: Nursing Home Reform, 1987.

61. Rader, H., Dolan, J., and Schwab, M., How to decrease wandering, a form of agenda behavior, *Geriat. Nursing*, 6(4), 196, 1985.

62. Burnside, I. M., Wandering behavior, in *Psychosocial Nursing Care of the Aged*, 2nd ed., Burnside, I. M., Ed., New York, McGraw Hill, 1980.

63. McGrowder-Lin, R. and Bhatt, A., A wanderer's lounge program for nursing home residents with Alzheimer's disease, *Gerontologist*, 28(5), 607, 1988.

64. Rader, J., A comprehensive staff approach to problem wandering, *Gerontologist*, 27(6), 756, 1987.

65. Rosswurm, M. A., Zimmerman, S. L., Schwartz-Fulton, J., and Norman, G. A., Can we manage wandering behavior?, *J. Long-Term Care Admin.*, 14, 5, 1986.

66. Sawyer, J. C. and Mendlovitz, A. A., A Management Program for Ambulatory Institutionalized Patients with Alzheimer's Disease and Related Disorders. Paper presented at the Annual Scientific Meeting of the Gerontological Society of American, Boston, 1982.

67. Birchmore, T. and Clague, S., A behavioural approach to reduce shouting, *Nursing Times*, 79, 37, 1983.

68. Mentes, J. C. and Ferraro, J., Calming aggressive reactions: a preventive program, *J. Gerontol. Nursing*, 15(2), 22, 1989.

69. Ryden, M. B. and Feldt, K. S., Goal-directed care: caring for aggressive nursing home residents with dementia, *J. Gerontol. Nursing*, 18(11), 35, 1992.

70. Butler, F. R., Burgio, L. D., and Engel, B. T., Neuroleptics and behavior: a comparative study, *J. Gerontol. Nursing*, 13(6), 15, 1987.

71. Billig, N., Cohen-Mansfield, J., and Lipson, S., Pharmacological treatment of agitation in a nursing home: one possible role of sub-typing, *J. Am. Geriat. Soc.*, 39(10), 1002, 1991.

72. Schneider, L. S., Pollock, V. E., and Lyness, S. A., A Meta-analysis of controlled trials of neuroleptic treatment in dementia, *J. Am. Geriat. Soc.*, 38, 553, 1990.

73. Fritz, J. and Stewart, J. T., *Am. J. Psychiat.*, 147(9), 1250, 1990.

74. Colenda, C. C., Buspirone in treatment of agitated demented patients, *Lancet*, May 21, 1168, 1988.

75. Pinner, E. and Rich, C. L., Effects of trazodone on aggressive behavior in seven patients with organic mental disorders, *Am. J. Psychiat.*, 145(10), 1295, 1988.

76. Herrera, C., Treatment of nocturnal agitation in a patient with Alzheimer's disease, *Gerontologist*, 25(special issue), 84, 1985.

77. Risse, S. C. and Barnes, R., Pharmacologic treatment of agitation associated with dementia, *J. Am. Geriat. Soc.*, 34(5), 368, 1986.

78. Maletta, G. J., Treatment of behavioral symptomatology of Alzheimer's disease with emphasis on aggression: current clinical approaches, *Int. Psychogeriat.*, 4(1), 117, 1992.

79. Marin, D. B. and Greenwald, B. S., Carbamazepine for aggressive agitation in demented patients during nursing care, *Am. J. Psychiat.*, 146, 805, 1989.

80. Petrie, W. M. and Ban, T. A., Propranolol in organic agitation, *Lancet*, 1, 324, 1981.

81. Yudofsky, S., Williams, D., and Gorman, J., Propranolol in the treatment of rage and violent behavior in patients with chronic brain syndrome, *Am. J. Psychiat.*, 138, 218, 1981.

82. Kyomen, H. H., Nobel, K. W., and Wei, J. Y., The use of estrogen to decrease aggressive physical behavior in elderly men with dementia, *J. Am. Geriat. Soc.*, 39, 1110, 1991.

83. Greenwald, B. S., Marin D. B., and Silverman, S. M., Serotoninergic treatment of screaming and banging in dementia (abstract), *Lancet*, December 20/27, 1986.

84. Hottin, P., Pharmacotherapy to control agitation in patients with cognitive deficits (in French) *Can. J. Psychiat.*, 35, 270, 1990.

85. Carlyle, W., Killick, L., and Ancill, R., ECT: an effective treatment in the screaming demented patient, *J. Am. Geriat. Soc.*, 39, 637, 1991.

Chapter 25

MANAGING PROBLEMS IN DEMENTIA PATIENTS: DEPRESSION AND AGITATION

Linda Teri

CONTENTS

I. INTRODUCTION

This chapter focuses on the treatment of two behavioral problems known to be prevalent and pervasive in patients with Alzheimer's disease (AD): depression and agitation. Depression in patients with dementia represents a debilitating combination of emotional, functional, cognitive, and behavioral difficulties. Agitation is one of the most common causes of patient institutionalization and reasons for the use of pharmacological or physical restraints. Consequently, both of these problems represent major health care needs for patients, family, and health care providers.

Depressed demented patients may suffer from dysphoric mood, loss of interest in previously enjoyable activities, trouble sleeping and eating, social and physical withdrawal, fatigue, complaints of worthlessness, guilt, and self-reproach.[1,2] They have been shown to have higher rates of behavioral and functional problems, and their caregivers report higher levels of distress, burden, and depression.[3-9]

Agitated patients with dementia may evidence a variety of problematic behaviors including verbal or physical aggressiveness, restlessness, irritability, hallucinations, delusions, paranoia, and catastrophic reactions. These problems are often cited among the primary reasons caregivers discontinue home care of demented patients and seek long-term institutionalization.[10-12] Whether in home or institutional settings, pleasant social interactions become impossible, day-to-day care becomes unmanageable, and quality of life is severely impoverished.

Depression and agitation in patients with dementia represent significant, prevalent, and pervasive behavioral problems with which caregivers must cope. Despite this, little empirical information is available to aid the clinician in treatment decisions. By far, much of the available literature is clinical in nature and centers on the use of various pharmacological approaches to care (e.g., see Reference 13). For depressed demented patients, antidepressant medications and ECT are often recommended.[14,15] For agitation, neuroleptics are the mainstay of care with nonneuroleptics rapidly gaining in popularity.[16,17] Thus far, only one placebo-controlled study has investigated the use of an antidepressant in this population[1,18] and only two placebo-controlled studies have been reported with neuroleptics in the treatment of agitation in dementia.[19,20] Reviews of these and associated studies are consistent in finding treatment effects of modest size and advising caution.[21,17] Indeed, some have suggested that pharmacological treatment be considered only *after* nonpharmacological strategies have failed.[17,22]

Nonpharmacological approaches, however, fare no better. In fact, far fewer clinical papers exist addressing nonpharmacological approaches and the empirical information available is scant.[23] Psychoeducational programs which attempt to educate and support caregivers using a broad-based approach are the most common nonpharmacological approach reported thus far.[24-28] The efficacy of these programs has been limited and increasing attention is being given to more direct behavioral approaches with some effectiveness demonstrated. Wandering, delusional verbalizations, agitation, aggression, depression, paranoid speech, anger, and physical violence have each been decreased using highly focused behavioral strategies such as shaping, stimulus control, and social reinforcement systems.[29-52] These reports, however, are often on small samples in highly constrained situations.

In summary, depression and agitation are common problems in AD that significantly effect patient and caregiver alike. While pharmacological and nonpharmacological strategies are commonly employed and frequently recommended, controlled clinical trials are seriously lacking. Two nonpharmacological approaches will now be described which are being evaluated as part of two randomized controlled clinical trials. While outcome data are not yet available, the systematic nature of these approaches and the availability of structured, detailed treatment manuals make these approaches particularly amenable to empirical study and clinical application.

II. THE SEATTLE PROTOCOL

The two nonpharmacological treatment programs described here combine specific behavioral techniques with caregiver education and training. One program was directed to careproviders of depressed demented patients.[1,43,53,54] The other focused on training careproviders of agitated demented patients.[55] Both interventions are based on social-learning and gerontological theory. Depression and agitation are viewed as a series of behaviors which are initiated and maintained by person-environment interactions that can be observed and modified. Such modifications alter the frequency and severity of the depressed or agitated behaviors under consideration. For patients with AD, many of the critical person-environment interactions revolve around the patient-caregiver dyad. Thus, the intervention seeks to alter the dyadic interpersonal interaction to decrease the problem behaviors. Treatment is individualized and systematic, focusing on the current observable interactions of direct relevance to the problem under consideration.

This is not to imply that behavioral intervention ignores the complex affective and cognitive aspects of the disease. The disease itself, the patient's individuality and that of their careprovider, their relationship and interaction with each other, the nature of their environment, and their inter-action with it are all factors which may affect and, in turn, be affected by behaviors and behavioral treatment. Consequently, while the focus of assessment and treatment is on individual behaviors, the larger biopsychosocial behavioral context is also taken into account.

Similar to other caregiver education programs, behavioral treatment incorporates providing basic education about AD, information about community and family resources to assist with caregiving responsibilities, and developing short- and long-term care plans. More unique, behavioral treatment involves teaching methods of behavior observation and change, identifying and develop-ing strategies to maximize patient function, and teaching effective problem-solving skills for day-to-day difficulties in patient care.

Teaching methods of behavior observation and change involves introducing the caregiver to the importance of behavioral observation and analysis and teaching them how to identify individual behavior problems and the antecedents and consequences of each behavior. Once the chain of behavior occurrence and response is understood, careproviders are guided through a systematic approach to change either the antecedents or the consequences in order to change the problem behavior. This process has been called the A-B-Cs of behavior change: A is the antecedent or triggering event that precedes the problem behavior; B, is the behavior of concern; and C is the consequence of that behavior. (This strategy of problem identification and treatment is detailed in a video training program by the author, entitled "Managing and Understanding Behavior Problems in Alzheimer's Disease and Related Disorders".[56])

Identifying and developing strategies to maximize patient cognitive function requires a careful analysis of the individual patient's relative abilities and disabilities in order to teach caregivers and patients how to maximize the former while minimizing the latter. Dementia reduces the day-to-day abilities of the afflicted individual. These reductions have far-reaching effects and can be hypothesized to be directly associated with depression and agitation in two basic ways. First, cognitive impairments reduce the availability of enjoyable activities to the patient. Figure 1 dem-onstrates the strong relationship between pleasant events and depression in one patient with depres-sion and AD.[51] As can be seen, days with higher rates of pleasant activity were days with higher levels of patient mood. Patient mood significantly correlated to both the duration of pleasant activity ($r = 0.89$) and its frequency ($r = 0.72$). Because depression is directly related to the rate and availability of enjoyable activity and so much a part of our enjoyment is related to what we can and cannot do, maximizing the patient's cognitive function is essential to improving patient depres-sion. Second, cognitive impairments and their functional correlates increase the potential for conflict between the caregiver and patient. Disagreements about how and when to do certain activities, added chores on the caregiver, and decreased functional independence of the patient can each contribute to depression and agitation.

Training careproviders in effective problem-solving skills to aid in managing the day-to-day difficulties in patient care occurs throughout treatment. Strategies are developed for identifying and confronting behavioral disturbances that are associated with the targeted behaviors, interfere with engaging in planned pleasant activities or otherwise cause conflict between the patient, caregiver, and others. Using the skills of behavior observation and analysis taught and reinforced throughout

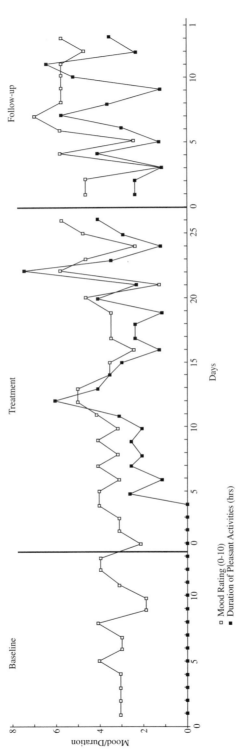

FIGURE 1   Association and treatment of depressed mood and pleasant events. (From Teri, L. and Uomoto, J., *Clin. Gerontol.*, 10, 49, 1991. With permission.)

TABLE 1   Revised Memory and Behavior Problem Checklist

Item	% of patients in whom behavior occurred at least once weekly	Mean[a] frequency x (s.d.)	Mean reaction[b] x (s.d.)
Depression			
Appears anxious	69	2.3 (1.5)	1.9 (1.2)
Appears sad or depressed	58	2.1 (1.6)	2.5 (1.3)
Comments about hopelessness	47	1.7 (1.7)	2.5 (1.1)
Comments about being a burden	34	1.2 (1.5)	2.0 (1.3)
Comments about loneliness	32	1.1 (1.5)	2.2 (1.2)
Crying	26	1.0 (1.3)	2.1 (1.1)
Comments about death	26	0.9 (1.4)	2.5 (1.3)
Comments about being a failure	18	0.6 (1.2)	2.0 (1.1)
Suicidal threats	9	0.3 (0.9)	2.6 (1.3)
Disruption			
Arguing	43	1.7 (1.6)	2.2 (1.2)
Waking caregiver up	23	0.8 (1.3)	1.7 (1.3)
Verbal aggression	21	0.7 (1.3)	2.1 (1.3)
Embarrassing behavior	20	0.8 (1.2)	1.7 (1.1)
Behavior dangerous to self or others	15	0.6 (1.1)	2.4 (1.4)
Talking loudly or rapidly	10	0.4 (1.0)	1.6 (1.3)
Threats to hurt others	6	0.2 (0.8)	2.9 (1.2)
Destroying property	5	0.2 (0.7)	1.9 (1.4)
Memory related			
Repeated questions	90	3.2 (1.2)	2.0 (1.1)
Forgetting recent events	85	2.7 (1.7)	1.5 (1.3)
Losing things	82	2.9 (1.4)	2.0 (1.1)
Forgetting the day	73	2.7 (1.7)	1.5 (1.3)
Reduced concentration	68	2.4 (1.7)	1.6 (1.7)
Forgetting past events	59	2.1 (1.4)	1.3 (1.0)
Hiding things	34	1.3 (1.7)	2.1 (1.3)

[a]   Includes behaviors that have never occurred.
[b]   Computed only for behaviors that occurred in the last week (1 or above on the rating scale).

each session, caregivers use the A-B-C approach described earlier to devise strategies for modifying problems. For depressed patients, problem behaviors include depressive behaviors, such as crying and self-deprecatory statements. For agitated patients, problem behaviors include wandering and aggression. The therapist introduces behavioral strategies for decreasing problem behaviors and increasing incompatible behaviors, as appropriate. To aid caregivers and therapists in identifying observable and potentially modifiable behaviors, the Revised Memory and Behavior Problems Checklist (RBMPC)[57] is used to evaluate the frequency of dementia-related problems and the caregiver's reaction to each behavior. Three domains of problems are assessed: memory-related, depression, and disruption problems. Table 1 shows the RMBPC items, then rates of occurrence, and their level of caregiver reactivity.

Caregivers of demented patients play an essential role throughout treatment. Each session actively trains caregivers in the systematic behavior management techniques just described. Care-providers are taught to assume a direct and active role in patient care and throughout treatment. Because patients are often limited in their ability to learn new skills, remember treatment content, and understand explanations and techniques, caregivers are essential in helping plan and implement treatment strategies.[58] The patient also plays an important role in treatment. As much as possible, considering the patient's level of understanding and ability to participate, they are involved in all aspects of treatment design and decision making.

Both nonpharmacological approaches are now being subjected to rigorous controlled clinical outcome trials. Seventy-two patient-caregivers have enrolled in the depression treatment trial. Over

200 subjects are expected to enroll in the agitation trial. The former will provide information on the efficacy of the Seattle Protocol as compared to a wait list control. The latter, conducted as part of the Alzheimer's Disease Cooperative Study Unit (L. Thal, P.I), will involve 21 sites across the country and compare behavioral treatment to pharmacotherapy and placebo. These and other studies will help determine how best to manage demented patients with depression and agitation.

ACKNOWLEDGMENT

Preparation of this paper was supported in part by grants MH-43266 from the National Institute of Mental Health and AG-10845 and AG-10483 from the National Institute of Aging.

REFERENCES

1. Teri, L., Baer, L., and Reifler, B., Depression in Alzheimer's patients: Investigation of symptom patterns and frequency, *Clin. Gerontol.*, 11, 47, 1991.
2. Weiner, M. F., Edland, S. D., and Luszczynska-Halina, Prevalence and incidence of major depression in Alzheimer's disease, *Am. J. Psychiat.*, 151, 1006, 1994.
3. Drinka, J. K., Smith, J. C., and Drinka, P. J., Correlates of depression and burden for informal caregivers of patients in a geriatrics referral clinic, *J. Am. Geriat. Soc.*, 35, 522, 1987.
4. Logsdon, R. and Teri, L., Neuropsychological and Behavioral Assessment in the Identification and Treatment of DAT, paper presented at the meeting of the Association for Advancement of Behavior Therapy, New York, 1988.
5. Pearson, J., Teri, L., Reifler, B., and Raskind, M., Functional status and cognitive impairment in Alzheimer's disease patients with and without depression, *J. Am. Geriat. Soc.*, 37, 1117, 1989.
6. Rovner, B. W., Broadhead, J., Spencer, M., Carson, K., and Folstein, M. F., Depression and Alzheimer's disease, *Am. J. Psychiat.*, 146, 350, 1989.
7. Teri, L., Borson, S., Kiyak, A., and Yamagishi, M., Behavioral disturbance, cognitive dysfunction, and functional skill, *J. Am. Geriat. Soc.*, 37, 109, 1989.
8. Pearson, J. L., Teri, L., Wagner, A., Truax, P., and Logsdon, R., The relationship of problem behaviors in dementia patients to the depression and burden of caregiving spouses, *Am. J. Alzheimer's Dis. Relat. Disord. Res.*, 8, 15, 1993.
9. Fitz, A. G. and Teri, L., Depression, cognition, and functional ability in patients with Alzheimer's disease, *J. Am. Geriat. Soc.*, 42, 186, 1994.
10. Chenowith, B. and Spencer, B., Dementia: the experience of family caregivers, *Gerontol. Soc. Am.*, 26, 267, 1986.
11. Colerick, E. and George, L. K., Predictors of institutionalization among caregivers of Alzheimer's patients, *J. Am. Geriat. Soc.*, 34, 493, 1986.
12. Cohen, C. A., Gold, D., Shulman, K., and Wortley, J., Factors determining the decision to institutionalize dementing individuals: a prospective study, *Gerontologist*, 33, 714, 1993.
13. Katzman, R. and Jackson, J. E., Alzheimer's disease: basic and clinical advances, *J. Am. Geriat. Soc.*, 39, 516, 1991.
14. Small, G. W., Psychopharmacological treatment of elderly demented patients, *J. Clin. Psychiat.*, 49, 8, 1988.
15. Raskind, M. A., Organic mental disorders, in *Geriatric Psychiatry*, Busse, E. and Blazer, D., Eds., American Psychiatric Press, Washington, DC, 1989, 313.
16. Weiner, M. F., Debus, J. R., and Goodkin, K., Pharmacological management and treatment of dementia and secondary symptoms, in *The Dementias: Diagnosis and Management*, Weiner, M. F., Ed., American Psychiatric Press, Washington, DC, 1991, 137.
17. Smith, D. A. and Perry, P. J., Non neuroleptic treatment of disruptive behavior in organic mental syndromes, *Ann. Pharmacother.*, 1400, 1992.
18. Reifler, B. V., Teri, L., Raskind, M., Veith, R., Barnes, R., White, E., and McLean, P., Double-blind trail of imipramine in Alzheimer's disease patients with and without dementia, *Am. J. Psychiat.*, 146, 45, 1989.
19. Barnes, R., Veith, R., Okimoto, J., and Raskind, M., Efficacy of antipsychotic medications in behaviorally disturbed dementia patients, *Am. J. Psychiat.*, 147, 1640, 1982.
20. Petrie, W. M., Ban, T. A., Berney, S., Fujimori, M., Guy, W., Ragheb, M., Wilson, W. H., and Schaffer, J. D., Loxapine in psychogeriatrics: a placebo-and standard-controlled clinical investigation, *J. Clin. Psychopharmocol.*, 139, 1170, 1982.
21. Schneider, L. S., Pollock, V. E., and Lyness, S. A., A meta-analysis of controlled trials of neuroleptic treatment in dementia, *J. Am. Geriat. Soc.*, 38, 553, 1990.
22. Rabins, P. V., Non-cognitive symptoms in Alzheimer's disease, in *Alzheimer's Disease*, Terry, R. D., Katzman, R., and Bick, K. L., Eds., Raven Press, New York, 1994, 419.
23. Zarit, S.H. and Teri, L. Interventions and services for family caregivers, *Annu. Rev. Gerontol. Geriat.*, 11, 241, 1991.

24. Gallagher, D. and Thompson, W., Depression, in *Clinical Geropsychology: New Directions in Assessment and Treatment,* Lewinsohn, P. M. and Teri, L., Eds., Pergamon Press, Elmsford, NY, 1993, 7.

25. Aronson, M. K., Levin, G., and Lipkowitz, R., A community based family/patient group program for Alzheimer's disease, *Gerontologist*, 24, 339, 1984.

26. Zarit, S. H., Orr, N. K., and Zarit, J. M., *The Hidden Victims of Alzheimer's Disease: Families under Stress,* New York University Press, New York, 1985.

27. Haley, W. E., Brown, S. L., and Levine, E. G., Family caregiver appraisals of patient behavioral disturbance in senile dementia, *Clin. Gerontol.*, 6, 25, 1987.

28. Toseland, R.W., Rossiter, C. M., and Labrecque, M. S., The effectiveness of peer-led and professionally led groups to support family caregivers, *Gerontologist*, 29, 465, 1989.

29. Baltes, M. M. and Zerbe, M. B., Independence training in nursing home residents, *Gerontologist*, 16, 419, 1976.

30. Blackman, D. K., Howe, M., and Pinkston, E. M., Increasing participation in social interaction of the institutionalized elderly, *Gerontologist*, 16, 69, 1976.

31. McDonald, M., Environmental programming for the socially isolated aging, *Gerontologist*, 18, 350, 1978.

32. Konarski, E. Q., Johnson, M. R., and Whitman, T. L., A systematic investigation of resident participation in a nursing home activities program, *J. Behav. Ther. Exp. Psychiat.*, 11, 249, 1980.

33. Carlsen, L. L. and Fremouw, W. J., The demonstration of a behavioral intervention for late life paranoia, *Gerontologist*, 21, 329, 1981.

34. Hussian, R. A. and Lawrence, P. S., Social reinforcement of activity of problem-solving training in the treatment of depressed institutionalized elderly patients, *Cognit. Ther. Res.*, 1, 57, 1981.

35. Patterson, R. and Jackson, G. M., Behavioral approaches to gerontology, in *Future Perspectives in Behavior Therapy,* Michelson, L., Hersen, M., and Turner, S., Eds., Plenum Press, New York, 1981, 292.

36. Hussian, R. A., A combination of operant and cognitive therapy with geriatric patients, *Int. J. Behav. Geriat.*, 1, 57, 1983.

37. Rosberger, Z. and McLean, J., Behavioral assessment and treatment of "organic" behaviors in an institutionalized geriatric patient, *Int. J. Behav. Geriat.*, 1, 33, 1983.

38. Schnelle, J. F., Traugber, B., Morgan, D. B., Embry, J. E., Binion, A. F., and Coleman, A., Management of geriatric incontinence in nursing homes, *J. Appl. Behav. Anal.*, 16, 235, 1983.

39. Linsk, N. L. and Pinkston, E. M., Training gerontological practitioners in home-based family interventions, *Educa. Gerontol.*, 10, 289, 1984.

40. Pinkston, E. M. and Linsk, N., Behavioral family intervention with the impaired elderly, *Gerontologist*, 24, 576, 1984.

41. Hussian, R. A. and Davis, R. L., *Responsive Care: Behavioral Intervention with Elderly Persons*, Research Press, Illinois, 1985.

42. Panella, J., Toileting strategies in day care programs for dementia, *Clin. Gerontol.*, 4, 61, 1986.

43. Teri, L. and Uomoto, J., Treatment of Depression in Alzheimer's disease: Helping Caregivers to Help Themselves and their Patients, presented to Gerontological Society of America, Illinois, 1986.

44. Hussian, R. A. and Brown, D. C., Use of two-dimensional grid patterns to limit hazardous ambulation in demented patients, *J Gerontol.*, 42, 558, 1987.

45. Burgio, K. L. and Engel, B., Urinary incontinence, in *Handbook of Clinical Gerontology*, Carstensen, L. L. and Edelstein, B. A., Eds., Pergamon Press, Elmsford, NY, 1987, 252.

46. Burgio, L. D. and Burgio, K. L., Behavioral gerontology: application of behavioral methods to the problems of older adults, *J. Appl. Behav. Anal.*, 19, 321, 1988a.

47. Burgio, L. D., Engel, B. T., McCormick, K., Hawkins, A., and Scheve, A., Behavior treatment for urinary incontinence in elderly inpatients: initial attempts to modify prompting and toileting procedures, *Behav. Ther.*, 19, 345, 1988b.

48. Pinkston, E. M., Linsk, N., and Young, R. N., Home based behavioral family treatment of the impaired elderly, *Behav. Ther.*, 19, 331, 1988.

49. Vaccaro, F. J., Application of operant procedures in a group of institutionalized aggressive geriatric patients, *Psychol. Aging*, 3, 22, 1988.

50. Vaccaro, F. J., Application of social skills training in a group of institutionalized aggressive elderly subjects, *Psychol. Aging*, 5, 369, 1990.

51. Teri, L. and Uomoto, J., Reducing excess disability in dementia patients: training caregivers to manage patient depression, *Clin. Gerontol.*, 10, 49, 1991.

52. Uomoto, J. M. and Brockway, J. A., Anger management training for brain injured patients and their family members, *Arch. Phys. Med. Rehab.*, 73, 1992.

53. Teri, L., Treating Depression in Alzheimer's Disease: Teaching the Caregiver Behavioral Strategies, Presented to American Psychological Association, Washington, DC, 1986.

54. Teri, L. and Logsdon, R., Assessment and management of behavioral disturbances in Alzheimer's disease patients, *Compreh. Ther.*, 16, 36, 1990.

55. Teri, L., Raskind, M., Weiner, M., Logsdon, R., Whitehouse, P., Peskind, E., Grundman, M., Thal, L., and Hill, R., Haloperidol, Trazodone, and Behavior Management techniques in Alzheimer's Disease Patients with Disruptive Agitated Behaviors: A Controlled Clinical Trial, funded by National Institute of Aging, Washington, DC, 1994.

56. Teri, L., Managing and Understanding behavior Problems in Alzheimer's Disease and Related Disorders, Training program with video tapes and written manual, Washington, DC, 1990.

57. Teri, L., Truax, P., Logsdon, R., Uomoto, J., Zarit, S., and Vitaliano, P. P., Assessment of behavioral problems in dementia: the revised memory and behavior problems checklist, *Psychol. Aging*, 7, 622, 1992.
58. Teri, L., Logsdon, R., Wagner, A., and Uomoto, J., The caregiver role in behavioral treatment of depression in dementia patients, in *Stress Effects on Family Caregivers of Alzheimer's Patients*, Light, B., Lebowtiz and Niederehe, G., Eds., Springer Press, New York, 1994, 185.

Chapter 26

OVERVIEW OF PSYCHOSOCIAL FACTORS CONTRIBUTING TO STRESS OF FAMILY CAREGIVERS

Kathleen C. Buckwalter

CONTENTS

I. THE FAMILY AS PRIMARY CARE PROVIDER

Persons with Alzheimer's disease (AD) and related disorders present many difficult care problems and management issues because of their progressive cognitive and physical deterioration. The family is the primary care provider for persons with AD.[1,2] More than 70% of all dementia patients are cared for at home by family members, and spouses are usually the primary caregivers. This trend is expected to continue with projected cutbacks in services such as respite for this population[3,4] Although caring for a relative with AD is among the most difficult forms of family responsibility, caretakers often receive inadequate support and training for the task. Thus, they may become physically and emotionally exhausted or face social deprivation and financial ruin.[5] Indeed, the burdens of care placed on families and society at large has emerged as one of the most serious health care delivery issues facing our society today.[6]

The costs of caring for persons with dementia are enormous and are expected to rise even further with anticipated increases in the oldest-old cohort. In 1994, the estimated costs of caring for 1.6 million persons with AD was $82.7 billion[7] and the Alzheimer's Association[8] has projected future costs of caring for an estimated 4 to 5 million victims of dementing illness at $1.75 trillion. It has also been estimated that, if family care of demented relatives were to be replaced by paid caregivers, the cost nationally would exceed $26 billion.[9] At present only about 10% of these expenses are covered by third-party payers or the government, with federal agencies paying for less than 4% of care provided.[10] Costs associated with the provision of in-home care are estimated at $13 billion annually, compared to $41 billion for nursing home costs.[11] Therefore, containment of long-term care costs will depend on the care provided by American families.

The financial costs of caring for persons with dementia are staggering, but the human costs of this devastating illness can also be overwhelming, and should not be underestimated. Although caregivers vary greatly in terms of the amount and type of stress or burden they experience as a result of caring for a loved one with dementia, the effects can be both financially and personally devastating, as they watch their family member become increasingly confused, incapable of communicating or carrying out everyday activities, undergoing personality and emotional changes, and losing control of elementary physical functions over an unpredictable clinical course averaging 8 to 10 years.

A number of converging societal trends suggest that demands on family caregivers will only continue, including increased longevity, geographic dispersion of the family, the need for many caregivers (especially women) to enter the work force, and changing patterns of marriage and child care.[12] An ever-increasing number of "old-old" requires care from adult children and spouses who themselves may be elderly and infirm. The increasing mobility of our society also diminishes access to family care, and increases in maternal age at the birth of the first child means that more and more caregivers are experiencing "double dependency", that is, caring for both a parent and child simultaneously, a situation Brody[13] has labeled "the Sandwich Generation."

The growing volume of caregiver literature has identified a number of factors that impact on functioning of the family care provider. Among the most prominent are coping styles of the caretaker, past relationship with the patient, gender, socioeconomic status, and the accessibility of support networks, both formal and informal.[13-16] Although attitudes toward the use of formal services and informal support vary greatly, family caregivers report they need assistance obtaining information regarding community resources, dealing with their feelings of grief, depression, and anger, and may benefit from educational, emotional/supportive, and problem solving interventions in addition to the provision of direct care services such as in-home companions and respite/day care.[17]

Geographic location also appears to impact on the caregiving process in terms of different patterns of health service utilization and use of informal vs. formal support systems by families.[18,19] In general, caretakers in rural environments tend to rely more on informal support networks, whereas their urban counterparts utilized formal organizations more frequently for tasks such as homemaking, personal care, and meal preparation.

II. OVERVIEW OF CAREGIVER BURDEN AND STRESS

As noted earlier, family caregivers of persons with Alzheimer's disease often experience significant emotional stress and extreme physical and financial burdens, in addition to apathy or hostility from the care recipient.[5] Thus, caregivers may themselves become "hidden patients", needing outside assistance and support to maintain their own health and functioning.[20] A vast amount of research and literature, including entire books, has been written on the caregiving experience.[21-23] However, few studies, with the notable exceptions of the work of Vitaliano and associates,[24] and Pearlin and colleagues,[24a] have examined caregiver burden using theoretical models of distress to guide the research effort. Fewer still have examined in detail the cultural and ethnic issues related to Alzheimer's disease.[25]

Despite these gaps in the literature and inconsistencies in the research methods used, studies overwhelmingly point to the adverse effects of caregiving for a person with dementia. Of particular note are the large number of methodologically rigorous studies citing caregiver depression as a major outcome. Other replicated findings include high levels of caregiver hostility, caregiver ill health and physical and emotional strain, increased psychotropic drug use and stress-related symptoms among caregivers, higher rates of health care utilization including more physician visits and prescription medications, and development of asocial behaviors.[23,26] Space limitations of this chapter preclude a thorough review of the literature in this domain. Therefore, the following section provides an abbreviated overview of caregiver burden and stress, the physical and psychosocial morbidity associated with caregiving, social and financial responses of family caregivers, and cultural issues related to caregiving.

A. CAREGIVER BURDEN AND STRESS

Burden, stress, and strain have emerged as important concepts in caregiver research. Caregiver stress has been defined by George and Gwyther[15] as "the physical, psychological or emotional, social and financial problems that can be experienced by family members caring for impaired older adults" (p. 243). Spouses of persons with dementia may be at greatest risk for caregiver stress as they are often themselves elderly and are likely to have physical problems that limit their ability to respond to caregiving demands.[21,27] Major findings from the literature on caregiver stress suggest that psychological morbidity (especially depression) is a frequent negative outcome associated with the caregiving experience. Decline in health status as a result of caregiving is also frequently reported by caregivers, but data on the physical health consequences of caregiving are equivocal and inconclusive.[23]

B. CARE-RECIPIENT BEHAVIORS THAT PROMOTE STRESS

Over the past decade, several researchers have concluded that catastrophic reactions, waking at night, incontinence, suspiciousness, and poor communication are most problematic for caregivers of persons with AD.[26,28,29] Other reported troublesome behaviors include repetitive questions, wandering, embarrassing, dangerous and hostile behaviors, and difficulty bathing, cooking, and managing money.[17,30] The more rapid the perceived rate of the AD patient's decline, the older the spouse caregiver, the greater their reported level of fatigue, and the more restless and less verbal the care recipient, the more likely the family caretaker is to institutionalize. These variables, along with ease of food preparation, were predictive of institutional vs. home-based care in the majority of AD patients and their families studied.[31]

C. FACTORS THAT PROMOTE ASSISTANCE SEEKING AND INSTITUTIONALIZATION

Patients with AD and their caretakers require assistance at several levels, including the opportunity to receive a clear diagnosis and explanation of the problem, help in assessing changing care needs throughout an unpredictable and changing clinical course, and in sorting through various care options, including when home care is no longer appropriate.[12] Attention to long-range planning issues, and legal and financial advice regarding such matters as conservatorships, advanced directives, and estate planning, are also needed. Chenoweth and Spencer[28] found that the most common symptoms prompting over half of the family members they surveyed to seek assistance included memory loss and problems related to personality changes, physical functional losses, work, driving, money management, and drinking. The inadequate response of health care professionals to families at the time of diagnosis is reflected in the fact that 54% of the family members were told that their situation was hopeless and that nothing could be done for them and another 20% received no explanation or information. Only 28% of those surveyed reported that they received a factual, adequate explanation of the disease, and a mere 16% received any advice on caregiving needs or how to cope with the stressful behavioral problems associated with AD. Family members also noted that they sought and found most helpful the physician's advice regarding institutional placement of their loved one.

The decision to place a loved on in a care facility is a difficult one, often plagued by feelings of guilt, inadequacy, and abandonment. Wilson[32] identified the primary social-psychological problem experienced by family caretakers as confronting negative choices, which she defined as "different degrees of impossibility" and "undesirable alternatives" (p. 95). Other psychosocial problems reported by family caregivers in counseling include concerns over their relationship with the care recipient, the need for better coping skills and more effective strategies to manage their loved one's diverse care needs, and dealing with other family members, in addition to feelings of guilt and inadequacy mentioned earlier.[32a]

The care recipient's level of cognitive dysfunction is only one factor in the family's decision to institutionalize. Many researchers have cited the demands associated with the constant care of a person with dementia as a precipitating factor in the placement decision,[33] although patient disability or severity of patient problems has only been weakly correlated with burden among dementia caregivers.[15,34]

The long-term care system must reflect a multiplicity of entry points for care along the continuum from diagnosis to death. Most studies indicate that families prefer in-home care[9] and yet current federal policies and financing mechanisms clearly favor institutional care.

D. RELATIONSHIP BETWEEN PSYCHOLOGICAL STRESS AND PHYSICAL MORBIDITY

Alterations in physiological functioning as a result of exposure to stress have been found to increase the probability of disease or illness.[35] Similarly, psychological stress and major life events can increase vulnerability to illness by compromising the integrity of the immune system.[36] The exact mechanism by which immunologic function moderates the effects of stress on health is not known. Most of the literature examining the physical effects of caregiving has used one or more of the following indicators of caregiver health: (1) self-reported health status, (2) self-reported incidence of illness-related symptoms; (3) self-reported utilization of health care services, (4) self-reported medication use; and (5) biological indicators as a measure of susceptibility to disease.[37] Findings from selected studies in this area are summarized below.

Numerous studies[38,39] have found that both male and female caregivers perceive themselves in poorer health and report more chronic illness than age-matched peers. Interestingly, these same caregivers also reported lower family incomes than controls, which may explain, in part, the lower reported health level. Similarly, Baumgarten et al.[40] found that caregivers reported lower levels of well being on all measures of health status, and higher levels of depression than matched controls, suggesting that the consequences of caring for a person with dementia are expressed in a number of somatic symptoms frequently associated with stress (e.g., chronic fatigue, headache, etc.).

E. MENTAL HEALTH RESPONSES

The chronic stresses associated with taking care of persons with AD has significant consequences for the caretakers' mental health, especially with regard to the risk of developing depression.[41,42] Several studies[43-45] have established high rates of depression among caregivers using stringent diagnostic criteria. Additionally, Goldman and Luchins[46] documented three cases of severe clinical depression requiring hospitalization, which they attributed directly to the caregiving relationship, and Barusch[47] reported that 67% of the caregivers surveyed responded that they had been depressed during their caregiving careers, although most had coped fairly well with the depression. However, 16% of those questioned were unable to cope with their depressive feelings.

Gallagher and colleagues[48] have extensively studied depression and other negative emotions such as anxiety, anger, and hostility in family caregivers. Their research supports previous work that has identified depressive disorders as common among caregivers, but differs in that they identified anger as the most common negative effect among AD caregivers, with 67% of their sample expressing frequent feelings of anger. A number of other studies[49,50] have found that wives are significantly more likely to report symptoms of depression than husbands, which the investigators attributed to demoralization and a sense of powerlessness over the disease, rather than true depression.

Some of the most complex and interesting research in this area has been conducted by Kiecolt-Glaser and associates, who have examined depression and distress as immunological modifiers. These researchers have documented poorer immune response, in particular changes in the percentages of helper T-lymphocytes and natural killer (NK) cells, in caregivers of persons with dementia, while controlling for nutritional intake and illness-related variables.[51] Caretakers in this study also reported about three times as many stress-related symptoms and higher rates of psychotropic drug use than controls, especially those caretakers living with the patient.

In summary, although depression is consistently reported as a consequence of caregiving, it is often difficult to ascertain if many of the symptoms associated with depression are, in fact, a response to physical illness, a direct manifestation of an illness, or represent a coexisting psychological illness. Research by Pruchno et al.[52] supported a model that suggests a "wearing out" of caregivers, such that high levels of depression left them vulnerable to decline in physical health over time. This finding makes intuitive sense, as many people who are depressed fail to eat and sleep well, and tend to ignore their health status in general, thus increasing their vulnerability to illness. Interestingly, studies comparing caregivers of persons with dementia and caregivers of persons with other diagnoses continue to support a pattern of poorer perceived health among the dementia caregivers and more use of psychotropic medications.[53]

A few studies have identified variables related to positive well-being rather than strain among caretakers. For example, Gilhooly[54] found that none of the caregivers in her study exhibited psychiatric impairments and that perceived satisfaction with social support, which was associated with good mental health and high morale, was common in her sample. The nature of the relationship between the AD patient and the caretaker may be a critical factor, in that those relationships defined as very close seemed to have more negative impact on the caretaker's mental health and overall well-being. The 1982 Long Term Care study also considered the positive benefits of caregiving as part of their data collection. Results suggest that many caregivers feel useful as a result of their caretaking role. For some, caregiving improved their sense of self-worth, as well as providing an important source of companionship. Clearly, not enough is known about the positive consequences of caregiving for family members and the relationship between positive experiences and caretaker health outcomes.

Thus, characteristics of the family caretaker, such as age, gender, and the nature of the relationship with the care recipient may be more important in understanding caregiver burden and well-being than symptoms manifested by the patient with AD. The relationship between caregiver coping and health outcomes deserves more investigation focusing on differences in physical, psychological, and physiologic (immune and neuroendocrine) status.

F. SOCIAL AND FINANCIAL RESPONSES

A chronic illness such as AD taxes the family's social, emotional, and financial resources. Caregivers consistently report less time for their own activities and interests as care demands increase over time with progression of the disease. George and Gwyther[15] also reported that caregivers who provided continuous at-home care over a 1-year period experienced decreased satisfaction with the amount of time available for social participation. Further, although caretakers need supportive relationships to ease their burden, the time available for such relationships often diminishes in relation to the increasing time devoted to care management. Friends and family may stop visiting because the person with AD insults them or engages in bizarre behaviors. For similar reasons, as well as for considerations of safety, family caretakers may stop taking their loved one outside the home for programs, activities, and social events.[55]

In addition, the financial resources of the caretaker often become seriously strained by the caregiving experience. Especially older caretakers are often reluctant to spend their limited reserves on home care services or respite care, preferring instead to save what little they have to be eligible for "a good nursing home" and to support institutionalization, which lasts on average 3 years.

G. CULTURAL AND ETHNIC ISSUES

The minority elderly population is estimated to be growing at least twice as rapidly as the general elderly population,[56] and many of these culturally diverse elderly are presenting with dementia. The NIMH Epidemiological Catchment Area Studies reported relatively high levels of cognitive impairment among Black and Hispanic populations, almost double the level found among the general Anglo population. Insufficient attention has been paid to the role of culture in the area of family care in Alzheimer's disease, especially in light of the fact that help-seeking and help-accepting behaviors, caretaking practices, and responses to the disease itself vary based on culturally normative outlooks.[25] For example, Black caregivers emphasize religiosity as a coping mechanism and report higher use of internal cognitive coping strategies, whereas Anglos are more likely to attend support groups and take action-oriented problem solving approaches.[57] Blacks also tend to maintain larger caregiver households and to use a broader range of informal social supports than their Anglo counterparts.[58]

III. SUMMARY

Dementia is unquestionably a family affair, as families today provide more care to a greater number of older people than at any other time in our history.[12] The length of the illness, behavioral symptoms, and often overwhelming expenses can result in family crises. Families are often ill equipped to understand symptoms and progression of the disease, basic care and behavioral management techniques, crisis intervention strategies, long-term care planning, and strategies for self-preservation. As discussed in this section, these family caregivers may suffer consequences such as social isolation, stress-related illness, abuse, impoverishment, and mental health problems including depression. Support of caregiving families through education, research, and the provision of AD-capable and -friendly services is thus a primary mission of those concerned with the care of persons with dementia and their families.

ACKNOWLEDGMENT

Preparation of this chapter was supported in part by a grant from the National Institute of Nursing Research, #5R01NR03234-02.

REFERENCES

1. Daniels, M. and Irwin, M., Caregiver stress and well-being, in *Alzheimer's Disease Treatment and Family Stress: Directions for Research*, Light, E. and B.D. Lebowitz, Eds., Hemisphere Publishing Corporation: New York, 1990, 292.
2. Miller, B., McFall, S., and Montgomery, A., The impact of elder health, caregiver involvement, and global stress on two dimensions of caregiver burden, *J Gerontol.*, 46(1), 59, 1991.
3. Grant, I., Patterson, T., Hauger, R., and Irwin, M., Current research on dementia & Alzheimer's disease, *Arch. Psychiat.*, 4(Suppl.), 77, 1992.
4. Neundorfer, M., Coping and health outcomes in spouse caregivers of persons with dementia, *Nursing Res.*, 40(5), 260, 1991.
5. Hall, G. R., Buckwalter, K. C., Stolley, J. M., Gerdner, L. A., Garand, L., Ridgeway, S., and Crump, S., Standardized care plan: managing Alzheimer's patients at home, *J. Gerontol. Nursing*, 21 (1), 37, 1995.
6. Buckwalter, K. C., Report of the advisory panel on Alzheimer's Disease, *Arch. Psychiat. Nursing*, 3(6), 358, 1989.
7. Ernst, H. and Hayes, S., The U.S. economic and social costs of Alzheimer's disease revisited, *Am. J. Public Health*, 84(8), 1261, 1994.
8. Alzheimer's Association, Advances in Alzheimer's *Research*, 4 (1), 4, 1994.
9. Office of Technological Assessment, *Losing a Million Minds: Confronting the Tragedy of Alzheimer's Disease and other Dementias*, U.S. Congress, Washington, DC, 1987.
10. Doty, P., Liu, K., and Wiener J., An overview of long term care, *Health Care Fin. Rev.*, 6, 69, 1985.
11. Young, H. M., The transition of relocation to a nursing home, *Holistic Nursing Pract.*, 4(3), 74, 1990.
12. Advisory Panel on Alzheimer's Disease, First Report of the Advisory Panel on Alzheimer's Disease, DHHS Publ. No. (ADM) 89-1644, U.S. Government Printing Office, Washington, DC, 1989.
13. Brody, E. M., Patient care as a normative family stress, *Gerontologist*, 125(1), 19, 1985.
14. Cantor, M. H., Strain among caregivers: a study of experience in the U.S., *Gerontologist*, 23, 597, 1983.
15. George, L. K. and Gwyther, L. P., Caregiver well-being: a multidimensional examination of family caregivers of demented adults, *Gerontologist*, 26(3), 253, 1986.
16. Zarit, S. H. and Zarit, J. M., Familes under stress: Interventions for caregivers of senile dementia patients, *Psychotherapy, Theory, Res. Pract.*, 19, 461, 1982.
17. Grunow, J. L., An In-Home Intervention Program for Caregivers of Persons with Dementia, Symposium presented at the Gerontological Society of America, Washington, DC, 1987.
18. Blieszner, F., McAuley, W., Newhouse, J., and Mancim, J., Rural-urban differences in service use by older adults, in *Aging Health and Family: Long Term Care*, Burbaker, T.H. Ed., Sage Publications, Newbury Park, CA, 1987.
19. Scott, J. P. and Roberto, K. A., Use of informal and formal support networks by rural elderly poor, *Gerontologist*, 25(6), 624, 1985.
20. National Institute on Aging, Proposed initiatives of FYs 1991-1993: Advisory Council Mailing, Washington, DC, 1992.
21. Kuhlman, G. J., Wilson, H. S., Hutchinson, S. A., and Wallhagen, M., Alzheimer's disease and family caregiving: critical synthesis of the literature and research agenda, *Nursing Res.*, 40(6), 331, 1991.
22. Light, E. and Lebowitz, B. D., Eds., *Alzheimer's Disease Treatment and Family Stress: Directions for Research*, National Institute of Mental Health, Rockville, MD, 1989.
23. Schultz, R., Visintainer, P., and Williamson, G. M., Psychiatric and physical morbidity effects of caregiving, *J. Gerontol.*, 45, 181, 1990.
24. Vitaliano, P., Maiuro, R. D., Ochs, H., and Russo, J., A model of burden in caregivers of DAT patients, in *Alzheimer's Disease Treatment and Family Stress: Directions for Research*, Light, E. and Lebowitz, B. D., Eds., National Institute of Mental Health, Rockville, MD, 1989, 267.
24a. Pearlin, L., Mullan, J., and Semple, S., et al., Caregiving and the stress process: an overview of concepts and their measures, *Gerontologist*, 30(5), 583, 1990.
25. Valle, R., Cultural and ethnic issues in Alzheimer's disease family research, in *Alzheimer's Disease Treatment and Family Stress: Directions for Research*, Light, E. and Lebowitz, B. D., Eds., National Institute of Mental Health, Rockville, MD, 1989, 122.
26. Rabins, P. V., Mace, H. L., and Lucas, M. S., The impact of dementia on the family, *JAMA*, 248, 333, 1982.
27. Pruchno, R. A. and Resch, N. L., Aberrant behaviors and Alzheimer's disease: mental health effects on spouse caregivers, *J. Gerontol.*, 44, 5177, 1989.
28. Chenoweth, B. and Spencer, B., Dementia: The experience of family caregivers, *Gerontologist*, 26, 267, 1986.
29. Gmeiner, C., Patient behavior, care needs, personalized community resources of both institutionalized and non-institutionalized Alzheimer's patients, in *Proceedings of a National Conference on AD and Dementia*, Altman, H. J., Ed., Plenum Press, New York, 1987.
30. Quayhagen, M. P., and Quayhagen, M., Alzheimer's stress: coping with the caregiving role, *Gerontologist*, 28, 391, 1988.

31. Maas, M. and Buckwalter, K. C., Nursing research in Alzheimer's disease, *Annual Review of Nursing Research*, Springer, New York, 1991.

32. Wilson, H. S., Family caregivers: the experience of Alzheimer's disease, *Appl. Nursing Res.*, 2, 40, 1989.

32a. Smith, G., Smith, M., and Toseland, R., Problems identified by family caregivers in counseling, *Gerontologist*, 31 (1), 15, 1991.

33. Stevens, G. L., Walsh, R. A., and Baldwin, B. A., Family caregivers of institutionalized and noninstitutionalized elderly individuals, *Adv. Clin. Nursing Res.*, 28(2), 349, 1993.

34. Zarit, S. H., Todd, P. A., and Zarit, J. M., Subjective burden of husbands and wives as caregivers; a longitudinal study, *Gerontologist*, 29, 260, 1986.

35. Brantley, P. J. and Garrett, V. D., Psychobiological approaches to health and disease, in *Comprehensive Handbook of Psychopathology*, 2nd ed., Sutker, P. B. and Adams, H. E., Eds., Plenum Press, New York, 1993, 647.

36. Kiecolt-Glaser, J. K. and Glaser, R., Psychosocial moderators of immune function, *Ann. Behav. Med.*, 9, 16, 1987.

37. Garand, L., Physical Morbidity Associated with Giving Care to a Person with Dementia, unpublished paper, University of Iowa College of Nursing, Iowa City, 1993.

38. Stone, R., Cafferata, G. L., and Sangl, J., Caregivers of the frail elderly: a national profile, *Gerontologist*, 27(5), 616, 1987.

39. Haley, W. E., Levine, E. G., Brown, S. L., Berry, J. W., and Hughes, G. H., Psychological, social, and health consequences of caring for a relative with senile dementia, *J. Am. Geriat. Soc.*, 35, 405, 1987.

40. Baumgarten, M, Battista, R. N., Infante-Rivard, C., Hanley, J. A., Becker, R., and Gauther, S., The psychological and physical health of family members caring for an elderly person with dementia, *J. Clin. Epidemiol.*, 45(1), 61, 1992.

41. Crook, T. H. and Miller, N. E., The challenge of Alzheimer's disease, *Am. Psychol.*, 40, 1245, 1985.

42. Eisdorfer, C. and Cohen, D., Management of the patient and family coping with dementing illness, in *Aging*, 3rd ed., Cox, H., Ed., Bushkin Publishing Group, Guilford, CT, 1983.

43. Cohen, D. and Eisdorfer, C., Depression in family members caring for a relative with Alzheimer's disease, *J. Am. Geriat. Soc.*, 36, 885, 1988.

44. Coppel, D. B., Burton, C., Becker, J., and Fiore, J., Relationships of cognitions associated with coping reactions to depression in spousal caregivers of Alzheimer's disease patients, *Cognitive Ther. Res.*, 9, 253, 1985.

45. Fiore, J., Becker, J., and Coppel, D. B., Social network interactions: a buffer to stress, *Am. J. Commun. Psychol.*, 11, 423, 1983.

46. Goldman, L. S. and Luchins, D., Depression in spouses of demented patients, *Am. J. Psychiat.*, 141(11), 1467, 1984.

47. Barusch, A. S., Problems and coping strategies of elderly spouse caregivers, *Gerontologist*, 28, 677, 1988.

48. Gallagher, D. E., Intervention strategies to assist caregivers of frail elders: current research status and future research directions, in *Annual Review of Gerontology and Geriatrics*, Vol. 5, Lawton, M. P. and Maddox, G., Eds., Springer, New York, 1985, 249.

49. Anthony-Bergstone, C. R., Zarit, S. H., and Gatz, M., Symptoms of psychological distress among caregivers of dementia patients, *Psychol. Aging*, 3, 245, 1988.

50. Fitting, M., Rabins, P., Lucas, M. J., and Eastham, J., Caregivers for dementia patients: a comparison of husbands and wives, *Gerontologist*, 26, 248, 1986.

51. Kiecolt-Glaser, J. K., Glaser, R., Shuttleworth, E. C., Dyer, C. S., Orocki, P., and Speicher, C. E., Chronic stress and immunity in family caregivers of Alzheimer's disease victims, *Psychosoma. Med.*, 49, 523, 1987.

52. Pruchno, R. A., Kleban, M. H., Michaels, J. E., and Dempsey, N. P., Mental and physical health of caregiving spouses: development of a causal model, *J. Gerontol.*, 45(5), 192, 1990.

53. Grafstom, M., Fratiglioni, L., Sandman, P. O., and Winbald, B., *J. Clin. Epidemiol.*, 45(8), 861, 1992.

54. Gilhooly, M., The impact of caregiving on care-givers: factors associated with the psychological well-being of people supporting a dementing relative in the community, *Br. J. Med. Psychol.*, 57, 35, 1984.

55. Barnes, R. F., Raskind, M. A., Scott, M. A., and Murphy, C., Problems of families caring for Alzheimer's patients: use of a support group, *J. Am. Geriat. Soc.*, 29(2), 80, 1981.

56. Manuel, R. C., Ed., *Minority Aging: Sociological and Social Psychological Perspectives*, Greenwood Press, Westport, CT, 1982.

57. Wykle, M. and Segal, M., A comparison of Black and White family caregivers experience with dementia, *J. Black Nurses Assoc.*, 5(1), 29, 1991.

58. Wood, J. B. and Parham, I. A., Coping with perceived burden: ethnic and cultural issues in Alzheimer's family caregiving, *J. Appl. Gerontol.*, 9(3), 325, 1990.

Chapter **27**

THE INFLUENCE OF SOCIAL CONTEXT ON THE CAREGIVING EXPERIENCE

_____ Rhonda J. V. Montgomery

CONTENTS

I. DIVERSITY OF CAREGIVING AND CAREGIVERS

Although a vast literature has emerged in the past 2 decades describing caregivers and the costs of caregiving in terms of health, social, and psychological consequences, this literature is marked by numerous inconsistencies. For example, there have been dramatic inconsistencies regarding (1) descriptive characteristics of the caregiver,[1] (2) the type of care normally provided,[2] (3) the consequences of caregiving for caregivers and elders,[3] and (4) the impact of interventions designed to assist caregivers.[4] Indeed, the empirical literature has led some reviewers to conclude that caregiving can be characterized by a diversity of processes and outcomes.[5]

An understanding of social factors that create this diversity among caregivers and the implications of this diversity for meeting caregivers' needs are critical for practitioners charged with developing and implementing support services. The diversity of caregiving and of its consequences reflect two basic characteristics of the caregiver role. First, there is no generic caregiver role; rather the caregiving role for any given individual emerges from a prior role relationship between the caregiver and the elder, e.g., spouse or son or daughter.[6-8] As such the actions of the caregiver are governed by the norms of the initial role relationship and influenced by the unique values, beliefs, and circumstances of the role occupant. Consequently, as with other social roles, there are both consistencies in the caregiving process and unique adaptations to these consistencies. Second, caregiving is a dynamic process that unfolds and changes over time. It has been likened to a career of variable length.[9-11] As such, each caregiving history has (1) a beginning, (2) some definable temporal extension or duration, and (3) an end or resolution (e.g., recovery, death, or nursing home placement).

Because the caregiving role is an emergent role that evolves out of another preexisting familial role, individuals assume the caregiver role and perform in that role in a manner that is consistent with the expectations and obligations that accompany the initial role the caregiver has in relationship to the elder (e.g., the role of spouse, son daughter, or other relative). Consequently, both the obligations and expectations that a caregiver has as a spouse, a daughter, or a son influence how and to what extent he or she assists the impaired relative and the consequences that a caregiver experiences as a result of his or her caregiving behaviors.

Clearly, within our society, the marital relationship is fundamentally different from the parent-child relationship in its history, expectations, level of commitment, patterns of costs and rewards, and duration. Spousal caregiving emerges out of a reciprocal relationship where two persons have historically shared responsibility for the other's welfare and have voluntarily made a personal and legal commitment to care for one another. In contrast, parent-child relationship have historically been asymmetrical in terms of responsibility with the parent having a moral and legal obligation to care for the child. Although this relationship shifts from one of dependency for the child as the child becomes an adult, parent-child relationships throughout the life cycle tend to remain asymmetrical with care and assistance going down generation until the parent becomes impaired.[11] In combination with gender norms regarding the division of household labor and kin care, these differences in the initial dyadic relationship are reflected in consistent patterns that have been observed in (1) prevalence of different types of caregivers,[12-14] (2) the types of tasks performed,[14-18] (3) the length of time that care is provided,[19,20] and (4) variations in the experience of caregiver stress and burden.[20-23]

II. PREVALENCE AMONG TYPES OF CAREGIVERS

There is a general consensus within the literature that, most often, one family member serves as the primary source of care for an impaired elderly person although others in the family and friend network may serve as "secondary caregivers". It has also become widely recognized that a principle of substitution operates in the selection of the primary caregiver. When available, a spouse provides the majority of care. In the absence of spouse, a daughter is most likely to assume the role. In the absence of a daughter, a son will assume the role although there is considerable evidence that sons transfer many care tasks to their spouses. In the absence of offspring other more distant family members become responsible.[12,13,24] This principle of substitution is consistent with both the stronger personal and legal obligation that is characteristic of spousal relationships as opposed to adult child-parent relationships and the role expectations for women in our society to assume responsibility for kin care and household tasks. [15,18,25] It also is reflected in the findings from numerous studies that report caregivers to be primarily women and spouses.[14,26]

III. PATTERNS IN TASK PERFORMANCE

Although a child might serve as a substitute source for care, there is considerable evidence that there are dramatic differences between the types of tasks that children perform as caregivers and those that spouses perform. There are also differences between spouses and children in the intensity of tasks and the length of time that care tasks are performed. Spouses who identify themselves as caregivers report between 40 and 60 hours performing caregiving tasks depending upon the sample.[23,27] Moreover, the majority of these hours are devoted to household chores, meal preparation, and personal care such as bathing, dressing, and toileting. In contrast, studies that have included significant numbers of adult children report that the average amount of time that children spend performing care tasks is one third to one half as much time as reported for spouses. In addition children tend to concentrate more of their time doing care management tasks and assisting with transportation and shopping.[23] Children not only provide less care and less intensive care, they tend to provide assistance for shorter periods of time.[14,19,27-29]

IV. CARE SHARING

Spouses and adult children who are primary caregivers also differ in the way they share care responsibilities with other family members who may participate in the caregiving process as back-up or secondary sources of care.[28-31] When the primary caregiver is a spouse, secondary caregivers are most likely to be adult-children. When the primary caregiver is a child, secondary caregivers tend to be the spouse or sibling of the primary caregiver.

Regardless of who the second caregiver is, spouses tend to perform 80% or more of the care tasks.[20,27,29] The care provided by second caregivers tends to account for a smaller proportion of the overall care and tends to complement the care tasks of the spouse which are usually concentrated on personal care and household chores. As secondary caregivers, children concentrate their efforts on tasks that are more role appropriate such as help with transportation, banking, and paper work or sporadic household and yard maintenance activites. There is, however, some variation with the sex of the child who is a second caregiver. Daughters tend to provide more care of every type except help with legal and banking tasks than do sons; daughters also tend to provide more routine care and distribute their hours more evenly across the various types of tasks.[27-31] Sons tend to concentrate their efforts on tasks that are more circumscribed and sporadic such as occasional shopping trips or annual yard and house maintenance activities.[2,28] This pattern is most pronounced for sons who are second caregivers for their mothers. Sons as second caregivers provide less assistance to mothers than to fathers and they provide almost no help for mothers with personal care. Montgomery and colleagues report that the assistance provided by sons accounted for only 3.2% of the care that their mother received in contrast to the 22.4% of care that daughters provided as second caregivers.[28]

Despite their greater work load, spouses are also the least likely caregivers to seek and use formal support services.[20] This tendency is most pronounced for wives who tend to resist outside support to a greater degree than do husbands.[14,20,30]

In contrast to the care-sharing patterns observed for spouses who are primary caregivers, adult children who are primary caregivers tend to share care tasks more equally with second caregivers. In this family constellation second caregivers tend to do similar tasks as primary caregivers and distribute their caregiving time among the various tasks in a similar manner. Consequently, the assistance provided by second caregivers in families where the primary caregiver is an adult child tends to supplement the care provided by the primary caregivers.[20,28,30]

Again, however, the sex of the caregivers involved tends to be associated with the patterns of care sharing. As primary caregivers, daughters provided a greater percentage of total care than did son primary caregivers. Primary and secondary caregivers tend to share the care load almost equally when the primary caregiver is a son. Moreover, second caregivers tend to provide the greatest proportion of the elder's total care and the greatest amount of personal care when they are assisting primary caregivers who are the opposite sex of the elder.[28]

V. CULTURAL DIFFERENCES

The differences in care constellations between families with spouse primary caregivers vs. adult-children likely account for cultural differences that have been observed in care patterns and use of support services. The prevalence of daughters as the primary caregiver is considerably greater among Black and Hispanic populations than among white populations. The limited number of studies of these cultural groups suggest that adult children account for almost 75% of the caregivers vs. the 40 to 60% that have been found in studies of white populations.[33-35] Consequently, the daughters providing care for minority elders tend to provide more household and personal care than is true in white samples and they tend to express a need for and use of more in-home services and adult day care when it is available.[34,35] At the same time minority families tend to include a larger number of persons in the caregiving constellation, probably reflecting the greater equality in care sharing observed for adult children.[33-35]

VI. CAREGIVING TRAJECTORIES

The greater propensity for spouses to provide more and more intense care than do adult children is not solely a consequence of different levels of felt obligation, but is also a consequence of different trajectories in caregiving careers. Even though caregiving can be described in temporal units, the passage of time per se is unlikely to be an adequate descriptor of the caregiving situation. The careers of adult children and spouse are likely to differ both in terms of the factors that define the onset of the role and the factors that contribute to the abdication of the role. Many of the tasks that children consider a part of their caregiving role (e.g., assistance with transportation, banking, and household chores) are assumed by spouses as part of their marital role. Therefore, spouses tend not to recognized their caregiving role as unique from their spousal role until they begin providing personal care. For many spouses, then, caregiving has an almost imperceptible onset. In contrast, providing a parent with transportation and assistance with banking or shopping can represent a major role change for children. Consequently, children tend to identify themselves as caregivers at an earlier point in the caregiving process than do spouses and the point of transition to the caregiver role tends to be more easily recognized.

The earlier self-identification by children into the caregiving role has two consequences. First, children are likely to experience strain in their lives and associate this strain with the caregiving role earlier in the care process. This experience of strain earlier in the elder's dependency cycle accounts for research findings that indicate children reporting a greater or equal sense of burden than do spouses although children are performing fewer care tasks.[25,27,36] Second, children are more likely to leave the caregiving role when the impaired elder is at earlier stages in the disease and dependency process.[19] For children, the structural conditions that keep the person in the caregiving role are decidedly weaker. Since there are no legal obligations and limited familial expectations for adult children to provide care, those children for whom caregiving would be an extremely difficult proposition are unlikely to assume the caregiving role in the first place. When caregiving interferes with other familial and work obligations, there are generally fewer normative and psychological sanctions (e.g., guilt) for abdicating the role. [25,37]

These differences in caregiving patterns are illustrated by the work of Montgomery and Kosloski,[19] who reported that the decision to place a parent in a nursing home was associated with greater cognitive and physical impairment of the parent and greater objective burden. Notably, a sense of duty or obligation was not associated with placement, but children reporting greater affection were less likely to place their parent in a nursing home.

Not recognizing early care tasks as unique from the marital role, spouses are not likely to experience the caregiving role as burdensome or stressful until their afflicted mate is very dependent. Even then, their greater commitment appears to make them persist and endure in the caregiving role even if it involves extensive personal care.[19,24,38] This greater endurance is demonstrated by the findings of Montgomery and Kosloski which indicate that the level of functioning of the impaired elder and the level of objective burden of the spouse were not related to nursing home placement. However, spouses reporting a greater sense of obligation were less likely to place an elder. Also, the presence of cognitive impairment was associated with nursing home placement. It appears that, when the elder becomes sufficiently impaired to substantially alter the basic marital relationship, spouses are more likely to abdicate their caregiving role.

In summary, the caregiving experience of adult children tends to differ from that of spouses in several important ways. First, children have greater volition in their choice of the caregiving role and their choice of leaving the role than do spouses who express and demonstrate a greater obligation to this role.[20,38] Second, the caregiving role of children tends to be more circumscribed and occurs in the earliest phases of the elder's impairment. Children tend to concentrate their efforts on transportation, assistance with money matters and shopping, and some household chores. Spouses do not define themselves as caregivers until the elder has reached a level of impairment at which most children abdicate the caregiving role.[39] Consequently, spouses provide more care of all types and are far more likely to be providing personal care and extensive household care. Third, when spouses assume the caregiving role they tend to shoulder the majority of the care burden, while children, especially sons, tend to share the work load more equally with their siblings or spouses. Finally, spouses tend to find the role more emotionally stressful while children report that the role impacts on their time, energy, and other familial relationships.[19,20,28]

VII. IMPLICATIONS FOR EFFECTIVE SUPPORT SERVICES

Differences in caregiving roles often translate to different needs for and willingness to use support services.[10,40,41] The support services for caregivers that are most commonly available are educational programs, support groups, and respite services which include volunteer programs, adult day care centers, and in-home chore and personal care services. Despite considerable consensus about the value of such services for alleviating caregiver stress and burden, a consistent research finding and lament of providers has been that support services designed to alleviate caregiver burden and stress go unused, especially by spouses, who have been shown to seek formal assistance relatively late in the caregiving career.[24,42] This lack of service use has been attributed to (1) lack of perceived need on the part of the caregiver,[43] (2) inappropriate targeting of services to caregiver's needs,[24,42] and (3) barriers created by providers in the way in which services are offered.[43-47] Simply put, caregivers will not use services for which they perceive no need or for which the monetary, emotional, or physical costs of using the service outweigh the perceived benefits.

VIII. EDUCATIONAL PROGRAMS

Clearly, for a caregiver to benefit from an educational program, the information provided must match the caregiver's current need for information. Since children who provide care identify themselves as caregivers far earlier in the care process, their needs for information are going to be quite different from those of spouses who are unlikely to seek help for themselves until they are in later stages of the caregiving career. In the earliest phases of caregiving (i.e., the phase when children are mostly likely to seek help), caregivers are most likely to be seeking information about the disease process, the availability of community services, and legal and financial information. In the later phases of caregiving, the point at which spouses are more likely to self-identify as caregivers, there is a greater need for behavior management support, coping skills, and information about in-home support services. This variation in caregiver needs and caregiver trajectories likely explains the limited impact that shotgun approaches to information dissemination through group education, materials development, and media have had. [50-52] Such approaches tend to overwhelm families with information that may not be relevant to their immediate situation and, at the same time, fail to reach caregivers with critical information until it is too late. [11,39,50,52] Recent evidence suggests that caregivers are more receptive to educational programs and benefit from these programs when they are appropriately targeted to the different contexts and when information is dispensed throughout the caregiving experience. [49,50,53,54]

IX. SUPPORT GROUPS

Educational programs are often linked with support groups for caregivers. In the past, caregivers have been shown to benefit from support groups through decreases in stress and subjective burden and increases in active coping strategies and knowledge of community resources.[50,51,55] Again, however, there is some evidence that spouses benefit from support groups in different ways than do adult children. In particular, support groups can help spouses cope with changes in their marital relationship, encourage them to seek outside help, and to set aside time for themselves. Children benefit from support groups by extending their support network and gaining better knowledge of community services. The different needs and concerns of the two groups again suggest the need for targeted programs. There is also some evidence that support groups are more difficult for spouses to attend due to lack of transportation, lack of respite care, and greater dependence of the care receivers.[55] Support groups have also been predominantly attended by white and middle-class caregivers.[52]

X. RESPITE

Perhaps the most controversial finding in the caregiver intervention literature has been the failure of respite to impact either caregiver burden or nursing home placement.[39,41,42] While this has prompted some observers to dismiss respite as a useful support, more recent research suggest that the original negative findings stemmed from lack of use of respite services by a substantial portion of the eligible caregivers in the samples.[56] This failure to use services becomes understandable when differences in caregiving trajectories are acknowledged. In early phases of caregiving, respite is not really appropriate since these caregivers tend not to be performing intense care tasks and, in the case of children, are often not living with the care receiver. Therefore, many children do not perceive a need for respite. At the same time, spouses may not identify themselves as caregivers until the very late stages of their mate's dependency. Consequently spouses are likely to perceive information about respite programs directed toward "caregivers" as being largely irrelevant to them. Only when caregivers are providing extensive care *and* have identified themselves as caregivers will they reach the point of full receptivity to respite programs. At this juncture, respite programs can be expected to have their greatest impact.[42,56]

Frequently, however, caregivers have gone beyond the optimal point of receptivity when they seek respite. Often, when spouses seek assistance through formal providers, they may already be considering relinquishing the caregiving role due to the elder's the consistent decline and increasing caregiver burden. This is when respite programs become "too little too late" and fail to serve a preventive function.[19,39]

Clearly the social context of caregiving dyads has significant impact on the caregiving experience and its consequences. In the future, providers will be far more effective in their support efforts if they acknowledge and target both the diversity and the consistencies that social contexts create.

ACKNOWLEDGMENT

Preparation of this paper was supported in part by grant 5U01-AG1-318-04 from the National Institute on Aging.

REFERENCES

1. Stone, R., Defining family caregivers of the elderly: implications for research and public policy, *Gerontologist*, 31, 616, 1991.
2. Matthews, S. H. and Rosner, T. T., Shared filial responsibility: the family as the primary caregiver, *J. Marriage Fam.*, 50, 185, 1988.
3. Schulz, R. Theoretical perspectives on caregiving: concepts, variables, and methods, in *Aging and Caregiving: Theory, Research, and Policy*, Biegel, D. E. and Blum, A., Eds., Sage Publications, Newbury Park, CA, 1990, 27.
4. Zarit, S., Interventions with frail elders and their families: are they effective and why?, in *Stress and Coping in Later-Life Families*, Stephens, M., Crowther, J., Hobfo, S., and Tennenbaum, D., Eds., Hemisphere Publishing, New York, 1990.
5. Kahana, E. and Young, R., Clarifying the caregiving paradigm: challenges for the future, in *Aging and Caregiving*, Biegel, D. and Blum, A., Eds., Sage, Newbury Park, CA, 1990.
6. Dwyer, J. W. and Seccombe, K., Elder care as family labor: the influence of gender and family position, *J. Fam. Issues*, 12, 1991.
7. Kosloski, K. D. and Montgomery, R. J. V., Caregiving Career Lines: Markers and Determinants, 30th Meeting of the International Institute of Sociology, Paris, 1993.
8. Stoller, E. P., Forster, L. E., and Duniho, T. S., Systems of parent care within sibling networks, *Res. Aging*, 14, 313, 1992.
9. Montgomery, R. J. V. and Hatch, L. R., The feasibility of volunteers and families forming a partnership for caregiving, in *Family and Long-Term Care*, Brubaker, T. H., Ed., Sage Publications, Beverly Hills, CA, 1987, 143.
10. Knight, B. G., Lutzky, S. M., and Macofsky-Urban, F., A meta-analytic review of interventions for caregiver distress: recommendations for future research, *Gerontologist*, 33, 240, 1993.
11. Pearlin, L. I., The careers of caregivers, *Gerontologist*, 32, 647, 1992.
12. Cantor, M., Neighbors and friends: an overlooked resource in the informal support system, *Res. Aging*, 1, 434, 1979.
13. Cicirelli, V. G., Siblings as caregivers in middle and old age, in *Gender, Families, and Elder Care*, Dwyer, J. W. and Coward, R. T., Eds., Sage, Newbury Park, CA, 1992, 84.
14. Stone, R., Cafferata, G., and Sangl, J., Caregivers of the frail elderly: A national profile, *Gerontologist*, 27, 616, 1987.
15. Finley, N. J., Theories of family labor as applied to gender differences in caregiving for elderly parents, *J. Marriage Fam.*, 51, 79, 1989.
16. Lee, G., Gender, families and elder care, in *Gender and Family Care of the Elderly*, Dwyer, J. W. and Coward, R. T., Eds., Sage Publications, Newbury Park, CA, 1992, 120.
17. Walker, A. J. and Pratt, C. C., Daughter's help to mothers: intergenerational aid vs. caregiving, *J. Marriage Fam.*, 53, 3, 1991.
18. Montgomery, R. J. V., Gender differences in patterns of child- parent caregiving relationships, in *Gender and Family Care of the Elderly*, Dwyer, J. W. and Coward, R. T., Eds., Sage Publications, Newbury Park, CA, 1992, 65.
19. Montgomery, R. J. V. and Kosloski, K. D., A longitudinal analysis of nursing home placement for dependent elders cared for by spouses vs. adult children, *J. Gerontol. Soc. Sci.*, 49(Suppl.), 62, 1994.

20. Stoller, E. P., Gender differences in the experiences of caregiving spouses, in *Gender and Family Care of the Elderly*, Dwyer, J. W. and Coward, R. T., Eds., Sage Publications, Newbury Park, CA, 1992, 49.

21. Stoller, E. P. and Pugliesi, K. L., Other roles of caregivers: competing responsibilities or supportive resources, *J. Gerontol.* 44(Suppl.), 231, 1989.

22. Kleban, M. H., Brody, E. M., Schoonover, C. B. and Hoffman, C., Family help to the elderly: perceptions of sons-in-law regarding parent care, *J. Marriage Fam.*, 51, 303, 1989.

23. Montgomery, R. J. V. and Datwyler, M. M., Women and men in the caregiving role, *Generations*, 34, 1990.

24. Horowitz, A., Family caregiving to the frail elderly, *Annu. Rev. Gerontol. Geriat.* 194, 1985.

25. Montgomery, R. J. V. and Borgatta, E. F., Values, costs and health care policy, in *Critical Issues in Aging Policy: Linking Research and Values*, Borgatta, E. F. and Montgomery, R. J., Eds., Sage Publications, Beverley Hills, CA, 1987, chap. 1.

26. Dwyer, J. W. and Coward, R. T., *Gender, Families, and Elder Care*, Sage Publications, Newbury Park, CA, 1991.

27. Johnson, C. L. and Catalano, D. J., A longitudinal study of family supports to impaired elderly, *Gerontologist*, 23, 612, 1983.

28. Montgomery, R. J. V., Kosloski, K. D., and Datwyler, M. M., Factors defining caregivers. Final Report to the National Institute on Aging, Grant No. R01-AG05702; 1993.

29. Montgomery, R. J. V. and Kamo, Y., Parent care by sons and daughters, in *Aging Parents and Adult Children*, Mancini, J. A., Ed., Lexington Books, Lexington, MA, 1989, 213.

30. Tennstedt, S., McKinlay, J., and Sullivan, L. M., Informal care for frail older persons: the role of secondary caregivers, *Gerontologist*, 29, 677, 1989.

31. Coward, R. T. and Dwyer, J. W., The association of gender, sibling network composition, and patterns of parent care by adult children, *Res. Aging*, 12, 158, 1990.

32. Miller, B. and McFall, S., Stability and change in the informal task support network of frail older persons, *Gerontologist*, 31, 735, 1991.

33. Chatters, L. M., Taylor, R. J., and Neighbors, H. W., Size of informal helper network mobilized during a serious personal problem among black americans, *J. Marriage Fam.*, 51, 667, 1989.

34. Hinrichsen, G. A. and Ramirez, M., Black and white dementia caregivers: a comparison of their adaptation, adjustment, and service utilization, *Gerontologist*, 32, 375, 1992.

35. Wallace, S. P., Snyder, J. L., Walker, G. K., and Ingman, S. R., Racial differences among users of long-term care: the case of adult day care, *Res. Aging*, 14, 471, 1992.

36. Young, R. and Kahana, E., Specifying caregiver outcomes: gender and relationship aspects of caregiving strain, *Gerontologist* 29, 660, 1989.

37. Miller, B. and Montgomery, A., Family caregivers and limitations in social activities, *Res. Aging*, 12, 72, 1990.

38. Doty, P., Family care of the elderly: the role of public policy, *Milbank Q.*, 64, 34, 1986.

39. Montgomery, A., Rhonda, J. V. and Borgatta, E. F., The effects of alternative support strategies on family caregiving, *Gerontologist* 29, 457, 1989.

40. Haley, W. E. and Pardo, K. M., Relationship of severity of dementia to caregiving stressors, *Psychol. Aging*, 4, 389, 1989.

41. Lawton, M. P., Brody, E. and Saperstein, A., A controlled study of respite service for caregivers of Alzheimer's patients, *Gerontologist*, 29, 8, 1989.

42. Montgomery, R. J. V. and Kosloski, K. D., Respite revisited: re-assessing the impact, *Adv. Long Term Care*, in press.

43. Caserta, M. S., Lund, D. A., Wright, S. D., and Redburn, D. E., Caregivers to dementia patients: the utilization of community services, *Gerontologist*, 27, 209, 1987.

44. Gwyther, L. P., Overcoming barriers: home care for dementia patients, *Caring*, 8, 12, 1989.

45. Gwyther, L. P., Ballard, E., and Hinman-Smith, E., Overcoming Barriers to Appropriate Service Use: Effective Individualized Strategies for Alzheimer's Care, Duke Family Support Program, Durham, NC, 1990.

46. Kosloski, K. D. and Montgomery, R. J. V., Perceptions of respite service as predictors of utilization, *Res. Aging*, 15, 399, 1993.

47. Wallace, S. P., Campbell, K., and Lew-Ting, C. Y., Structural barriers to the use of formal in-home services by elderly Latinos, *J. Gerontol. Soc. Sci.*, 49(Suppl.), 253, 1994.

48. Yeatts, D. E., Crow, T., and Folts, E., Service use among low- income minority elderly: strategies for overcoming barriers, *Gerontologist*, 32, 24, 1992.

49. Gwyther, L. P., Gold, D. T., Hinman-Smith, E. A., and Poer, C. M., A low-cost educational intervention for caregivers of memory-impaired older adults, 47th Annual Scientific Meeting of the Gerontological Society of America, 1994.

50. Toseland, R. W. and Rossiter, C. M., Group interventions to support family caregivers: a review and analysis, *Gerontologist*, 29, 438, 1989.

51. Toseland, R. W., Labrecque, M. S., Goebel, S. T., and Whitney, M. H., An evaluation of a group program for spouses of frail elderly veterans, *Gerontologist*, 32, 382, 1992.

52. Toseland, R. W., Rossiter, C., and Labrecque, M. S., The effectiveness of peer-led and professionally led groups for caregivers, *Gerontologist*, 29, 465, 1989.

53. Zarit, S. H. and Toseland, R. W., Current and future direction in family caregiving research, *Gerontologist*, 29, 481, 1989.

54. Mittelman, M. S., Ferris, S. H., Steinberg, G., Shulman, E., Mackell, J. A., Ambinder, A., and Cohen, J., An intervenion that delays institutionalization of Alzheimer's Disease patients: treatment of spouse-caregivers, *Gerontologist*, 33, 730, 1993.
55. Haley, W. E., Group intervention for dementia family caregivers: a longitudinal perspective, *Gerontologist*, 29, 478, 1989.
56. Kosloski, K. D. and Montgomery, R. J. V., The impact of respite use on nursing home placement, *Gerontologist*, 35, 67, 1995.

Chapter 28

CARE FOR FAMILIES FACING ALZHEIMER'S DISEASE: PRIMARY CARE PRACTICE IMPLICATIONS FROM RESEARCH

Lisa P. Gwyther

CONTENTS

0-8493-8997-6/97/$0.00+$.50

I. FAMILY RESPONSES TO ALZHEIMER'S CARE

Families continue to provide the bulk of chronic care over the course of Alzheimer's disease.[1] Family care is preferred, based in strong family values that cross cultural/ethnic lines, intimate, individualized, dignified, but unrelenting. Despite the research emphasis on objective and subjective measures of caregiver stress and burden, not all family caregiving outcomes are negative or burdensome.[2] Feelings always intensify with increasing dependency and families are increasingly caring for more dependent members for longer periods of time than at any time in our history.[3]

Some families rise to the challenge, feel effective, competent, and proud to leave a legacy of commitment to family values. Some family caregivers derive a sense of meaning in living up to obligations or an enhanced self worth in their positive influence on the quality of life for an Alzheimer's patient despite a difficult situation. Other families recognize previously unknown strengths, new family bonding, or feelings of connectedness.

II. THE ROLE OF PRIMARY CARE

Regardless of the outcomes of caregiving for families, Alzheimer's disease forces families to make a set of decisions about tasks and the degree to which they will accept help and from whom. The quality of those decisions will determine the quality of care and life for both patient and family. The primary care clinician is usually the first and only professional families turn to for help with decision making.[4] As such, the primary care professional can have the greatest influence on critical family care decisions.

III. FAMILY CARE RESEARCH

The impact of Alzheimer's disease on the patient and family is a dynamic process that changes over time but invariably creates a permanent imbalance in the normal give-and-take of family relationships.[5] Patient and family responses vary with race, ethnicity, culture, expectations, beliefs, values, socioeconomic status, education, gender, relationship, family history or conflict, living arrangements, and somewhat inconsistently by functional impairment, severity, or duration of the patient's symptoms.[6] Despite this heterogeneity and the often fragile complexity of Alzheimer's family care arrangements, research findings document the predominance of informal or unpaid family care, sources of family stress, burden and satisfaction, predictors of use of formal and informal help, and limited evidence of effectiveness of interventions to support family care.[7] The clinical literature identifies expectable transitions and decision points.[8] These research findings and clinical literature have significant implications for primary care practice. This chapter provides a research-based chronological clinical framework for family-friendly or -centered primary care.

IV. GOALS OF FAMILY-CENTERED PRIMARY CARE

An estimated 30% of persons with moderate to severe dementia live alone, perhaps having outlived all available informal support from family and friends.[9] Often, however, the patient is able to live independently *because of* considerable help from family members who personally provide care or arrange for care from a distance. When family caregivers are involved, family-centered primary care has the potential to:

- Increase the effectiveness of family care (competency) and family coping.
- Decrease the negative consequences of caregiving on individual family members' health, mental health, financial resources, personal time, and satisfaction with time for other activities.[10]

- Reduce the overall level or potential for family conflict, neglect, abuse, or exploitation.
- Enhance family satisfaction with preferred levels of involvement in caregiving.
- Find an equitable balance between quality of life for family care providers and quality of care for the person with dementia.

In essence, it is in the best interest of both patient and multiple affected family members for the primary care clinician to pay attention to families. Family informants will generally demand attention but they are also more likely to insure compliance with prescribed care routines. If the clinician can prevent or treat excess disability in patients, he or she may prevent or minimize secondary disability in family members and extend the potential for preferred family involvement in care.

V. THREE EXPECTABLE TRANSITION POINTS IN PRIMARY CARE

Families, and more recently patients themselves, turn to a primary care provider when they begin to question whether they are dealing with a primary cognitive impairment, a psychiatric illness, another medical condition, or normal aging. Although the process of evaluation, diagnosis, and interpretation may occur over several visits, because there is greater public and professional awareness, more Alzheimer's patients are seeking diagnosis earlier and living longer with it.[11]

The second major transition leading to primary care visits occurs when the patient becomes more apathetic, resistive, functionally dependent, unable to safely stay or live alone, use or answer the telephone, handle money, or leave the house without creating a significant danger to himself or others. At this point, the living situation may no longer meet his/her needs or meet the competing or conflicting needs of other members of a shared household. This is the point at which most families are forced to decide whether to accept outside or paid help, what kind, how much, and at what cost. Families may turn to aging services, delivered meals, congregate or assisted living, agency, private, or volunteer home care, homemaker or chore programs, group respite programs, an adult day center, or a permanent or temporary move to another family member's home or residential facility. Often behavioral and psychiatric manifestations of the illness are prominent at this point, and families also turn to primary care clinicians for help in managing these challenging or disruptive symptoms.

The third and final expectable transition occurs when the patient requires full-time nursing care or becomes totally dependent in physical activities of daily living such as eating, toileting, and moving around the house. At this point families turn to primary care physicians as gatekeepers to institutional care and as authority figures to legitimize the need to "let go" of physical care responsibilities.

All three of these primary care decision points have the potential to create conflict between and among patient and family and carry the potential for neglect, abuse, or exploitation of vulnerable patients and their often well-intentioned but uninformed family caregivers. Problems arise at all three points from partial, incorrect, or missing information, inappropriate expectations of the patient, family or service delivery system, conflict arising from differing perceptions of the patient's needs, or lack of access to available, acceptable services.[12]

The primary care provider is well positioned for timely intervention to support family and community care and to minimize costly or inappropriate use of scarce emotional, physical, financial, and acute care resources.

VI. HELPING PATIENTS AND FAMILIES THROUGH DIAGNOSIS

Families, and more often patients, report difficulty in getting primary care physicians to take seriously memory or cognitive complaints. Often friends, neighbors, employers, and other family members notice the hallmark insidious changes before these symptoms would be identified in a routine outpatient visit. Changes in function, mood, initiative, or behavior of the Alzheimer's patient may be attributed somewhat cavalierly to depression, relationship or communication problems, or anxiety. Even if the primary care physician suspects early dementing changes, he or she may not take the time to get a good family informant history. If a thorough diagnostic evaluation is offered, families may be discouraged from talking with the patient about the diagnosis because "nothing can be done".

The primary care approach to a presenting problem of cognitive decline can set a positive tone for effective long-term care. The diagnosis of Alzheimer's has devastating implications for a patient's self-esteem, dignity and control, and a family's interdependent future. Patients and families appreciate leaving no stone unturned in a search for treatable or reversible causes of dementing symptoms or excess disabilities.

Alzheimer's patients may be reluctant to seek evaluation, resistive to testing, or deny their impairments. Often, however, they are relieved to be told it is not a personality or character flaw, laziness, psychosis, or "hopeless".

This is the time to correct misconceptions about etiology and specificity of diagnosis. The primary care clinician can acknowledge predictable changes in need for help as well as the unpredictable course and development of symptoms. It is the time to encourage families to enjoy things they can still do together, to structure routines, simplify or break down tasks into doable segments, and slow down the pace of activities and environmental demand to match the patient's abilities.[13]

A wise primary care clinician will immediately initiate discussions of financial and legal precautions to protect the patient's assets, income, and right to decide on a trusted surrogate decision maker.[14]

Often patients and families are overwhelmed at the time of diagnosis and unable to integrate all needed explanations. Because many family members become aware of symptoms at the time of a traumatic event such as a spouse's death, a hospitalization, illness of the caregiver, vacation, or job change, they may attribute the patient's symptoms to grief or a time-limited stress reaction to an event for which they feel responsible (a daughter's divorce).

This is also a key time to protect patient self-esteem and dignity, reminding the family of what he/she can still do and why it is important to remain open minded, flexible, and responsive to the patient's need to be heard, involved, and feel appreciated. Information should be reassuring, repeated, timed, and dosed to address only questions of immediate relevance to the patient and family. Families should be told that much more is known about Alzheimer's disease and there are sources of available information and help when they determine they are "ready" for it.

A continuing source of primary care is often the critical variable in timing and dosing of information to enhance compliance. A primary care clinician can offer an informed, consistent explanation to all affected family members. To buffer potential family conflict at this point, it is often helpful to give the family a common enemy — the disease is the enemy, not the patient, other family members, family events, or the diagnostician. Family members living at a distance from the patient may minimize the patient's symptoms and need for assistance and exacerbate the primary caregiver's sense of frustration, isolation, and lack of support. Clinical help in reappraising symptoms, behavior, and etiology can bring families together for support and care planning.

Patients and families are especially fearful of medical abandonment or nihilism at the time of diagnosis.[15] For this reason, families may interpret well-meaning service referrals as hopeless medical abandonment. Even though a diagnosis may confirm their worst fears, families and patients take hope from a clinician's positive expectations of their capacity to adapt and cope with change over time. They want the primary care clinician to "stand by" them, by offering routine follow-up and referral to treatment or research options, just as they would expect with any other chronic illness.

VII. ACCEPTING OUTSIDE HELP

Although successive generations are becoming more comfortable in accepting the need for professional or paid services, dementia care poses unique decision dilemmas for family acceptance of outside help.[16] Some families expect this help from family members, church, and community as "earned credits".

Unfortunately, by the time the patient cannot safely be left alone, he or she may be less aware of the extent of his/her dependency and more resistant to any changes, new people, or places. Families are forced to make lonely decisions, often in direct opposition to the expressed wishes of the person they are caring for. Also, the patient's inappropriate or uncharacteristic behavior at this point may be a source of embarrassment to the family who then may be unwilling to expose him/her to public or professional scrutiny.

Research findings on Alzheimer's families' use of community-based services document four major trends:[17]

1. Families are reluctant to use any formal agency help other than physicians, private house-keepers, or sitters, and only after available family help is used first.
2. Families delay seeking help. Although they may reach out fleetingly and often for reassurance that services are available, the fear of future nursing home costs keeps many families from paying out-of-pocket for respite services.[18]
3. Families use less help than professionals would recommend or that their objective requirements for task assistance would indicate.
4. Families who delay help seeking to a final year before death or institutionalization of the patient may find inappropriate or inadequate help relative to their need. In general, Medicare pays only for diagnosis, primary care visits, and skilled hospital and home care benefits, not the long-term personal care assistance that Alzheimer's patients need. Medicaid is available only to those who have limited assets and income. Public sources for community-based care are extremely limited, even for veterans.

Families look to primary care for generalists who learn over time to be "expert" in the individual family's unique needs and preferences. Families do not want to be treated like dependent patients or used like "physician extenders". They want clinicians to acknowledge that the family has an adaptational challenge in caring for someone with Alzheimer's disease, without defining the family as the problem. Families look to physicians to be ultimately accountable, to monitor the patient's condition, and to help the family set limits on what they can realistically do given competing obligations to other family members, jobs, or themselves.

Routine primary care visits provide opportunities to monitor changes in patient function, family tolerance, or capacity to care, and to make timely referrals before a crisis limits options. Families who resist asking for help for themselves may respond positively if it comes in the form of a recommendation from a trusted professional. Referrals to support groups, adult day care, and in-home help are better accepted if the clinician describes the services in terms of benefits for the patient as well as the family. Families should be encouraged to seek consumer input from the Alzheimer's Association in locating and evaluating quality care and programs.

Again, the key is limiting the scope of recommendations to enhance compliance. Too many recommendations for changes in patient or family routines, living arrangements, or care may overwhelm a burdened primary family caregiver and reduce overall compliance with referral recommendations.[19] People under stress are often poor decision makers or easily discouraged or distracted by initial searches for services that may not be available to them.

Sometimes it is helpful to enlist the services of a social worker, nurse, or private care manager who can help the family assess their needs, preferences, and options, and limit the time and energy demands on the family caregiver.

At this point it is helpful to remind families of some axioms of Alzheimer's family care:

- Families will be forced to modify expectations of the patient, themselves, and the limits of medical treatment. Primary care providers can help by being available, tolerant, and practical.
- Negative feelings of sadness, anger, fear, frustration, guilt, and grief are inescapable. Knowledge and skills to enhance effective coping and care buttress family strength and capacity and limit the impact of inevitable negative feelings.
- Family care is not always natural, fragile, overly romantic, neurotic, or beyond clinical tinkering. Most families provide care based on values or obligation, not choice, and many families never identify themselves as caregivers.
- Family care is not limited to spouses and daughters — nieces, parents, in-laws, grandsons, and even unrelated friends who have been granted familial status (fictive kin) may step in and should be included in planning.
- There are no right or wrong decisions, care strategies, or places to provide care. Home care may be preferred, but it is not, ipso facto, of better quality or without cost. Decisions must be based on consensus, advanced directives if available, and informed judgment. Unconventional care strategies may be culturally sanctioned and more acceptable to minority families.
- There are no perfect saints or martyrs among family caregivers. Most family members have limits and need professional support in accepting them.
- There is rarely a fair or equal division of responsibility for continuous care of someone with Alzheimer's. Although primary family responsibility may rotate among siblings, one family member is usually the primary caregiver at any one time. This does not preclude equitable division of secondary support.
- Defense mechanisms are neither good nor bad. Professionals may be quick to label a family caregiver's response as "unhealthy denial", but husband caregivers, in particular, may provide quality care with greater satisfaction or confidence by remaining hopeful that their wives will respond and improve. Accepting a poor prognosis is not a prerequisite for effective family care.
- There is no perfect control or risk-free environment for someone with Alzheimer's. Some unpredictable behavioral disruptions and consequent risks are likely enough to justify contingency plans.
- No one can care for an Alzheimer's patient alone. Outside help supplements or complements personalized care, rarely substitutes for family involvement,[20] and enhances family capacity to sustain preferred levels of involvement.
- Coping skills for handling acute crises do not transfer well to the prolonged loss, grief, and wear and tear of Alzheimer's care. The critical variable is the family's flexibility in adjusting expectations of themselves and the patient to unmet realistic dependency needs and the limits of family capacity.

VIII. ENHANCING COMPLIANCE WITH REFERRALS

- Anticipate resistance or anxiety about unfamiliar services. Explore questions, fears of intrusive or impersonal treatment, or family reservations based on previous caregiving experience.
- Refer to culturally or linguistically acceptable services. Cultural, educational, or social difference may affect whether a caregiver accepts a referral.[21] Be aware of negative connotations of labels like day care, mental health, aging, welfare, and even Alzheimer's.
- Is the recommended service timely, appropriate, convenient, useful, dependable, prohibitively expensive, appropriately skilled in terms of trained staff, and does it meet the expressed preferences and needs of the family?
- Check or have someone check for you eligibility, costs, waiting lists, limits on duration, frequency or intensity of service, alternative providers, contact names, telephone numbers,

and hours of operation. Be sure the family understands their obligations or responsibility in accepting a specific service.
- Monitor service use and satisfaction. Was the service delivered as promised with dignity, skill, and by qualified providers? If the family is disappointed in the quality, dependability, cost, or convenience in using the service, they are unlikely to try again.

IX. LATE STAGE DECISIONS

Contrary to what is listed on death certificates, most Alzheimer's patients eventually die from declines set in motion by the progressive dementia. However, given adequate nutrition, skin care, hydration, and aggressive treatment of the effects of immobility or infections, the terminal care period may extend for years at considerable out-of-pocket and public costs. Families generally delay institutionalization, often waiting for an event like an accident, illness, or hospitalization of the patient or primary caregiver to prompt a crisis placement.

In the later stages of dementia, the primary care physician becomes even more actively involved. Families need guidance on options and consequences of artificial feeding or hydration, the consequences of swallowing difficulties, skin breakdown, incontinence, treatment of infections or comorbidities, and the need for hospitalization. The primary care clinician can be especially helpful in sorting out symptoms of disease progression from treatable or reversible comorbidities, excess disabilities, or effects of medications. Again, the Alzheimer's Association has clinical and products information useful to home care, day care, and nursing home staff.

Families may need primary care help in rehearsing predictable decision points or a clinician's support should they change their decisions about terminal care given unforeseen situations or emotions. If a solid primary care relationship is established, this can be an ideal time to talk about autopsy options so that families are not disappointed when an opportunity to confirm a diagnosis is lost to insufficient planning.

The major and most difficult decision for most families is where to provide terminal care. Family stress, burden, and responsibility do not stop at the door of the nursing home. Many families continue to provide personal care and extensive emotional support to institutionalized relatives. However, families need realistic guidance about what is involved in terminal care and the lost economies of scale in turning one's home into a 24-hour, 7-day-a-week skilled facility. Hospice options are technically open, but generally unavailable for home care and nursing home care, despite recent evidence that palliative care models are easily adapted for late-stage dementia patients.[22]

Because these decisions are costly, emotionally difficult, and imply irreversible losses for the patient and family, placement decisions should be well informed. Again, consumer input from the Alzheimer's Association and experienced local family caregivers is invaluable. Few incentives (financial, religious, or motivational) will make an unwilling family assume care. Few, if any, disincentives will keep a determined family (particularly older spouses in long-term marriages) from honoring a commitment to care. If families are unwilling to explore options, they should receive full primary care support in providing care in a preferred setting.

Many families will "try" a nursing home or several levels of group care, before their dissatisfaction with the quality or lack of individualization precipitates a patient's move back to the family home. Other families will maintain home care long after it is in the best interests of the patient or family. In these situations, primary care providers must be particularly alert to neglect, abuse, or exploitation and refer to Adult Protective Services as necessary.

Neglect, abuse, and exploitation can also happen in nursing home, board and care, and assisted-living facilities. Elegant physical environments and amenities have little to do with overall quality of care. The human environment, staffing, training, and consistency of staff relationships with patients are better predictors of quality care and family satisfaction, but these criteria are more difficult to measure in brief primary care visits.

Families should be prepared for the fact that institutions cannot offer the same personalized care, but there are trade-offs in terms of benefits and losses with institutional resources. Families are well advised to stay involved and visible in the facility to encourage staff interest.

X. PRIMARY CARE: IN SEARCH OF A CLINICIAN FOR ALL SEASONS

Change is inevitable with a degenerative dementia and family dynamics change over the trajectory of chronic care. Families differ in their capacity, interest, and willingness to work with a primary care clinician in caring for a family member with dementia. The continuity of primary care and the skills in managing common geriatric syndromes are ideally suited to needs of persons with dementia.[23]

Ideally, primary care clinicians maintain sustained interest and hope, take a proactive preventive, pharmacologic, and nonpharmacologic approach to the management of the most troubling memory, behavioral, and psychiatric manifestations of the illness, and make skilled use of consultants and informal sources of support. Skilled primary care clinicians know how to manage scarce care resources, work with families, and maximize compliance with referrals. A comprehensive understanding of normal aging, common geriatric problems, dementia, and family counseling skills help primary care providers buffer family conflict, manage family crises, and prepare families for the prolonged anticipatory bereavement and losses associated with Alzheimer's care.

Individual assets for a primary care clinician working with Alzheimer's families include flexibility, a problem-solving approach, a sense of humor, a capacity for interdisciplinary collaboration, and an understanding of how cultural beliefs and values associated with care outcomes influence family decision making.

XI. SUMMARY

The primary care physician can be helpful to Alzheimer's families by taking a strong consumer focus and listening to what the patient and family need and prefer. Families look for continuity of primary care from clinicians who encourage second opinions, acknowledge limits, and offer proactive medical treatment. Families turn to primary care clinicians for reassurance, validation, and absolution that they have done their best in a difficult situation with no right answers. They look to primary care for information to make sense of what is happening to the patient, but that information must be translated in culturally and linguistically sensitive terms, timed and dosed for immediate use, and repeated often. Families want primary care clinicians who will not be neutral, will acknowledge trade-offs in care, and offer recommendations based on predictors of expectable outcomes. Finally, families want primary care clinicians to support them and help them gain confidence in the effectiveness of their care without usurping family control.

ACKNOWLEDGMENT

Preparation of this paper was supported in part by a grant from the National Institute on Aging #5 P50 AG 05128-09.

REFERENCES

1. McConnel, S. and Riggs, J. A., A public policy agenda: supporting family caregiving, in *Family Caregiving: Agenda for the Future*, Cantor, M. H., Ed., American Society on Aging, San Francisco, 1994, 25.
2. Gwyther, L. P., Clinician and family: a partnership for support, in *Dementia Care: Patient, Family and Community*, Mace, N. L., Ed., The Johns Hopkins University Press, Baltimore, 1990, 202.
3. Stone, R., Cafferata, G., and Sangl, J., Caregivers of the frail elderly: a national profile, *Gerontologist*, 27, 616, 1987.

4. George, L. K. and Gwyther, L. P., Caregiver well-being; a multidimensional examination of family caregivers of demented adults, *Gerontologist*, 26, 253, 1986.

5. George, L. K. and Gwyther, L. P., Caregiver well-being; a multidimensional examination of family caregivers of demented adults, *Gerontologist*, 26, 253, 1986.

6. Wright, L. K., Clipp, E. C., and George, L. K., Health consequences of caregiver stress, *Med. Exer. Nutrit. Health,* 2, 181, 1993.

7. Schulz, R. and Williamson, G. M., Health effects of caregiving; prevalence of mental and physical illness in Alzheimer's caregivers, in *Stress Effects on Family Caregivers of Alzheimer's Patients*, Light, E., Niederehe, G., and Lebowitz, B. D., Eds., Springer Publishing Company, New York, 1994, Chap. 3.

8. Gwyther, L. P., Clinician and family: a partnership for support, in *Dementia Care: Patient, Family and Community*, Mace, N. L., Ed., The Johns Hopkins University Press, Baltimore, 1990, 202.

9. Webber, P. A., Fox, P., and Burnette, D., Living alone with Alzheimer's disease: effects on health and social service utilization patterns, *Gerontologist*, 34, 8, 1994.

10. George, L. K. and Gwyther, L. P., Caregiver well-being; a multidimensional examination of family caregivers of demented adults, *Gerontologist*, 26, 253, 1986.

11. Beard, C. M., Kokmen, E., O'Brien, P. C., and Kurland, L. T. The prevalence of dementia is changing over time in Rochester, MN, *Neurology*, 45, 75, 1995.

12. Gwyther, L. P., Ballard, E., and Hinman-Smith, E. A., Overcoming Barriers to Appropriate Service Use: Effective Individualized Strategies for Alzheimer's Care, Duke Center for Aging, Durham, NC, 1990.

13. Goldstein, M. K., Gwyther, L. P., Lazaroff, A. E., and Thal, L. J., Managing early Alzheimer's disease, *Patient Care*, 44, 1991.

14. Advisory Panel on Alzheimer's Disease, Alzheimer's Disease and Related Dementias: Legal Issues in Care and Treatment, U.S. Department of Health and Human Services, Bethesda, 1994.

15. McCann, J. J., Long term home care for the elderly: perceptions of nurses, physicians and primary caregivers, *QRB*, 66, 1988.

16. Gwyther, L. P., Service delivery and utilization: research directions and clinical implications, in *Stress Effects on Family Caregivers of Alzheimer's Patients*, Light, E., Niederehe, G., and Lebowitz, B. D., Eds., Springer, New York, 1994, 293.

17. Gwyther, L. P., Service delivery and utilization: research directions and clinical implications, in *Stress Effects on Family Caregivers of Alzheimer's Patients*, Light, E., Niederehe, G. and Lebowitz, B. D., Eds., Springer, New York, 1994, 293.

18. Gwyther, L. P., Overcoming barriers: home care for dementia patients, *Caring*, 8, 12, 1989.

19. Gold, D. T., George, L. K., Weinberger, M., et al. Easing caregiver burden: an intervention to overcome barriers to service utilization, *Gerontologist*, 30, 32A, 1990.

20. Alzheimer's Association, Time out! The Case for a National Family Caregiver Support Policy, Alzheimer's Association; Washington, DC, 1991.

21. Valle, R., U.S. ethnic minority group access to long-term care, in *Caring for an Aging World: International Models for Long-Term Care, Financing and Delivery*, Schwab, T., Ed., McGraw-Hill, New York, 1989, 339.

22. Volicer, L., Collard, A., Hurley, A., Bishop, C., Kern, D., and Karon, S., Impact of special care unit for patients with advanced Alzheimer's disease on patients' discomfort and costs, *JAGS*, 42, 597, 1994.

23. Warshaw, G. A., Gwyther, L. P., Phillips, L., and Koff, T. H., *Alzheimer's Disease: An Overview for Primary Care,* The University of Arizona Health Sciences Center, Tuscon, AZ, 1996.

RESOURCES

ALZHEIMER'S ASSOCIATION

The Alzheimer's Association issues regular reports on its research grants and occasional research updates, as well as on many materials for families and caregivers. A library provides reference service. Information on participation in drug trials is also available. Contact a local chapter or the Alzheimer's Association, 919 North Michigan Avenue, Suite 1000, Chicago, Illinois 60611-1676; Telephone: 312-335-8700 or 800-272-3900; Web site: http://www.alz.org

BENJAMIN B. GREEN-FIELD NATIONAL LIBRARY AND RESOURCE CENTER

The Green-Field Library is part of the national offices of the Alzheimer's Association. The Resource Center is available to provide information for those involved in patient care, research, or those who simply want to know more about the disease. Professional librarians provide reference assistance to those seeking information. The library contains thousands of books, videotapes, reports, and articles on Alzheimer's disease, related disorders, and aging. In addition, there is access to the information in hundreds of online databases. Information requests may be made in person, over the telephone, or by mail, fax, email, or through the World Wide Web. The facility is open to all during the Association's business hours, Monday through Friday from 8:30 a.m. to 5:00 p.m, central time. Telephone: 312-335-9602; FAX: 312-335-0214; email: greenfld@alz.org; Web site: http://www.alz.org

ALZHEIMER'S DISEASE EDUCATION AND REFERRAL CENTER (ADEAR)

Sponsored by the National Institute on Aging, ADEAR is a national resource center for information on Alzheimer's disease including research findings and participation in clinical trials. ADEAR publishes *Connections*, a quarterly newsletter for professionals. Write or call ADEAR Center, P.O. Box 8250, Silver Spring, Maryland 20907-8250; Telephone: 800-438-4380.

SOCIETY FOR NEUROSCIENCE

With more than 23,000 members, the Society is one of the world's largest organizations for basic scientists and clinicians who study the brain and nervous system. Its annual meeting, held in the fall, includes many presentations on Alzheimer's disease research. Abstract volumes are available for purchase. For information about obtaining publications, write or call Office of Public Affairs, Society for Neuroscience, 11 Dupont Circle NW, Suite 500, Washington, DC 20036; Telephone: 202-462-6688.

NATIONAL INSTITUTE OF NEUROLOGICAL DISORDERS AND STROKE (NINDS)

Part of the National Institutes of Health (NIH), NINDS conducts and sponsors research on Alzheimer's disease and other neurological disorders. Its Alzheimer's research focuses on the basic biology and genetics of the disease and its diagnosis and clinical management. Write or call NINDS, Public Inquiries, Building 31, Room 8A-16, Bethesda, Maryland 20892; Telephone: 301-496-5751.

NATIONAL INSTITUTE OF MENTAL HEALTH (NIMH)

Part of the NIH, NIMH studies Alzheimer's disease in three prinicipal areas: genetics and neurobiology, clinical research, and psychosocial research on the stress associated with caregiving.

Write or call NIMH, Public Inquiries, Parklawn Building, Room 7C02, 5600 Fishers Lane, Rockville, Maryland 20857; Telephone: 301-443-4513.

NATIONAL INSTITUTE OF NURSING RESEARCH (NINR)

Part of NIH, NINR supports and conducts research related to the diverse caregiving responsibilities of nurses including the development of ways to enhance mental functioning and independence. Write or call NINR, Building 31, Room 5B-13, Bethesda, Maryland 20892; Telephone: 301-496-0207.

NATIONAL INSTITUTE ON AGING (NIA)

Part of NIH, NIA leads the federal effort on Alzheimer's disease and aging research. NIA conducts and sponsors research on the epidemiology, cause, diagnosis, and management of Alzheimer's disease. Write or call NIA, Building 31, Room 5C-27, Bethesda, Maryland 20892; Telephone: 301-496-1752.

INDEX